Culture and Panic Disorder

Culture and Panic Disorder

Edited by Devon E. Hinton and Byron J. Good

Stanford University Press
Stanford, California

Stanford University Press
Stanford, California

Printed in the United States of America on acid-free, archival-quality paper

Library of Congress Cataloging-in-Publication Data

Culture and panic disorder / edited by Devon E. Hinton and Byron J. Good.
    p. cm.
 Includes bibliographical references and index.
  ISBN 978-0-8047-6108-6 (cloth : alk. paper)--ISBN 978-0-8047-6109-3 (pbk. : alk. paper)
  1. Panic disorders--Diagnosis--History. 2. Panic disorders--Cross-cultural studies. 3. Cultural psychiatry. 4. Ethnopsychology. 5. Medical anthropology. I. Hinton, Devon E. II. Good, Byron.
  RC535.C88 2009
  362.196'85223--dc22   2008047519

Designed by Bruce Lundquist
Typeset at Stanford University Press in 10/14 Adobe Garamond

Contents

Contributors   vii

Foreword
   David H. Barlow   xiii

Preface
   Alan Harwood   xvii

Acknowledgments   xxi

1. Introduction:
   Panic Disorder in Cross-Cultural and Historical Perspective
   Byron J. Good and Devon E. Hinton   1

PART I THEORETICAL APPROACHES TO THE STUDY OF PANIC DISORDER

2. Theoretical Perspectives on the Cross-Cultural Study
   of Panic Disorder
   Laurence J. Kirmayer and Caminee Blake   31

3. A Medical Anthropology of Panic Sensations:
   Ten Analytic Perspectives
   Devon E. Hinton and Byron J. Good   57

PART II   HISTORICAL PERSPECTIVES ON WESTERN PANIC

  4. The Irritable Heart Syndrome in the American Civil War
      Robert Kugelmann   85

  5. Twentieth-Century Theories of Panic in the United States:
      From Cardiac Vulnerability to Catastrophic Cognitions
      Devon E. Hinton and Susan D. Hinton   113

PART III   CULTURAL VARIATIONS IN PANIC DISORDER

  6. Comparative Phenomenology of 'Ataques de Nervios,'
      Panic Attacks, and Panic Disorder
      Roberto Lewis-Fernández, Peter J. Guarnaccia,
      Igda E. Martínez, Ester Salmán, Andrew B. Schmidt,
      and Michael Liebowitz   135

  7. Dizziness and Panic in China:
      Organ and Ontological Disequilibrium
      Lawrence Park and Devon E. Hinton   157

  8. Gendered Panic in Southern Thailand:
      'Lom' ("Wind") Illness and 'Wuup' ("Upsurge") Illness
      Pichet Udomratn and Devon E. Hinton   183

  9. 'Ihahamuka,' a Rwandan Syndrome of Response to the Genocide:
      Blocked Flow, Spirit Assault, and Shortness of Breath
      Athanase Hagengimana and Devon E. Hinton   205

10. Panic Illness in Tibetan Refugees
      Eric Jacobson   230

      Index   263

Contributors

DAVID H. BARLOW is professor of psychology and psychiatry, and founder and director emeritus of the Center for Anxiety and Related Disorders at Boston University. He received his doctorate from the University of Vermont in 1969 and has published more than five hundred articles and chapters, as well as sixty books, mostly on the nature and treatment of emotional disorders. He was editor of *Behavior Therapy*, *Journal of Applied Behavior Analysis*, and *Clinical Psychology: Science and Practice*, and is currently editor-in-chief of the Treatments That Work series for Oxford University Press.

CAMINEE BLAKE, a clinical psychologist, is a staff psychologist in the Youth Service, Department of Psychiatry, Jewish General Hospital, and at the Home Ventilation Unit, Montreal Chest Hospital. She completed a postdoctoral fellowship in transcultural psychiatry at McGill University and another at Yale University, and she has a master of arts degree in experimental social psychology from Carleton University. She does research and clinical work in culture and mental health, with a special interest in the Caribbean community.

BYRON J. GOOD is professor of medical anthropology in the Department of Social Medicine, Harvard Medical School. He received his doctorate in anthropology from the University of Chicago in 1967. He is author of *Medicine, Rationality, and Experience: An Anthropological Perspective* (Cambridge University Press, 1994). Among his edited works, with colleagues, are *Postcolonial Disorders*, with Mary-Jo

DelVecchio Good, Sandra Teresa Hyde, and Sarah Pinto (University of California Press, 2008); *Subjectivity: Ethnographic Investigations*, with João Biehl and Arthur Kleinman (University of California Press, 2007); *Pain as Human Experience*, with Mary-Jo DelVecchio Good, Paul Brodwin, and Arthur Kleinman (University of California Press, 1994); and *Culture and Depression*, with Arthur Kleinman (University of California Press, 1985). He was editor-in-chief of *Culture, Medicine, and Psychiatry* from 1986 to 2005, and chair of the Department of Social Medicine at Harvard Medical School from 1999 to 2006.

PETER J. GUARNACCIA is professor in the Department of Human Ecology at Cook College and investigator at the Institute for Health, Health Care Policy, and Aging Research. He earned his doctorate in anthropology from the University of Connecticut in 1984. His research interests include cross-cultural patterns of psychiatric disorders, family strategies for coping with mental illness, and cultural competence in mental health organizations. Recent publications include "Are *Ataques de Nervios* in Puerto Rican Children Associated with Psychiatric Disorder?," published in the *Journal of the American Academy of Child and Adolescent Psychiatry* (2005, with Igda Martinez, Rafael Ramirez, and Glorisa Canino), and "It's Like Going Through an Earthquake: Anthropological Perspectives on Depression Among Latino Immigrants," published in the *Journal of Immigrant and Minority Health* (2007, with Igda M. Pincay).

ATHANASE HAGENGIMANA, a psychiatrist, attended medical school at the National University of Rwanda and completed his psychiatry residency at the University of Nairobi, Kenya. He currently works as an International Civil Servant with the United Nations, acting as chief staff counselor in the Ivory Coast. He was senior lecturer in psychiatry and psychology at the National University of Rwanda. He did postdoctoral studies at Harvard Medical School, where he was also an instructor and research fellow in psychiatry. He has been awarded fellowships from the Educational Commission for Foreign Medical Graduates, the Social Science Research Council, the Center for Advanced Holocaust Studies, and the John W. Kluge Center at the Library of Congress. His research interests include the psychological causes and consequences of violent conflict, specifically posttraumatic stress reactions.

ALAN HARWOOD is professor emeritus of anthropology at the University of Massachusetts, Boston. He received his doctorate in anthropology from Columbia University in 1967. In addition to authoring articles on medical anthropology, he is also author of the monographs *Witchcraft, Sorcery, and Social Categories Among the Safwa* (Oxford University Press, 1970) and *Rx: Spiritist as Needed: A Study of a*

Puerto Rican Community Mental Health Resource (Wiley Interscience, reprinted by Cornell University Press, 1987). He also edited the pioneering volume *Ethnicity and Medical Care* (Harvard University Press, 1981). In 1983 he received the Wellcome Medal of the Royal Anthropological Institute of Great Britain and Ireland for his research on the application of anthropology to medical problems. He was founding editor of the *Medical Anthropology Quarterly* and has edited series of books in medical anthropology for both Cambridge and Rutgers University Presses.

DEVON E. HINTON is a psychiatrist and medical anthropologist, and associate professor of psychiatry at Harvard Medical School and Massachusetts General Hospital. The subject of his doctoral thesis (Harvard University, 1999) was a panic syndrome occurring in Northeastern Thailand. He is fluent in Cambodian and Thai; conversant in Lao, Spanish, and Vietnamese; and director of a Southeast Asian Refugee Clinic in Lowell, Massachusetts. He is first author of more than fifty articles, most on panic disorder and related cultural syndromes among traumatized Southeast Asian refugees. He has also been editor of five special journal issues: on panic disorder, on sleep paralysis, on the medical anthropology of sensations, on music-based healing rituals, and on trauma-related nightmares. He is principal investigator of a National Institute of Mental Health–funded grant to develop a culturally sensitive treatment for Cambodian refugees with posttraumatic stress disorder and comorbid panic attacks.

SUSAN D. HINTON has a bachelor's degree in anthropology and English from the University of California at Berkeley, and a master's degree in comparative literature with an emphasis on Latin American culture and literature, also from the University of California at Berkeley. She and her husband have three years of field research experience in Northeastern Thailand. She has coauthored several articles on cultural syndromes and panic disorder among Southeast Asian refugees.

ERIC JACOBSON received his doctorate in anthropology from Harvard University and is a medical anthropologist on the faculty of the Department of Social Medicine, Harvard Medical School. He investigates placebo phenomena and classical Asian medicines at the Osher Research Center and at Harvard Medical School. He has published articles and book chapters on placebo response in clinical trials, psychiatric aspects of Tibetan medicine, diagnostic reasoning in traditional Chinese medicine, and alternative therapies.

LAURENCE J. KIRMAYER is James McGill Professor and director of the Division of Social and Transcultural Psychiatry at McGill University and editor-in-chief of

Transcultural Psychiatry. He directs the Culture and Mental Health Research Unit at the Sir Mortimer B. Davis–Jewish General Hospital in Montreal, where he conducts research on the mental health of indigenous peoples, on mental health services for immigrants and refugees, and on the cultural basis of psychiatric theory and practice. He is coeditor of *Understanding Trauma: Integrating Biological, Clinical, and Cultural Perspectives* (Cambridge University Press, 2007), *Healing Traditions: The Mental Health of Aboriginal Peoples in Canada* (University of British Columbia Press, 2008), and *Encountering the Other: The Practice of Cultural Consultation* (Springer Science and Business Media, in press).

ROBERT KUGELMANN has a doctorate in psychology and is professor of psychology at the University of Dallas in Irving, Texas. He is author of two books, *The Windows of Soul* (Bucknell University Press, 1983) and *Stress: The Nature and History of Engineered Grief* (Praeger, 1992). His current research includes a book in progress, "Contested Boundaries: Psychology and Catholicism," and phenomenological research, both empirical and historical, on pain. Other areas of research and publication are critical health psychology and the history of psychology.

ROBERTO LEWIS-FERNÁNDEZ is director of the New York State Cultural Competence Center of Excellence and of the Hispanic Treatment Program at New York State Psychiatric Institute, and associate professor of clinical psychiatry at Columbia University. His research focuses on the sociocultural determinants of illness experience, on symptomatology, on help-seeking behavior, and on treatment outcome among U.S. Latinos diagnosed with anxiety, depressive, and dissociative disorders. Other research areas include the relationship between psychiatric diagnoses and Latino popular syndromes, sociocultural factors associated with treatment dropout, misdiagnosis of psychosis as a result of folk idioms of distress, symptom presentations of trauma-related disorders among Latino patients, and collaboration models between mental health and primary care medicine to increase access to culturally competent care for consumers with psychiatric disorders.

MICHAEL LIEBOWITZ is professor of clinical psychiatry at Columbia University and managing director of the Medical Research Network, a private clinical trials facility. He graduated from Yale College and Medical School and did his psychiatric training at the Medical Center Hospital of Vermont and Columbia University. At Columbia he started the Anxiety Disorders Clinic, which he directed from 1982 until 2006. His research interests include classification and treatment of atypical depression, social anxiety disorder, panic disorder, and obsessive-compulsive disorder. He chaired the *DSM-IV* workgroup on anxiety disorders and developed the Liebowitz Social Anxiety Scale. He has authored or coauthored more than 250 peer-reviewed publications.

IGDA E. MARTÍNEZ is a doctoral candidate in clinical psychology at the Graduate School of Applied and Professional Psychology of Rutgers University. Her research interests in Latino mental health have led to several collaborations, including "Culture-Specific Diagnoses and Their Relationship to Mood Disorders," a chapter in *Diversity Issues in the Diagnosis, Treatment, and Research of Mood Disorders* (Oxford University Press, 2008, with Peter J. Guarnaccia); and "Mental Health in the Hispanic Immigrant Community: An Overview," a chapter in *Mental Health Care for New Hispanic Immigrants: Innovative Approaches in Contemporary Clinical Practice* (Haworth Press, 2005, with Peter J. Guarnaccia and Henry Acosta), among other recent publications.

LAWRENCE PARK is director of inpatient services at Massachusetts General Hospital (MGH) and lecturer at Harvard Medical School. He also serves as MGH site director of the International Training Program in Mental Health of the Department of Social Medicine at Harvard Medical School. He received a master's degree in cross-cultural psychiatry at the Committee on Human Development at the University of Chicago, and earned his doctorate in medicine at the University of Wisconsin Medical School. His research interests include mental illness and mental health policy in China.

ESTER SALMÁN graduated from Manhattan College with a bachelor of science degree in psychology and was inducted into Psi Chi (the National Honor Society in Psychology) and Sigma Xi (the Scientific Research Society). In 1990 she began working in clinical psychiatry at the Columbia University Clinic for Anxiety and Related Disorders, where she later founded the Hispanic Treatment Program. While at Columbia University she served as co-investigator for several National Institute of Mental Health–sponsored grants focusing on culture and psychiatric disorders, and as a result authored several peer-reviewed scientific journal publications as well as chapters in books devoted to Latino mental health issues.

ANDREW B. SCHMIDT received his master's degree in clinical social work from New York University and is enrolled in the doctorate in social work program at Hunter College, City University of New York. He works as a technical specialist in the Anxiety Disorders Clinic at the New York State Psychiatric Institute. In this role he provides oversight and technical supervision for all data-related activities associated with the multiple research studies conducted at the clinic. He is also coauthor of papers on obsessive-compulsive disorder, social phobia, and ethnic disparities of mental health care.

PICHET UDOMRATN received his doctorate in medicine from the Prince of Songkla University in Southern Thailand and is professor of psychiatry there. He is president of the Association of Southeast Asian Nations Federation for Psychiatry and Mental Health and of the Psychiatric Association of Thailand. He is a former editor of the *Journal of the Psychiatric Association of Thailand* and has authored more than one hundred publications, including books, research articles, reviews, and special articles. His major fields of interest and research are anxiety and mood disorders, particularly panic disorder; schizophrenia; sleep disorders; geriatric psychiatry; psychopharmacology; and medical education. He is the pioneering researcher on panic disorder as it presents in Thailand, and his book on panic disorder written in the Thai language is now a standard text in that country.

Foreword

ANY CONSIDERATION of the origins and functions of the emotions of anxiety and fear would presuppose that these must be universal phenomena. Since the time of Darwin we have assumed that evolution should favor members of a species who are anxious and fearful, and recent research has established that these two emotions are at least partially distinct, with different functions (Suárez et al. in press). Many theorists, such as Howard Liddell (1949), make the case that anxiety represents the ability of individuals to plan for the future and be vigilant for possible upcoming threats or challenges. Fear, on the other hand, is the more dramatic emotion, scientifically observed by Darwin as a "flight-fight" response to immediate and imminent threat or danger. Of course predispositions to experience anxiety and fear and the resulting action tendencies should be normally distributed across the population, meaning that certain numbers of individuals will present with excesses of these traits or, at the very least, lower thresholds for their expressions.

It has also become clear in the past thirty years that the fundamental and protective emotion of fear occurring at inappropriate times (when there is nothing to be afraid of) is a substantial problem in psychopathology. This inappropriate expression of fear has come to be called *panic* (or a *panic attack*) (Barlow 2002). Thus, it has been assumed that the experiences of anxiety and fear and their occasional excesses or inappropriate expressions such as panic exist in nearly all cultures and subcultures.

In fact, the excitement of a new, more objective study of anxiety and panic that began in the early 1980s is nicely described in this volume because one of the editors,

Byron Good, as well as the author of this foreword were both present at a National Institute of Mental Health–sponsored meeting on anxiety and the anxiety disorders in September 1983 (Tuma and Maser 1985). At that wide-ranging conference it was noted with some prescience that the 1980s would come to be the decade of anxiety from a clinical research perspective after a similar focus on depression in the 1970s and on schizophrenia in the 1960s. It was also at that conference that investigators explored the notion that the phenomenon of panic was far more ubiquitous in its occurrence than was assumed in the relatively narrow context of panic disorder. Indeed, it was noted that panic attacks were found across the full range of psycho-pathology. Panic then became a phenomenon that was given its own definition in *DSM-IV* and placed prior to descriptions of the anxiety disorders of which panic attacks were one of the building blocks.

At that conference it was also largely decided that the term *spontaneous*, used to modify panic attacks (and implying a purely biological origin of these attacks), was unscientific because it suggested (at one level of analysis) that no trigger or cause could be identified. This term was replaced by the modifiers *uncued* and *un-expected*, indicating that these attributions and perceptions were in the mind of the patient and did not imply the lack of existence of a clear trigger for panic attacks, which might often be outside of awareness (such as a subtle change in somatic homeostasis). Thus, unexpected and uncued panic attacks simply meant that the patient was not aware of the variety of triggers that might be operating, and that effective therapy would involve identifying these triggers and giving the patients coping mechanisms for dealing with them.

However, nowhere across the wide range of psychopathology is it more clear than in anxiety, fear, and panic that these experiences are expressed in culturally specific idioms, allowing for countless potential triggers, both cognitive and somatic. Furthermore, a given culturally specific idiom will affect the course of anxiety and fear, how it is interpreted by the individual, and the way it is presented to clinicians or healers. Accepted methods for clinicians to resolve these issues are also affected by culturally specific understandings.

Thus, if one takes a broad view, the prevalence of most anxiety disorders seems relatively consistent around the world, and this is particularly true for panic disorder (Horwath and Weissman 1997), although this assessment needs further empirical investigation. However, the source of fear and the specific attributions these individuals make are clearly culture specific, with substantial implications for classification, course, and treatment.

In this remarkable book, two of the world's leading scholars studying culturally specific idioms of psychopathology articulate a number of remarkable insights into the nature of fear and panic. On one level, the book presents the most scholarly and compelling account yet to appear of both cross-cultural and historical perspectives on panic disorder. This account alone is a broadening experience for several reasons. First, the phenomenon of panic is a relatively discrete event, unlike, for example, the very heterogeneous and wide-ranging set of symptoms and behaviors that constitute schizophrenia. Consequently, cultural variations seem more readily apparent and can be studied with a fair degree of certainty, revealing that the basic human phenomena of fear, panic, and the flight-fight response constitute the fundamental experience, regardless of the culture in which one is working. Second, because we have "officially" recognized panic attacks in our nomenclature only since the publication of *DSM-III* in 1980, integrating a historical perspective with a contemporary cross-cultural perspective provides a particularly enlightened context in which to look at various expressions of the phenomenon of panic. These two reasons alone are sufficient to make this volume invaluable.

This brings us to the third and perhaps most important accomplishment of this remarkable volume. In this book we find a well-articulated alternative methodological strategy for studying the phenomenon of panic, in addition to more traditional psychopathological and neurobiological approaches. To quote the editors, "this approach thus provides one model for making psychological and cultural processes central to investigations of culture and panic disorder, rather than focusing more narrowly on cultural variability in symptom criteria and diagnostic entities." Indeed, in articulating this model of panic disorder, the editors and their contributors are able to highlight the "wide range of cognitive and psychological processes that can trigger experiences of panic as well as anxiety about the likelihood and danger of future episodes" (Chapter 1). It seems clear from reading this volume that any study of panic attacks and panic disorder is incomplete without this informed perspective.

David H. Barlow
Boston, Massachusetts
April 2008

References

Barlow, D. H. 2002. *Anxiety and Its Disorders: The Nature and Treatment of Anxiety and Panic.* 2nd ed. New York: Guilford Press.

Horwath, E., and M. Weissman. 1997. Epidemiology of Anxiety Disorders Across Cultural Groups. In *Cultural Issues in the Treatment of Anxiety.* S. Friedman, ed. Pp. 21–39. New York: Guilford Press.

Liddell, H. S. 1949. The Role of Vigilance in the Development of Animal Neurosis. In *Anxiety.* P. Hoch and I. Zubin, eds. Pp. 183–196. New York: Grune & Stratton.

Suárez, L., S. Bennett, C. Goldstein, and D. H. Barlow. In press. Understanding Anxiety
Disorders from a "Triple Vulnerabilities" Framework. In *Oxford Handbook of Anxiety
and Related Disorders*. M. M. Antony and M. B. Stein, eds. New York: Oxford University Press.

Tuma, A. H., and J. D. Maser, eds. 1985. *Anxiety and the Anxiety Disorders*. Hillsdale, NJ:
Erlbaum.

Preface

SOME THIRTY YEARS AGO, Arthur Kleinman, along with his colleagues Byron and Mary-Jo Good, began a program of research built around the study of major psychiatric disorders from a meaning-centered, cross-cultural perspective. Their approach has been, in essence, to treat the nosology of the American Psychiatric Association's *Diagnostic and Statistical Manual of Mental Disorders (DSM)* as a cultural artifact— the culture-specific product of particular medical specialists in Western postindustrial society. Applying this heuristic, they have selected important *DSM* psychiatric categories for comparison with diagnostically and behaviorally similar conditions found in different parts of the globe. Their goal in doing this has not been to see if the *DSM* categories map onto each local manifestation, but to use the comparisons to clarify the underlying illness process. By examining each local manifestation in its epidemiological, social, and cultural (that is, meaning) context in relation to the *DSM* category, universal features of the condition become clarified, as do specific social and cultural features that contribute to producing the differences. In short, this method leads to a more sophisticated, less ethnocentric understanding of the general illness type. Applying this method, Kleinman and the Goods, and more recently their students, have provided anthropologists, psychologists, psychiatrists, and other interested scholars with enlightening and fruitful analyses of such major psychiatric conditions as depression (Kleinman and Good 1985), anxiety (Good and Kleinman 1985), pain (Good et al. 1994), schizophrenia (Jenkins and Barrett 2004), dementia (Leibing and Cohen 2006), and eating disorders (Becker 2007).

The present book, devoted to a cross-cultural, meaning-centered study of panic disorder, follows in the same research tradition. As such, it makes a number of significant contributions. First, we are provided with a comprehensive cultural history of panic-like disorders in Western medicine from the nineteenth century to the present, with a particular focus on how disagreements between psychoanalysts and biologically oriented psychiatrists in the 1980s shaped and changed the concept of panic disorder.

Once it was established as a "real" entity in the third edition of the *DSM*, panic disorder generated a spate of biologically oriented research and pharmacological treatment agendas that have only somewhat recently been supplanted by the more psychologically oriented agenda favored by the editors of this book. This agenda involves examining panic disorder from a psychosocial perspective, in particular that of *catastrophic cognitions*. This perspective goes beyond the more biological orientation of the *DSM–IV* and helps us understand why certain sensations are particularly meaningful and threatening in certain societies and therefore become amplified into a localized syndrome of panic. Chapter 3, by Devon E. Hinton and Byron J. Good, specifically catalogs how people's sensations might be shaped cognitively to provoke a full-blown panic attack. In this same vein, in Chapter 2, transcultural psychiatrist Laurence J. Kirmayer and Caminee Blake survey cultural, social, and psychological processes that generate panic attacks. The book thus redirects research attention to the cognitive processes and cultural contexts that play a key role in this disorder and lends considerable support for treatment strategies designed to alter the cognitions of panic sufferers.

In thinking about catastrophic cognitions as triggers of panic, the etymology of the word *panic* itself provides a fine example of the embeddedness of anxiety in a cognitive schema—specifically that of the ancient Greeks. Early uses of the term *panic* in English lead back to its origins in classical mythology. The word first appeared in the seventeenth century as an adjective, combined with the word *fear*: "panic [that is, Pan-ic] fear" or "panic terror," fear inspired by the god or earth spirit Pan (Skeat 1893:418; see also OED Online 2007). Part man and part goat, Pan was the son of Hermes and the nymph Penelope, who, according to Homeric Hymn 19, "sprang up and left the child" out of disgust at his animalistic appearance. Once abandoned, Pan inhabited mountainsides and forests, particularly in Arcadia, a region looked down upon by Athenians and other "cultivated" Greeks as less civilized. A swift runner and agile rock-climber, Pan became the embodiment of the mysterious noises that frighten travelers in remote and lonely places outside village boundaries. Shepherds and hunters, the denizens of these areas, paid homage to the god and were thus protected by him. However, for settled villagers, rough, rustic areas provoked the fear associated with Pan's name. In addition, as one of Dionysus's retinue, Pan was constantly on the prowl sexually, most famously after nymphs. Often unsuccessful in these pursuits because of the intervention of other nymphs or gods, Pan, like the satyrs, embodied uncontrolled, aggressive male sexuality. For ancient Greeks, then, panic was semantically associated with abandonment; uncivilized, remote mountains and forests; and unchecked male sexuality—surely a rich set of cognitions that might, under certain circumstances, precipitate a full-blown panic attack.[1]

As a key contribution, this anthology definitively establishes, particularly through the historical and descriptive ethnographic chapters, that panic symptoms and syndromes are and have been widespread and disabling to people across societies in many parts of the world. By comparing panic disorder, as conceived in the *DSM–IV*, with local, panic-like illness categories from various societies (and from previous historical periods in the United States), the collection shows that the two are not equivalent, although they are clearly related typologically. Specifically, the comparisons provide crucial evidence that many *DSM* markers or criteria for panic disorder do not apply in other cultural settings (for example, the sensation of panic does not always come out of the blue, does not always crescendo in a matter of minutes, and does not always have as its primary focus the particular physical symptoms described in the *DSM*). These comparisons thus yield greater clarity about the core symptoms of panic disorder, as well as the expansion of the concept of panic disorder to encompass related conditions found around the globe. This enlarged perspective raises new questions for cross-cultural research and, more practically, allows clinicians to view what have heretofore been considered localized, culture-bound syndromes as part of a larger set of panic-related conditions that may respond to similar but culturally appropriate treatment modalities.

Finally, this collection demonstrates that panic syndromes are often linked to memories of trauma and violence, and that panic symptoms are a conspicuous part of the psychological experience of persons who have suffered war, dislocation, and other major social catastrophes. This observation calls into question the *DSM* dictum ruling out a comorbid diagnosis of panic disorder and posttraumatic stress disorder (PTSD), and suggests a reconsideration of the *DSM* classification of the anxiety disorders in addition to further study of the specific relationship between panic disorder and PTSD. In view of the many people worldwide who in recent times have experienced the traumata of war and dislocation, reexamination of the anxiety disorders seems particularly useful and warranted. In suggesting questions for this task, *Culture and Panic Disorder* is an invaluable resource. It is also a fitting tribute to the heuristic value of the model pioneered by Kleinman and the Goods so many years ago.

Alan Harwood
Cambridge, Massachusetts
March 2008

Notes

1. As with many Greek gods, the myths about Pan are numerous and sometimes contradictory. The themes I have focused on here deal specifically with panic and dominate the accounts in Campbell (1949:81–82) and Hamilton (1940:40), and on the Web sites http://www.theoi.com/Georgikos/Pan.html and http://www.theoi.com/Cult/PanCult.html.

References

Becker, A. 2007. Culture and Eating Disorders Classification. *International Journal of Eating Disorders* 40(Suppl.):S111-116.

Campbell, J. 1949. *The Hero with a Thousand Faces*. New York: Meridian.

Good, B. J., and A. Kleinman. 1985. Culture and Anxiety: Cross-Cultural Evidence for the Patterning of Anxiety Disorder. In *Anxiety and the Anxiety Disorders*. A. H. Tuma and J. D. Maser, eds. Pp. 297-323. Hillsdale, NJ: Erlbaum.

Good, M. J., P. Brodwin, A. Kleinman, and B. J. Good, eds. 1994. *Pain as Human Experience*. Berkeley: University of California Press.

Hamilton, E. 1940. *Mythology: Timeless Tales of Gods and Heroes*. New York: Mentor Books.

Jenkins, J. H., and R. J. Barrett, eds. 2004. *Schizophrenia, Culture, and Subjectivity: The Edge of Experience*. Cambridge: Cambridge University Press.

Kleinman, A., and B. J. Good, eds. 1985. *Culture and Depression: Studies in the Anthropology and Cross-Cultural Psychiatry of Affect and Disorder*. Berkeley: University of California Press.

Leibing, A., and L. Cohen, eds. 2006. *Thinking About Dementia: Culture, Loss, and the Anthropology of Senility*. New Brunswick, NJ: Rutgers University Press.

Oxford English Dictionary (OED) Online. 2007. *Oxford English Dictionary*. Oxford, UK: Oxford University Press. http://dictionary.oed.com (accessed Dec. 10, 2007).

Skeat, W. W. 1893. *An Etymological Dictionary of the English Language*. Oxford, UK: Clarendon Press.

Acknowledgments

THE EDITORS would like to express their great gratitude to Alan Harwood, who served as a special editor for this volume. He provided expert advice on all chapters, as well as invaluable corrections, suggestions, and inspiration.

Culture and Panic Disorder

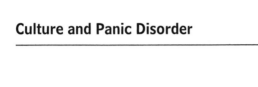

.

1

Introduction

Panic Disorder in Cross-Cultural and Historical Perspective

Byron J. Good and Devon E. Hinton

PANIC DISORDER (PD), as currently conceived, is a medical condition that may be diagnosed when a person experiences recurrent, unexpected attacks of panic or anxiety, followed by persistent concern about having additional attacks or about losing control, going crazy, or having a heart attack. Panic attacks are intense periods of fear or discomfort, feelings that sometimes seem quite irrational. They are described as "attacks" because they often develop rapidly and include such symptoms as palpitations, sweating, trembling, shortness of breath, a feeling of choking, chest pain, nausea, dizziness, derealization or depersonalization, and numbness or chills or hot flushes, as well as fear of losing control or fear of dying.

PD, according to contemporary psychiatric classification, belongs to a group of neuropsychiatric conditions for which anxiety is the hallmark symptom. Although anxiety disorders are often thought of as relatively mild conditions, researchers estimate that in the United States these disorders account for 32 percent of the total economic costs of psychiatric illness, exceeding the costs associated with schizophrenia (21 percent) and mood disorders, including depression (22 percent) (Taylor 2000:4). Within the costs of panic attacks are emergency room visits and extensive medical tests to determine whether those experiencing the panic are suffering a heart attack or some other life-threatening condition as they fear. PD most commonly begins when the sufferer is between fifteen and thirty years of age. Studies suggest that between 1.5 and 3.5 percent of members of a population will suffer PD sometime during their lifetime.

1

PD was first recognized—or invented—as a distinctive form of mental ill-ness in the 1970s; codified in 1980 as part of the third edition of the American Psychiatric Association's *Diagnostic and Statistical Manual,* or *DSM–III* (APA 1980); and popularized as a treatable clinical entity in the 1980s. Also in the 1980s, many researchers argued that PD had a largely physiological and genetic basis rather than a primarily psychological one. Since Freud, acute anxiety had been interpreted as resulting from unconscious feelings surfacing into partial aware-ness.[1] PD thus figures prominently in the history of the biological revolution in psychiatry. During the 1990s, PD was, to an important extent, reconceived by cognitive psychologists as spiraling episodes of anxiety arising from *catastrophic cognitions* that trigger physiological experiences of terror or panic. PD continues to be an important domain of research, clinical care, and pharmaceutical invest-ment within psychiatry, both in the United States and globally. The story of PD is thus an intriguing chapter in the contemporary sociology of psychiatric knowl-edge and practice.

Acute anxiety and panic, however, quickly escape the confines of current di-agnoses of anxiety disorders. They belong, on the one hand, to a long history of changing conceptualizations of neuropsychological distress in North American and European medical writing and practices, sharing complex relationships with categories such as cerebrocardiac neuropathy, irritable heart syndrome, neuras-thenia, agoraphobia, anxiety reaction, anxiety neurosis, and neurasthenic neu-rosis. On the other hand, as Jackie Orr (2006) has recently shown in her book *Panic Diaries: A Genealogy of Panic Disorder,* acute anxiety and panic belong to a much broader cultural domain of changing experience and understanding in the twentieth-century United States—from the social panic produced by the 1938 radio broadcast of H. G. Wells' *War of the Worlds,* to concerns about measur-ing and managing fears and anxieties in American society, to David Sheehan's popular book *The Anxiety Disease* (1983), to multiple pharmaceutical interven-tions, clinical trials, and research studies sponsored by the National Institute of Mental Health (NIMH) and the pharmaceutical industry. The story of PD thus belongs to a very broad range of social, political, cultural, and medical concerns in Western societies.

What is little recognized, however, in most accounts of PD, whether medical writing, historical analyses, or cultural studies, is that acute anxiety and panic-like conditions appear in local social and cultural worlds in many parts of the globe. Psychiatric research has investigated cross-cultural differences almost exclusively in epidemiological terms—asking whether PD, defined uniformly across cultures, is more or less prevalent in one society or social class or subculture or risk group than in another, and concluding simplistically that "prevalence, course, gender distribution, and age of onset of PD appear to be generally consistent throughout the world" (Taylor 2000:5). It is only recently that rich ethnographic research on acute anxiety and panic conditions has begun to provide real understanding of what *panic* and *panic disorder* may mean in local cultural worlds—for example, in the lives of Tibetan Buddhist refugees or contemporary Chinese psychiatric patients or Puerto Ricans suffering from *ataques de nervios*. Such research begins to provide a much deeper understanding of the relation of PD to culture, allowing questions to be asked, research to be conducted, and generalizations to be argued in ways that were impossible as recently as a decade ago.

This book is a collection of essays examining the complex relationships among culture, social conditions, and PD from three broad perspectives. The first chapters of the book are theoretical, developing a general framework for investigating the relationship of acute anxiety experiences to culture through an anthropology of the sensations, cultural phenomenology, theories of catastrophic cognitions, and ethnotheories of the body, illness, and healing. These essays make a strong argument that current psychological theories of panic attacks—which understand these attacks as resulting from an escalating cycle of catastrophic interpretations of bodily experience—provide a particularly rich basis for cross-cultural studies of panic and PD. The second set of chapters is historical, providing a partial cultural history of acute anxiety and panic in the West. The essays in this section make clear just how historically specific and contingent are current conceptualizations of PD, complicating enormously any effort to compare PD as an entity across time and space, as one might compare tuberculosis through social, cultural, and historical lenses. The third set of essays is positioned within cross-cultural psychiatry and medical anthropology, providing ethnographic and clinical accounts of PD and panic-like conditions in a number of specific settings. These chapters begin to answer questions about how panic attacks and PD may vary across cultures, and how PD as conceived by contemporary psychiatry relates to local idioms of distress, local categories of illness, and local moral worlds.

In this introduction we outline some of the critical issues and themes that emerge in the volume. We begin by reviewing the history of the professional biologization of PD, its conceptualization as a seizure-like entity minimally related to cultural or social context. We do so by tracing the history of the *DSM*, starting with the Sterling conference held in 1983. The next section describes the emergence of theories of the cause of PD that challenged this simple biologization, and outlines the theoretical ramifications of the most prominent of these theories: the catastrophic cognitions theory of panic. The final section gives an overview of the contributions of the current volume to advancing the study of PD in historical and cross-cultural perspective.

The Biologization of Panic Disorder in the 'DSM'

We begin by tracing the development of the *DSM–III* and *DSM–IV* conceptualization of PD, placing it in the context of theories of anxiety and panic in the 1980s and 1990s.

Reimagining Anxiety: From a Psychoanalytic to a Physiopsychological Perspective

In September 1983, nearly sixty researchers and administrators associated with the NIMH gathered in the Sterling Forest Conference Center in Tuxedo, New York, to discuss the state of the field of clinical and biological research about anxiety and anxiety disorders. Organized by the Clinical Research Branch of NIMH, the conference was designed to identify research issues, outline critical directions for new research, and stimulate broad scientific interest in the study of anxiety and anxiety disorders. The conveners of the conference argued that the major preoccupation of the psychiatric research community in the 1950s and 1960s was with schizophrenia, and in the 1970s, with affective disorders. They predicted confidently, however, that in the 1980s anxiety disorders would replace schizophrenia and affective disorders as the most critical site of progress in research in the neurosciences and psychiatry. The conference was designed both to stimulate and to give direction to that research, as a similar conference sponsored by NIMH had done for depression ten years earlier.

The edited book that resulted from the conference, *Anxiety and the Anxiety Disorders* (Tuma and Maser 1985), provides a sense of the field at the beginning of the 1980s. The initial chapters focus on basic biological and psychological research on anxiety, with papers on the neurobiology of anxiety and fear, on cognition and psychophysiology,[2] and on the use of animal models for research on fear and anxiety based in classic learning theory. The chapters that follow provide a broad picture of the state of clinical research on anxiety and anxiety disorders at that time. What the book fails to convey, however, is the excitement among participants at the meeting—the talk around the tables and in the corridors, the feeling of exhilaration about what emerging research was revealing, the powerful sense that the time was ripe for rapid progress in studying anxiety—and the place of PD in generating that excitement.[3]

It should be remembered that 1983 was only three years after the publication of the third edition of the *DSM* (APA 1980). In the context of psychiatric nosology, the *DSM–III* was a revolutionary document, purposely based in a *neo-Kraepelinian* or *descriptive* model of psychiatric classification and diagnosis, a model that eschewed efforts to classify disorders by their psychological causes in favor of establishing clear, symptom-based criteria that could be validated through empirical investigation. (For a critical description of the neo-Kraepelinian movement, see Good 1992:182–187; for apologists' accounts, see Blashfield 1984; Klerman 1978; Weissman and Klerman 1978). The *DSM–III* represented a rejection of the previous theoretical framing of psychiatric classification of disorders in psychoanalytic terms, as represented by the *DSM–II*. Although advocates for the so-called neo-Kraepelinian approach claimed that the *DSM–III* was "atheoretical," it was solidly grounded in a medical- or biological-psychiatry paradigm. The *DSM–III* represented psychopathology as a set of discrete, heterogeneous disorders or diseases, based on the hypothesis that such disorders would ultimately be shown to result from pathologies of structure and function at the level of human neurobiology. This view stands in stark contrast with the psychoanalytic assumptions about subjectivity, personality, and psychopathology that framed much of the previous diagnostic manual, the *DSM–II*, particularly in its classification of the neuroses. The *DSM–III* represented symbolically a major paradigm shift within psychiatry, with diagnosis and classification, neurobiology, and pharmaceutical treatments all assuming new importance.

The emergent paradigm reflected in the *DSM–III* provided the organizing frame and the context for the Sterling Forest Conference. The participants exuded a sense of confidence that research on anxiety and anxiety disorders had finally begun to catch up with other areas of the neurosciences, that enormous progress was under way, and that PD was a critical site for demonstrating the value of the neo-Kraepelinian approach. Studies of neurotransmitters and the neuroendocrine system supplemented the classic fight-or-flight-response understanding of anxiety as a distinctive physiological system based in human evolution. Studies had begun to demonstrate the role of specific neurotransmitters to explain how benzodiazepines and other anxiolytic medications function and to provide a deeper understanding of the hypothalamic-pituitary-adrenocortical system. Basic research on learning, studied experimentally in animal models, was helping to explain, at the level of molecular biology, classic observations about relations among stressful stimuli, fear responses, arousal, habituation, and inhibition or disinhibition. These studies were being linked through cognitive psychology to clinical phenomena and newly emerging cognitive therapies for the anxiety disorders.[4] There was strong support for the categorization of anxiety disorders into five basic types—phobias, panic, generalized anxiety disorder, obsessive-compulsive disorder, and posttraumatic stress disorder (PTSD). The organizers and most participants in the meeting took it for granted that these categories are based in natural reality and that it would prove most fruitful to pursue research and clinical approaches that focus primarily on one or another of these discrete disorders.

But why was PD seen as so important to this field? Why was there such excitement about PD, a sense that it would be *the* major "growth industry" in anxiety research in the 1980s, as Robert Spitzer, a driving force behind the *DSM–III*, predicted?[5] The discussion around the conference tables and in the dining room seemed to make clear what was only occasionally referred to in the scientific panels: not only was PD a newly recognized psychiatric disorder, especially promising for yielding scientific knowledge, but it also provided neo-Kraepelinian psychiatrists and neuroscientists with a unique opportunity to attack the stronghold of psychoanalysis. Whereas psychoanalysis had made little progress in decades of writing about anxiety and anxiety attacks, many at the conference felt that in a very short time biological psychiatry had made enormous scientific progress and promised far more to come. Only three of the forty-three scientific papers in the meeting addressed psychodynamic perspectives on anxiety, and the talk in the corridors was of psychoanalysts as dinosaurs, about to disappear.

PD provided a particularly powerful basis for arguing that the neo-Kraepelinian paradigm could advance understanding of acute anxiety, long considered the domain of the neuroses and psychoanalysis. There were three broad reasons for this claim. First, new evidence suggested that PD is a discrete, heterogeneous disorder, distinct from other anxiety disorders. Particularly interesting was the discovery that panic attacks do not respond to the benzodiazepines, typically used for anxiety, but respond specifically to the drug imipramine, usually considered an antidepressant (Klein 1980).[6] Klein had shown that imipramine was effective against spontaneous panic attacks but not against chronic anxiety, suggesting that panic attacks are a distinctive disorder (see Barlow 2002:125–126; McNally 1994:1–4).[7] Defining clear criteria for PD allowed researchers to investigate the specific biological, genetic, pharmacological, and epidemiological characteristics of this distinctive disorder.

In addition, Klein (1980) and Sheehan (1983) argued strongly that PD consisted of panic attacks that were largely *unprovoked* and experienced by sufferers as coming *out of the blue*. This formulation suggested that panic attacks are generated physiologically rather than psychologically, that they result from neurobiological processes rather than from the surfacing of unconscious psychological conflicts associated with seemingly unrelated stimuli. This argument was supported by findings of apparent physiological differences associated with PD, including intriguing research suggesting that infusion of sodium lactate would trigger panic attacks in persons suffering unmedicated PD, but not in normal populations.

Finally, a series of papers had recently argued that agoraphobia, a severe and little-understood condition, could be explained through conditioning-type learning theory as rooted in anxiety associated with those locations in which the person had suffered a terrifying panic attack, followed by the gradual development of an irrational fear that leaving his or her house, particularly without the support of another person, might provoke another anxiety attack (Klein 1980). PD was thus conceived as *discrete*, as *unprovoked*, as having symptoms that map directly onto a *physiological substrate*, and as producing *secondary elaborations* that make sense of other distinctive anxiety disorders (see Good 1992:188–189). This might be called a *physiopsychology*, in which a physiological event is primary (it causes panic) and psychology—namely, the psychological state of fear—is secondary; and in this model, psychological process is reduced to conditioning: the pairing of fear to a certain place.

This brief account of a moment in the history of American psychiatry provides insight into current dominant view of PD, with its strong attachment both to criteria that define *panic disorder* as a discrete, heterogeneous condition and to the idea that panic attacks are unprovoked. In the next part of this section, we briefly describe the emergence of PD within the APA's diagnostic and statistical manuals, and in the following sections we suggest how recent psychological research, cross-cultural studies, and historical research challenge this dominant model.

Panic Disorder in the Subsequent 'DSM' Tradition

In recent theory, anxiety and fear are considered distinct emotions (for a review, see Barlow 2002). Fear is a primitive alarm in response to a perceived immediate danger. It leads to arousal; to activation of both the sympathetic and parasympathetic nervous systems, experienced in bodily sensations such as palpitations and sweating; and to certain action tendencies (freezing or fleeing). In contrast, "anxiety is considered to be a future-oriented emotion, characterized by perceptions of uncontrollability and unpredictability over potentially dangerous events" (Barlow 2002:104).

According to current thinking, in the psychology and psychiatry enshrined in the *DSM–IV* (published in 1994), there are five general domains of distinct anxiety disorders:

- *Generalized anxiety disorder*, characterized by excessive worry about current life problems and future events, leading to muscular tension and other symptoms
- *Posttraumatic stress disorder*, marked by constant arousal and reactivity to any reminder of past traumas, as well as a tendency to reexperience past traumas as though they were current
- *Obsessive-compulsive disorder*, identified by contamination fears and a compulsion to repeat certain behaviors, especially checking behaviors
- *Phobias*, characterized by unreasonable levels of fear concerning objects, places, or situations, and anxiety about contact with these[8]

- *Panic disorder*, defined by episodes of acute fear or anxiety (with enough symptoms to constitute a "panic attack"), the fear often focusing on concerns of dying from internally arising bodily dysfunction.

Although PD first appeared as a diagnosis in *DSM–III* (1980), experiences of acute anxiety, with physical symptoms similar to those that serve as criteria for panic attacks, have a longer history in the APA's diagnostic manuals. In the *DSM–I*, published in 1952, what is now called PD was diagnosed most commonly as either an *anxiety reaction*, defined as a general state of fear with frequently associated somatic symptomatology, or as one of the *psychophysiologic autonomic and visceral disorders*. In *DSM–II*, published in 1968, the term *anxiety reaction* was replaced with *anxiety neurosis*, and *psychophysiologic autonomic and visceral disorders* was replaced by *psychophysiologic disorders*. Only in the *DSM–III*, published in 1980, did *panic disorder* become identified as a separate psychiatric entity. The diagnosis of *agoraphobia* first appeared in *DSM–III*, along with PD.

Table 1.1 outlines criteria for a PD diagnosis in the *DSM–III*. Criterion C specified that a PD diagnosis could not be made in the presence of other diagnostic entities. Thus, according to the *DSM–III's* hierarchical model of diagnosis, when PD co-occurred with another disorder, it was to be understood as an epiphenomenon,

Table 1.1   Diagnostic criteria for panic disorder in the *DSM–III*

A. At least three Panic Attacks within a three-week period in circumstances other than during marked physical exertion or in a life-threatening situation. The attacks are not precipitated only by exposure to a circumscribed phobic stimulus.

B. Panic Attacks are manifested by discrete periods of apprehension or fear, and at least four of the following symptoms appear during each attack:

(1) dyspnea

(2) palpitations

(3) chest pain or discomfort

(4) choking or smothering sensations

(5) dizziness, vertigo, or unsteady feelings

(6) feelings of unreality

(7) paresthesia (tingling in the hands or feet)

(8) hot or cold flashes

(9) sweating

(10) faintness

(11) trembling or shaking

(12) fear of dying, going crazy, or doing something uncontrolled during an attack

C. Not due to a physical disorder or another mental disorder, such as Major Depression, Somatization Disorder, or Schizophrenia.

SOURCE: *Diagnostic and Statistical Manual of Mental Disorders*. 3rd. ed. [*DSM–III.*] Pp. 231–232. Copyright 1980, American Psychiatric Association. Reprinted with permission.

a symptom of another condition and an indicator of illness severity rather than a unique entity (Baker 1989; Carey 1985). Major depressive disorder, for example, was higher in the hierarchy than PD, so PD could not be diagnosed in a person who had major depressive disorder.[9]

In the *DSM–III–R* (the revised edition of *DSM–III*, published in 1987), five major changes were made in the PD category (see Table 1.2):

1. No longer did three panic attacks have to be experienced in a period of three weeks to meet criteria; instead, a person was required to have suffered only one panic attack in the preceding month.

2. Nausea was added to the symptom list. The delay in including nausea in the list of panic attack symptoms reflects the dominance of cardiac symptoms and

Table 1.2   Diagnostic criteria for panic disorder in the *DSM–III–R*

A. At some time during the disturbance, one or more Panic Attacks (discrete periods of intense fear or discomfort) have occurred that were (1) unexpected, i.e., did not occur immediately before or on exposure to a situation that almost always causes anxiety, and (2) not triggered by situations in which the person was the focus of others' attention.

B. Either four attacks, as defined in criterion A, have occurred within a four-week period, or one or more attacks have been followed by a period of at least a month of persistent fear of having another attack.

C. At least four of the following symptoms developed during at least one of the attacks:

(1) shortness of breath (dyspnea) or smothering sensations

(2) dizziness, unsteady feelings, or faintness

(3) palpitations or accelerated heart rate (tachycardia)

(4) trembling or shaking

(5) sweating

(6) choking

(7) nausea or abdominal distress

(8) depersonalization or derealization

(9) numbness or tingling sensations (paresthesias)

(10) flushes (hot flashes) or chills

(11) chest pain or discomfort

(12) fear of dying

(13) fear of going crazy or doing something uncontrolled

D. During at least some of the attacks, at least four of the C symptoms developed suddenly and increased in intensity within ten minutes of the beginning of the first C symptoms noticed in the attack.

E. It cannot be established that an organic factor initiated and maintained the disturbance, e.g., amphetamine or caffeine intoxication, hyperthyroidism.

SOURCE: *Diagnostic and Statistical Manual of Mental Disorders*. 3rd ed., rev. [*DSM–III–R*.] Pp. 237–238. Copyright 1987, American Psychiatric Association. Reprinted with permission.

shortness of breath in twentieth-century Western scientific theories of panic etiology, and the neglect of dizziness-type complaints and nausea. The latter two complaints are particularly prominent in Asian populations, as essays in this volume demonstrate (see, for example, Chapters 7, 8, and 10).

3. It was specified that to be considered a panic attack, at least four symptoms must have developed suddenly, and increased in intensity to a state of panic within ten minutes.

4. A diagnosis of PD could be made even if another disorder was present; for example, a person could be diagnosed as suffering both PD and major depressive disorder. This represented a shift from a hierarchical to a comorbidity view of illness, a shift from a model in which one primary disorder generated all the other so-called secondary symptoms to a model of multiple, simultaneously occurring disorders. (However, as the next paragraph shows, the "cue" criteria led to PD not being diagnosed in the presence of PTSD.)

5. In *DSM–III–R*, the panic attacks in PD were defined as "uncued," that is, as unprovoked eruptions of anxiety. Only one type of panic attack in PD was thought to be provoked by a cue: agoraphobia-type panic attacks, in which being in certain external spaces, such as a mall, might trigger a panic attack, in essence constituting "place-caused" panic. This insistence on the uncued nature of panic attacks in PD implied that panic attacks in the context of PTSD could not be considered PD-type panic attacks. That is, if a patient feared death or insanity from the symptoms (for example, palpitations or racing thoughts) caused by encountering some reminder of a trauma event—that is, a trauma cue—such as someone resembling a perpetrator or a place similar to the location of the trauma, and if that fear escalated to panic, the panic attack could not be classified as PD in type.

In the *DSM–IV*, published in 1994, the criteria defining PD were minimally changed (see Tables 1.3 and 1.4). As in the previous edition, a person must experience "recurrent, unexpected panic attacks" that develop suddenly in less than ten minutes. Here we have the widely debated out-of-the-blue and rapid-crescendo criteria that configure panic as a sort of periodic seizure, unrelated to stimuli that awaken hidden conflicts or to cognitions about concurrent actions or bodily states. In *DSM–IV* (as in *DSM–III* and *DSM–III–R*) one type of triggering cue is allowed in defining panic attacks: the cue associated with agoraphobia. Being in certain places or situations, including being outside the home alone, being in a crowd, standing in a line, being on a bridge, or traveling in a bus, train, or automobile are considered *situationally predisposed panic attacks*. When these situations trigger panic attacks, the disorder is classified as PD with agoraphobia (see Table 1.5).

Table 1.3   Diagnostic criteria for panic disorder in the *DSM–IV*

A. Both (1) and (2):

(1) recurrent unexpected Panic Attacks

(2) at least one of the attacks has been followed by one month (or more) of one (or more) of the following:

(a) persistent concern about having additional attacks

(b) worry about the implications of the attack or its consequences (e.g., losing control, having a heart attack, "going crazy")

(c) a significant change in behavior related to the attacks

B. The Panic Attacks are not due to the direct physiological effects of a substance (such as a drug of abuse, a medication) or a general medical condition (such as hyperthyroidism).

C. The Panic Attacks are not better accounted for by another mental disorder, such as Social Phobia (e.g., occurring on exposure to feared social situations), Specific Phobia (e.g., on exposure to a specific phobic situation), Obsessive-Compulsive Disorder (e.g., on exposure to dirt in someone with an obsession about contamination), Posttraumatic Stress Disorder (e.g., in response to stimuli associated with a severe stressor), or Separation Anxiety Disorder (e.g., in response to being away from home or close relatives).

SOURCE: *Diagnostic and Statistical Manual of Mental Disorders.* 4th ed. [*DSM–IV.*] Pp. 401–402. Copyright 1994, American Psychiatric Association. Reprinted with permission.

Table 1.4   Diagnostic criteria for panic attack in the *DSM–IV*

A discrete period of intense fear or discomfort, in which four (or more) of the following symptoms developed abruptly and reached a peak within 10 minutes:

(1) palpitations, pounding heart, or accelerated heart rate

(2) sweating

(3) trembling or shaking

(4) sensations of shortness of breath or smothering

(5) feeling of choking

(6) chest pain or discomfort

(7) nausea or abdominal distress

(8) feeling dizzy, unsteady, lightheaded, or faint

(9) derealization (feeling of unreality) or depersonalization (being detached from oneself)

(10) fear of losing control or going crazy

(11) fear of dying

(12) paresthesia (numbing or tingling sensations)

(13) chills or hot flashes

SOURCE: *Diagnostic and Statistical Manual of Mental Disorders.* 4th ed. [*DSM–IV.*] P. 395. Copyright 1994, American Psychiatric Association. Reprinted with permission.

Table 1.5   Diagnostic criteria for agoraphobia in the *DSM–IV*

A. Anxiety about being in places or situations from which escape might be difficult (or embarrassing) or in which help may not be available in the event of having an expected or situationally predisposed Panic Attack or panic-like symptoms. Agoraphobic fears typically involve characteristic clusters of situations that include being outside the home alone; being in a crowd or standing in a line; being on a bridge; and traveling in a bus, train, or automobile.

B. The situations are avoided (e.g., travel is limited) or else are endured with marked distress or with anxiety about having a Panic Attack or panic-like symptoms, or require the presence of a companion.

C. The anxiety or phobic avoidance is not better accounted for by another mental disorder, such as Social Phobia (e.g., avoidance limited to social situations because of fear of embarrassment), Specific Phobia (e.g., avoidance limited to a single situation such as elevators), Obsessive-Compulsive Disorder (e.g., avoidance of dirt in someone with an obsession about contamination), Posttraumatic Stress Disorder (e.g., avoidance of stimuli associated with a severe stressor), or Separation Anxiety Disorder (e.g., avoidance of leaving home or relatives).

SOURCE: *Diagnostic and Statistical Manual of Mental Disorders*. 4th ed. [*DSM–IV.*] P. 396. Copyright 1994, American Psychiatric Association. Reprinted with permission.

As did the previous editions, the *DSM–IV* continues a sharp distinction between PD and PTSD, owing to the insistence on the untriggered nature of panic attacks in PD. Thus, if a panic attack is triggered by a trauma cue—for example, an experience that provokes a memory of a traumatic event, followed by physiological symptoms of anxiety and concerns about a heart attack—the episode is not considered a PD-type panic attack. According to the *DSM–IV*'s definition of PD, such hybrid entities do not meet PD criteria, but rather should be classified simply as PTSD.

One important change in the *DSM–IV* should be noted. The diagnosis of panic attacks was separated out from the diagnosis for PD. This reflected a growing realization that panic attacks were found in many disorders (for a discussion, see Chapter 6 in the present book), a realization that has continued to grow.

In the current edition of the psychiatric diagnostic manual, *DSM–IV–TR* (2000), the criteria for PD are unchanged from *DSM–IV*. The *DSM–V* Work Group on Panic Disorders has been meeting, but with no indication to date of any substantial changes from current criteria.

Recent Findings and Theories Challenging the 'DSM' Conceptualization of Panic Disorder

In this section we outline recent critiques of the *DSM–IV*'s biological conceptualization of PD, and the emergence of a psychological view of panic's origin. We discuss the important implications of a catastrophic cognitions theory in respect to historical and cross-cultural variations in panic.

Controversies Surrounding the Definition of Panic Disorder

Several elements in the *DSM* definition of PD have been particularly controversial. These elements relate in large measure to efforts to constitute PD as an autonomous, largely physiological disease entity. First, there remain important questions about the discrete set of anxiety symptoms listed as diagnostic criteria. In some cultural contexts, acute anxiety symptoms other than the thirteen listed in the *DSM–IV* take center stage. For example, among Cambodian refugee populations, tinnitus is called "*khyâl* shooting from the ears" (*khyâl choenh pii troechia*), and this somatic event is thought to indicate bodily weakness and a disorder in the "*khyâl* physiology." (According to the Khmer ethnophysiology, *khyâl* is a windlike substance that courses through blood vessels.) Tinnitus is a common—and personally and clinically important—complaint during anxiety and panic states in this group (Hinton et al. 2006a, in press). In addition, *DSM–IV* places certain symptoms together under a single criterion (such as feeling "dizzy, unsteady, lightheaded, or faint," or having "chills or hot flashes"), suggesting that they are somehow equivalent. Data suggest that these symptoms may be symbolically equivalent in one society but not in another, and that the experience and categorization of symptoms may differ across cultures in important ways.

Second, specific questions about the defining characteristics of panic attacks remain unresolved. For example, the research reported in this book suggests that it is arbitrary to require that for an experience of anxiety to qualify as a panic attack the anxiety must start abruptly and reach a peak in ten minutes. If a person feels increasingly anxious over a longer period—for example, over the course of an hour, finally reaching a state of panic—the *DSM–IV* would define this experience as not meeting the criteria for a panic attack. Findings presented in this book provide evidence that across cultures there are important variations in the pattern of onset of anxiety, raising serious questions about this criterion.

Third, in *DSM–IV*, the presence of PTSD excludes a diagnosis of PD. Criterion C (see Table 1.3) states that panic attacks should not be better accounted for by another disorder, specifying that the panic should not be a response to a "stimulus" associated with a traumatic event. If such a stimulus—for example, dizziness—both recalls a past traumatic event (such as being beaten on the head by police or soldiers in settings of conflict or torture) and causes thoughts about imminent bodily disaster, such as a stroke, the clinician should make the diagnosis not of PD but of PTSD. To this extent *DSM–IV* remains hierarchical, indicating that if one diagnosis (PTSD) is present, another diagnosis (PD) cannot be made. In respect to PD, the *DSM–IV* proscribes hybrid or comorbid entities. The relations among memories of trauma, panic attacks, PD, and PTSD raise important questions for empirical, cross-cultural research, and the exclusion of comorbid diagnoses of PTSD and PD remains controversial.

Fourth, in order to meet *DSM–IV* PD criteria, the panic attack should be "unexpected," that is, come out of the blue (see criterion A, number 1 in Table 1.3). Such a view, as we have suggested, aims to characterize a panic attack as an autonomous physiological process, a sort of seizure of the nervous system. In fact, most psychological researchers today think that panic is frequently triggered rather than unexpected; the anthropological data would also suggest this to be the case, as we note later and as the research reported in this book shows.

These rather straightforward controversies point to much more essential questions for the field. Are panic attacks indeed physiological eruptions, akin to a seizure, or are they (sometimes? always?) far more psychologically motivated and organized? Are there fundamental differences across cultures in the experience of panic attacks that raise important doubts about the universality of current diagnostic criteria? Can panic attacks be initiated by events or experiences that trigger fears or anxieties through hidden semantic networks or psychological associations that are out of awareness or unconscious? Indeed, are the panic attacks that occur in trauma disorders and PD (always? sometimes?) heterogeneous, or are they overlapping conditions? One of the goals of this book is to provide the best examples of cross-cultural, ethnographic, and clinical research that speak to questions such as these.

The Emergence of a Psychological Theory: Catastrophic Cognitions and Panic Disorder

There has long been a tension between theorizing panic attacks in neo-Kraepelinian terms—as a distinct pathological entity, largely understood as spontaneous biological events—and a more psychological interpretation of panic attacks. The Sterling Forest Conference, which occurred right after the publication of the *DSM–III*, represented a moment in which powerful claims were made about the adequacy of a biological understanding of panic attacks—claims that panic attacks are spontaneous physiological events in persons genetically predisposed to such a disorder. This noncultural, nonpsychological view of the core processes generating PD would continue in *DSM–IV*, as we have described.

Any modeling of panic attacks in PD also had to respond to observations that panic attacks occur in many *DSM*-defined disorders. Some panic attacks are "stimulus bound" (phobias) or "situationally predisposed" (social phobias), and memories (particularly traumatic memories) may trigger panic attacks or experiences of acute anxiety (PTSD). Modeling of panic attacks in PD required understanding the process of the rapid crescendo of panic symptoms, the focus on the body and fear of dying, or the worry that one was out of control and might be going crazy. Even the strongest proponents of a biological approach to understanding PD were required to introduce psychology—usually via behavioral learning theory and cognitive psychology, namely, *conditioning* theories—to understand the clinical phenomena, such as anticipatory anxiety and agoraphobia, even as they were claiming that biological psychiatry provided a clear, scientific alternative to psychoanalytic understandings of acute anxiety.

Over time, the hypothesis that panic attacks in PD were primarily unprovoked, seizure-like events was challenged empirically, leading to the development of more robust psychological theories of PD. The development of theories of catastrophic cognitions, in particular, has been extremely influential and has led to very different models for understanding and treating PD than were present in 1983.

Critiques of the Biological Explanations of the Laboratory Induction of Panic Attacks in Panic Disorder   Efforts to isolate physiological processes that cause panic have a long history, such as theories that focused on a heart etiology in the Civil War and World War I (see Chapters 4 and 5). One important hypothesis, which in 1983 was still referred to as evidence for a biological theory of PD, suggested that lactate might play a critical physiological role. In an influential research report, Pitts and McClure (1967) demonstrated that lactate caused panic among persons with what was called *effort syndrome:* when they injected those patients with lactate, acute episodes of headache, dizziness, faintness, weakness, and chest tightness, resulting in panic, followed. In the 1970s, researchers working within a cognitive paradigm challenged this purely biological formulation. In an article published in 1974, Ackerman and Sachar questioned the validity of the lactate theory of panic and hypothesized that panic was not produced by the effects of lactate (or of lactate-induced low calcium) in the brain, but rather by catastrophic cognitions about lactate-induced symptoms. Cold extremities associated with lactate injection could result in fear of stroke, they argued. Pitts and McClure and other cognitive theorists suggested that PD patients are hyperreactive to a wide spectrum of agents other than lactate, including carbon dioxide, yohimbine, and norepinephrine. According to cognitive theorists, the most parsimonious explanation for this broad reactivity was hypersensitivity to somatic sensations, irrespective of the method of induction (Barlow 2002:171, 178–179).

Panic Attacks as Triggered by Catastrophic Cognitions About Somatic Sensations   In the 1980s, cognitive theorists increasingly argued that the *DSM*'s out-of-the-blue criterion—that true panic attacks are unprovoked—should be eliminated (for reviews, see Beck 1988; Craske 1991; McNally 1994; Rapee et al. 1995; Street et al. 1989). Instead, they argued, catastrophic cognitions about bodily sensations constitute a core process in provoking panic attacks, and the feared bodily sensations that provoke panic may be induced by a wide range of "triggers." Clark (1986:462) summarized this catastrophic cognitions theory of panic as follows (see Figure 1.1):

The trigger for an attack often seems to be the perception of a bodily sensation which itself is caused by a different emotional state (excitement, anger) or by some

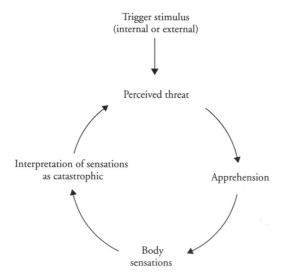

Figure 1.1   A cognitive model of the generation of a panic attack, as depicted by Clark (1986)

quite innocuous event such as suddenly getting up from the sitting position (dizziness), exercise (breathlessness, palpitations) or drinking coffee (palpitations). Once perceived, the bodily sensation is interpreted in a catastrophic fashion and then a panic attack results.

Other common ways in which sensations might be induced, and which then trigger panic attacks, were also explored, for example, hyperventilation, which causes a host of bodily sensations, including blurry vision and hand numbness (Beck 1988); and temperature and humidity changes (such as those resulting from entering a sauna or moving from a warm to a cold space), which cause somatic symptoms such as sweating or cold extremities (Rapee et al. 1995).

Theoretical Implications of the Catastrophic Cognitions Theory of Panic Disorder   If the catastrophic cognitions theory of panic (which is often called the *cognitive theory of panic disorder*) is valid, it has important implications in respect to the nature of PD and its historical and cross-cultural variability. Following are several hypotheses that emerge from a catastrophic cognitions theory of the generation of PD that have particular significance for investigating cross-cultural differences in the phenomenology and distribution of panic attacks and PD.

HYPOTHESIS 1: *The severity of catastrophic cognitions should predict panic severity and frequency.* According to the catastrophic cognitions theory of panic, the more severe a person's catastrophic cognitions about particular sensations are, the greater should be the frequency and severity of panic attacks. In support of this hypothesis, multiple studies demonstrate that the severity of catastrophic cognitions about panic sensations is strongly related to the severity and frequency of PD panic attacks (for a review, see Hinton et al. 2006b). This would suggest a close relationship between cultural interpretations of the danger of particular sensations and rates of PD associated with those sensations.

HYPOTHESIS 2: *Decreasing catastrophic cognitions should improve PD.* According to the catastrophic cognitions theory of panic, treatments that reduce a person's catastrophic cognitions about panic sensations should decrease the frequency and severity of PD panic attacks. In support of this hypothesis, multiple studies illustrate that reducing catastrophic cognitions of PD patients is at least as effective as medication in allaying the severity and frequency of PD panic attacks (for reviews, see Barlow 2002; McNally 1994; Taylor 2000). This finding provides further evidence that catastrophic cognitions occurring during PD panic attacks, which would be expected to vary by culture (see Hypothesis 3), are some of the very "cogs" of the disorder.

HYPOTHESIS 3: *The emphasized symptoms of PD panic attacks will vary across cultural groups and historical periods.* According to the catastrophic cognitions theory of panic, the sensations most prominent in PD panic attacks will vary depending on which sensations are viewed as potentially catastrophic by members of a society or social group. Given local illness concepts and syndromes, certain bodily sensations will be viewed with more fear, and those symptoms will form the critical symptoms associated with panic in those contexts.[10] The main symptoms focused on by persons suffering PD panic attacks should vary by cultural groups and historical periods, as well as across individuals within particular cultural groups and historical periods.

HYPOTHESIS 4: *The events or actions that trigger the sensations that cause PD panic attacks will vary across cultural groups and historical periods.* According to the catastrophic cognitions theory of panic, in different individuals, cultural groups, and historical periods what induces the feared sensations and triggers PD-type panic attacks may vary. Given local illness concepts and syndromes, specific bodily sensations will be viewed with more fear in certain situations, such as upon going into a crowded mall, upon engaging in worry, upon standing up, or upon going outside and being hit by a strong wind when feeling weak.[11] Put another way, the events and actions that trigger panic will vary radically by cultural group and historical period.

HYPOTHESIS 5: *PD catastrophic cognitions will vary across cultural groups and historical periods.* According to the catastrophic cognitions theory of panic, the catastrophic cognitions or modes of rationality associated with panic attacks may

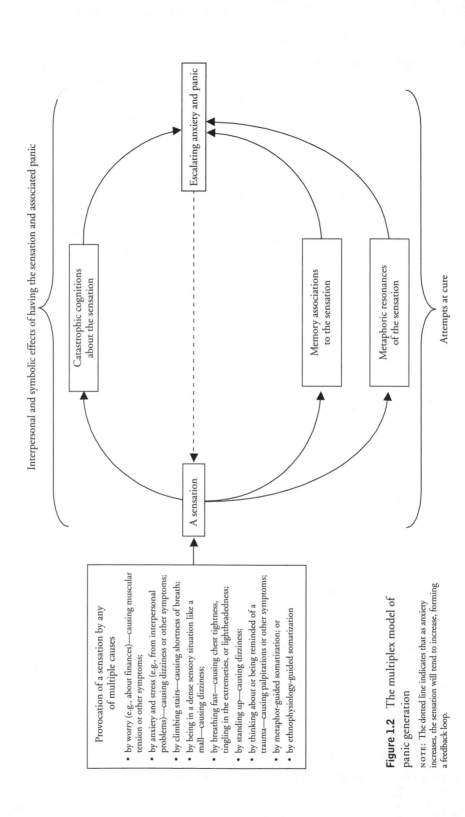

Interpersonal and symbolic effects of having the sensation and associated panic

Escalating anxiety and panic

Catastrophic cognitions about the sensation

Memory associations to the sensation

Metaphoric resonances of the sensation

A sensation

Attempts at cure

Provocation of a sensation by any of multiple causes

• by worry (e.g., about finances)—causing muscular tension or other symptoms;

• by anxiety and stress (e.g., from interpersonal problems)—causing dizziness or other symptoms;

• by climbing stairs—causing shortness of breath;

• by being in a dense sensory situation like a mall—causing dizziness;

• by breathing fast—causing chest tightness, tingling in the extremeties, or lightheadedness;

• by standing up—causing dizziness;

• by thinking about or being reminded of a trauma—causing palpitations or other symptoms;

• by metaphor-guided somatization; or

• by ethnophysiology-guided somatization

Figure 1.2   The multiplex model of panic generation

NOTE: The dotted line indicates that as anxiety increases, the sensation will tend to increase, forming a feedback loop.

vary depending on local ideas about human physiology and on local cultural syndromes. As conceptualizations of the body, its physiology, and illness syndromes have shifted, so too have the nature of catastrophic cognitions and the structure of the panic ontology. Catastrophic cognitions will thus vary significantly across cultures, cultural subgroups, and historical periods, depending on the regnant syndromes and ethnophysiologies.

HYPOTHESIS 6: *The onset of PD panic attacks may be relatively prolonged.* According to the catastrophic cognitions theory of panic, episodes of PD panic attacks are not seizure-like events. They may crescendo rapidly (in less than ten minutes, as specified in the *DSM–IV* criteria) or they may crescendo more slowly, even over several hours, worsening as the patient's catastrophic cognitions worsen. In fact, a recent study indicates that the ten-minute criterion should not even be applied to English-speaking North Americans (see Scupi et al. 1997).

HYPOTHESIS 7: *Hybrid panic attacks should occur that combine PTSD and PD characteristics.* According to the catastrophic cognitions theory of panic, PD panic attacks should frequently co-occur with trauma-related disorder. Encountering a trauma-related stimulus (such as conditions resembling the location of the original trauma) or thinking about a trauma may trigger various sensations. These sensations may in turn be cognized or interpreted as threatening and potentially catastrophic. For example, palpitations may recall a traumatic event in which the person experienced strong palpitations, and palpitations may concurrently evoke catastrophic cognitions (for instance, those of a heart attack). There is evidence that such hybrid panic attacks are common (see, for example, Hinton et al. 2006b). How these hybrid panic attacks occur can be depicted by a multiplex model such as that represented by Figure 1.2 (for further discussion of the components of this model, see Chapter 3).

Contributions of This Volume

Many of the chapters in the current volume draw on a catastrophic cognitions theory of panic and explore one or more of the hypotheses just outlined. The chapters provide support for these proposed hypotheses, illustrating the heuristic value of a catastrophic cognitions approach to the study of panic across cultural contexts and historical periods. Several chapters illustrate the great variability in the symptoms that form the core symptom of PD-type panic attacks; they demonstrate how historically and culturally varying syndromes and ethnophysiologies give rise to catastrophic cognitions that produce panic, and they demonstrate the hybrid nature of panic, linking panic and trauma symptoms. This approach thus provides one model for making psychological and cultural *processes* central to investigations of culture and PD, rather than focusing more narrowly on cultural variability in symptom criteria and diagnostic entities.

As we have already suggested briefly, the catastrophic cognitions approach may be integrated with an understanding of interpretive practices through which distinctive modes of reality are constituted (Good 1994), as well as with a cultural phenomenology and anthropology of sensations, as outlined by Hinton and Good in Chapter 3 of this book. An anthropological approach assumes that catastrophic cognitions are grounded in diverse symbolic forms, linked outwardly to social and political domains, and inwardly to bodily and psychological experience. Local bodily logics, networks of semantic or cultural associations, body metaphors, complex memory processes, and other symbolic forms are critical to the processes of appraisal and interpretation that produce responses to sensation that may trigger panic attacks (see Figure 1.2).

Theoretical Perspectives on Panic Disorder

The two chapters in Part I argue for the importance of studying PD from both a historical and a cross-cultural perspective, and they present some analytic tools for doing so: an anthropology of sensations (namely, sensations embedded in complex networks of meanings and within specific technological, political, and bodily practices); a catastrophic cognitions theory of panic; meaning-forming processes; and the link between power and knowledge (that is, an examination of who is empowered by a certain conceptualization of the cause of panic). They contend that the panic experience can be understood only when situated in the context of a particular life that exists in a specific cultural-historical moment, in a distinct environmental location (with a certain architecture, a certain range of sensory-scapes, a certain configuration of dangers), in a set sociological situation, and in a determined economic position.

Historical Perspectives on PD—Like Disorders

The second section of this collection provides contributions to a cultural history of PD. Any claim to studying the history of a disorder formally codified as recently as 1980 obviously falls prey to a presentist bias, raising questions about what phenomena should belong to such a history. Nonetheless, it is clear that broad categories of psychopathology have quite different cultural and civilizational histories. In European and American history, schizophrenia is embedded in ideas of genetic decline and degeneracy, dangerousness, incurability, and asylums, and these are in turn linked to ideas about human difference and evolution rooted jointly in colonial encounters with others and subsequent interpretations of these encounters. Depression has a quite different cultural history, being linked, on the one hand, to classical Hippocratic writings about melancholia and, on the other, to the Christian category *acedia*, one of the cardinal sins that affected early ascetics with a "weariness or distress of heart" "akin to dejection" (Jackson 1985). Anxiety has yet a different cultural trajectory—embedded in ideas of nerves and the depletion of nervous energy associated with industrialization, modernity, and the "age of anxiety," but also associated with danger and fear, linked to the battlefield and trauma as well as to acute experiences of cardiac distress; to debates about the role of physiological and functional sources of such distress; and to a broad range of irrational fears and phobias. Despite our ability to point to such broad cultural trajectories, isolating a cultural history of panic among these trajectories is particularly challenging.

The book's historical section aims to provide a genealogy[12] of current conceptualizations of PD—to identify phenomena that share a family resemblance to panic attacks; to trace epistemic shifts in understandings of these conditions; to note links between epistemic changes and other shifts in society; to look closely at diverse representations of acute fear and anxiety, particularly in medicine and psychiatry; and to observe debates and emerging ideologies about their causation. These chapters suggest that the acute onset of multiple symptoms, accompanied by fear of death or insanity, gave rise to multiple causal theories and to associated therapeutic practices and "technologies of the self" (Martin et al. 1988), providing PD with a distinctive cultural history.

Cross-Cultural Studies of Panic Disorder

For the Sterling Forest Conference, Byron Good and Arthur Kleinman were asked to provide a cross-cultural review of the literature on anxiety disorders, a review situated among the triumphalist claims of a universal biological psychiatry and neo-Kraepelinian understandings of psychiatric disorders. Their review (Good and Kleinman 1985) staked out a position in conversation with the neo-Kraepelinian views that were dominant at that conference. "Is there evidence that anxiety and disorders of anxiety exist in other cultures?" this review asks, and then poses the following questions. Are the five basic subcategories of anxiety disorders the same across cultures, or do subtypes of anxiety disorders differ by culture or by ethnomedical tradition? Are *DSM* symptom criteria universal, as the biological paradigm suggests, or does culture shape the symptoms associated with particular disorders? What is the relationship between particular local illness categories—for example, *ataques de nervios* among Puerto Ricans, or subtypes of neurasthenia in the Japanese Morita psychotherapy system—and *DSM* categories? What does the cross-cultural research tell us about these issues? Although it focused primarily on the cross-cultural literature, the review was intended to raise similar questions for diverse American ethnic groups, subcultures, and immigrant populations.

The Good and Kleinman review purposely challenged the assumptions of most researchers attending the Sterling Forest Conference as well as the architects of the

DSM system: that symptoms directly reflect physiological abnormalities and that categories of anxiety disorders are natural reflections of disordered human biology. It was also intended to raise questions about the relationship between culture and psychopathology that could be addressed only through research. Although in 1983 there was adequate evidence to raise these questions and to suggest substantial cross-cultural variation, for none of the anxiety disorders or particular cultures was the research strong enough to answer any of these questions in a convincing, empirical manner.

Over the past two decades, a wide-ranging literature based on both empirical research and clinical experience has begun to emerge, providing a basis for responding to many of these questions. The research reported in the chapters in the third section of this book goes considerably beyond the questions formulated by Kleinman and Good in 1983,[13] speaking to the controversies that have emerged in the past two decades. As we shall see, the studies also provide data relevant to new ways of thinking about PD.

To point forward, the ethnographic chapters in this book suggest the following:

- The data provide strong support for the relevance of using PD as a comparative category for research. Panic attacks are recognizable and widely reported in the cultures represented in this book.

- The studies presented here suggest that interdisciplinary research combining clinical, ethnographic, and epidemiological methods that draw on concepts from current psychiatry and critical social sciences is the most fruitful way to proceed.

- The ethnographic chapters in this book follow recent clinical investigations in raising serious doubts about a narrow focus of attention on those panic attacks that appear to be unprovoked or out of the blue. A clear distinction between panic attacks that are provoked and those that are not is often impossible to make. Basing a diagnostic approach on this distinction seems quite dubious. The cross-cultural research supports a far more social and psychological view of panic attacks than that represented by the narrow biological models.

- In many parts of the world and for many persons, a neat separation of panic attacks as found in PD and trauma experiences is not tenable. Several of the chapters suggest a rich and complex relationship between PD-type panic attacks and trauma experiences, which has clear implications for the *DSM* formulation of these as noncomorbid conditions.

- Some of the essays in this volume speak specifically to the question of the phenomenology of panic attacks, including both those symptoms that are most prominent and the pattern of emergence and crescendo of symptoms within the ten-minute period indicated by the *DSM* system. Clearly the *DSM* definitions do not adequately represent the empirical data obtained from cross-cultural studies.

- The chapters in this book provide extremely rich empirical data on the relationship between local illness categories and PD in settings as diverse as Puerto Rican mainland and island communities, Rwanda, Thailand, Tibetan refugee communities, and China. These chapters indicate that although there is a relationship between local illness categories and *DSM* categories, there is no one-to-one relationship between a particular local illness category and *DSM* categories. *Ataques de nervios* is not a Puerto Rican term for PD; *ataques* are culturally meaningful and phenomenologically consistent, but they are heterogeneous in terms of *DSM* disorders. There is now empirical evidence to indicate precisely the nature of the heterogeneity.

Overall, the ethnographic chapters in this book do not support the conceptualization of PD as a spontaneous, biological eruption with universal phenomenology. Instead, they open onto a more complex modeling of panic experiences. As such, they also suggest a more complex relationship between culture and PD than that represented by the 1983 formulation of Good and Kleinman (1985), which aimed to provide data relevant to the neo-Kraepelinian paradigm. The chapters here suggest that a wide range of cognitive and psychological processes may trigger experiences of panic as well as anxiety about the likelihood and danger of future episodes. They suggest that catastrophic cognitions play a significant role in panic attacks across diverse societies, and that culture is enormously significant in shaping which bodily sensations or internal experiences may be considered threatening or potentially catastrophic by individuals in these societies. They suggest that catastrophic cognitions are one type of "interpretive practice" (Good 1994), and therefore that interpretive cultural studies may be profitably linked to psychological studies in research on PD. The ethnographic studies further suggest that an anthropology of sensations may contribute significantly to understanding essential characteristics of panic attacks and PD.

Conclusion

This book provides a fundamental challenge to naturalizing accounts of PD that suggest that PD is a universal disease entity with relatively little variation across cultures. The essays in this collection show with great specificity that although panic experiences certainly exist widely across time and cultures, they belong to very different frames of social and cultural experience. Symptoms critical to panic attacks, the phenomenology of the panic experience, and the link to memories of trauma all vary by culture and individual history. These findings have great relevance for the development of culturally appropriate forms of clinical care, as well as for many of the most salient debates within anxiety disorder research. The essays suggest the enormous importance of an anthropology of sensations and detailed understandings of social and psychological experience for the basic science of anxiety and anxiety disorders, as well as for the development of therapeutics and mental health services. They suggest the importance for cultural and psychological anthropology of systematic, cross-cultural studies of panic attacks, PD, and anxiety disorders more broadly.

The chapters of this book represent a significant step forward in understanding panic and PD from a cross-cultural perspective. Simple epidemiological studies based on criteria derived from studies of middle-class American experiences of panic attacks can no longer be accepted as sufficient for making claims about PD being essentially invariant or generally consistent throughout the world (see, for example, Taylor 2000). At the same time, the research represented here is only the beginning of a rich understanding of anxiety, panic, and fear in social and cross-cultural contexts. Orr's *Panic Diaries* (2006) suggests the broad range of social and historical materials that may be relevant to a deeper understanding of PD. Linking such wide-ranging studies to investigations of individual lives in diverse local cultures remains a challenge to be taken up by new generations of scholarship.

Notes

1. In 1895, Freud gave one of the clearest descriptions of what we now call *panic attacks*, labeling them *anxiety attacks* (see McNally 1994). In Freud's view, accumulation of sexual tension, arising from abstinence, coitus interruptus, and the like, erupts into panic.

2. Here the term *psychophysiology* means the study of the physiological correlates of emotional states such as fear and joy: *autonomic arousal pattern*, as in palpitations, sweating, and muscle tension; and *endocrinal states*, as in elevation of cortisol or epinephrine levels. It might better be called an *emotion-physiology*.

3. The first author of this introduction, Byron Good, was one of the participants in the conference, where he presented the first draft of the paper "Culture and Anxiety: Cross-Cultural Evidence for the Patterning of Anxiety Disorders," which was published as Chapter 13 of the Tuma and Maser volume (Good and Kleinman 1985). The observations about the 1983 conference are his.

4. In the conference and in the resulting volume (Tuma and Maser 1985), the notion of *cognitive* was rather limited. In that conference and volume, the so-called cognitive theory of anxiety examined mainly how fear was represented in the mind, the most prominent model being Lang's (1985) associative network model, in which an emotional state was operationalized as a network consisting of a certain label of the emotion, an associated event, a certain

pattern of physiological arousal, and a certain posture. Cognitive-type treatment was conceptualized as "exposure" to a "fear network." These models focused on memory encoding, retrieval, and "extinction," which were linked to animal models of learning.

5. See Good 1992:187–193 for a more detailed description of the Sterling Forest Conference and its discussions of PD.

6. In fact, this is not the case. Benzodiazapines are effective for PD (Rosenbaum et al. 2005).

7. Imipramine does not have these specific effects, as later research would reveal. It is also effective for depression and chronic anxiety, as in its proven efficacy for generalized anxiety disorder (Rosenbaum et al. 2005).

8. Phobic disorders include *social phobia*, characterized by fear in social situations and anxiety about entering such situations; and *specific phobia*, characterized by fear of certain places or things, such as snakes.

9. The *DSM–III*'s hierarchical conceptualization of diagnosis had an unfortunate consequence: the neglect of PD as an object of inquiry by cross-cultural researchers who had a primary interest in other disorders, such as depression. As an example, in his study of neurasthenia patients, Kleinman (1986:203) found remarkably high rates of PD (in the one hundred patients diagnosed with neurasthenia, 35 percent suffered PD and 87 percent suffered major depressive disorder). Interestingly, in the follow-up study of these same patients who were treated for depression, 33 percent continued to meet criteria for major depressive disorder, 29 percent for PD (Kleinman 1986:219). In line with contemporary diagnostic views, Kleinman (1986: 75) suggested that "anxiety problems seemed secondary to depression," and panic never became a primary focus of his research. The fact that many of the patients in his study had experienced severe trauma associated with the Cultural Revolution in China, a major finding of Kleinman's research, suggests that panic symptoms linked to that trauma may have been quite significant complicating factors in the pathology of the sample he studied.

10. American panic attack sufferers have been shown to focus frequently on one symptom, presenting to the emergency room or to a physician's office with one somatic complaint, such as dizziness or chest pain, not mentioning the other symptoms of autonomic arousal (Katon 1984, 1989). If the physician does not ask about the presence of other autonomic arousal symptoms (such as palpitations, sweating, and shortness of breath), the complaint may be misdiagnosed either as a physical ailment (for example, chest pain as a heart attack, or dizziness as vestibular disorder), thereby resulting in inappropriate and expensive testing, or as a chronic symptom of simple somatization, thereby resulting in ineffective treatment.

11. As an example, Cambodian refugees fear dizziness upon standing; it indicates excessive *khyâl* surging in the body, which may cause "*khyâl* overload" (*khyâl koa*), an extreme and dangerous form of "*khyâl* attack" that may bring about syncope and various physical disasters (see Chapter 3). This "*khyâl* overload" must be treated by culturally indicated methods such as "coining" the body and "biting the ankles," or death may well result. Owing to syndrome-generated catastrophic cognitions, dizziness upon standing causes much greater fear for a Cambodian than for an American. The frequency with which certain sensation-inducers bring about panic varies by culture. Common triggers of panic among Cambodian refugees include standing and feeling dizzy, seeing a spinning object, and smelling car-exhaust fumes

(see Chapter 3); among Vietnamese refugees, triggers include standing and feeling dizzy, a cold wind hitting the body, and urination (see Chapter 3). Both Cambodian and Vietnamese refugees fear that "worry" can damage the body and mind, so if any sensations—particularly dizziness—occur during worry episodes, a spiral of panic may ensue.

12. For Foucault's notion of *genealogy*, see Gutting (1989) and Visker (1995).

13. See Good and Kleinman (1985).

References

Ackerman, S., and E. J. Sachar. 1974. The Lactate Theory of Anxiety: A Review and Re-evaluation. *Psychosomatic Medicine* 36:69–81.

American Psychiatric Association (APA). 1952. *Diagnostic and Statistical Manual of Mental Disorders.* 1st ed. [*DSM–I.*] Washington, DC: American Psychiatric Association.

———. 1968. *Diagnostic and Statistical Manual of Mental Disorders.* 2nd ed. [*DSM–II.*] Washington, DC: American Psychiatric Association.

———. 1980. *Diagnostic and Statistical Manual of Mental Disorders.* 3rd ed. [*DSM–III.*] Washington, DC: American Psychiatric Association.

———. 1987. *Diagnostic and Statistical Manual of Mental Disorders.* 3rd ed., rev. [*DSM–III–R.*] Washington, DC: American Psychiatric Association.

———. 1994. *Diagnostic and Statistical Manual of Mental Disorders.* 4th ed. [*DSM–IV.*] Washington, DC: American Psychiatric Association.

———. 2000. *Diagnostic and Statistical Manual of Mental Disorders.* 4th ed. [*DSM–IV–TR.*] Washington, DC: American Psychiatric Association.

Baker, R. 1989. Introduction: Where Does "Panic Disorder" Come From? In *Panic Disorder: Theory, Research, and Therapy.* R. Baker, ed. Pp. 1–12. New York: Wiley.

Barlow, D. H. 2002. *Anxiety and Its Disorders: The Nature and Treatment of Anxiety and Panic.* 2nd ed. New York: Guilford Press.

Beck, A. 1988. Cognitive Approaches to Panic Disorder: Theory and Therapy. In *Panic: Psychological Perspectives.* S. Rachman and J. Maser, eds. Pp. 33–54. Hillsdale, NJ: Erlbaum.

Blashfield, R. K. 1984. *The Classification of Psychopathology: Neo-Kraepelinian and Quantitative Approaches.* New York: Plenum Press.

Carey, G. 1985. Epidemiology and Cross-Cultural Aspects of Anxiety Disorders: A Commentary. In *Anxiety and the Anxiety Disorders.* A. H. Tuma and J. D. Maser, eds. Pp. 325–330. Hillsdale, NJ: Erlbaum.

Clark, D. 1986. A Cognitive Approach to Panic. *Behaviour, Research, and Therapy* 24:461–470.

Craske, M. C. 1991. Phobic Fear and Panic Attacks: The Same Emotional States Triggered by Different Cues? *Clinical Psychology Review* 11:599–620.

Good, B. J. 1992. Culture and Psychopathology: Directions for Psychiatric Anthropology. In *New Directions in Psychological Anthropology.* T. Schwartz, G. M. White, and C. A. Lutz, eds. Pp. 181–205. Cambridge, UK: Cambridge University Press.

———. 1994. *Medicine, Rationality, and Experience: An Anthropological Perspective.* Cambridge, UK: Cambridge University Press.

Good, B. J., and A. Kleinman. 1985. Culture and Anxiety: Cross-Cultural Evidence for the Patterning of Anxiety Disorder. In *Anxiety and the Anxiety Disorders.* A. H. Tuma and J. D. Maser, eds. Pp. 297–323. Hillsdale, NJ: Erlbaum.

Gutting, G. 1989. *Michael Foucault's Archaeology of Scientific Reason*. Cambridge, UK: Cambridge University Press.

Hinton, D. E., D. Chhean, V. Pich, S. G. Hofmann, and D. H. Barlow. 2006a. Tinnitus Among Cambodians: Relationship to PTSD Severity. *Journal of Traumatic Stress* 19:541–546.

Hinton, D. E., D. Chhean, V. Pich, K. Um, J. Fama, and M. H. Pollack. 2006b. Neck-Focused Panic Attacks Among Cambodian Refugees: A Logistic and Linear Regression Analysis. *Journal of Anxiety Disorders* 20:119–138.

Hinton, D. E., S. D. Hinton, D. Chhean, V. Pich, and M. H. Pollack. In press. The "Multiplex Model" of How Somatic Symptoms Generate Distress: Application to Tinnitus Among Traumatized Cambodian Refugees. *Transcultural Psychiatry*.

Jackson, S. W. 1985. Acedia the Sin and Its Relationship to Sorrow and Melancholia. In *Culture and Depression: Studies in the Anthropology and Cross-Cultural Psychiatry of Affect and Disorder*. A. Kleinman and B. J. Good, eds. Pp. 43–62. Berkeley: University of California Press.

Katon, W. 1984. Panic Disorder and Somatization: Review of Fifty-Five Cases. *American Journal of Medicine* 77:101–106.

———. 1989. *Panic Disorder in the Medical Setting*. Washington, DC: U.S. Department of Health and Human Services.

Klein, D. F. 1980. Anxiety Reconceptualized. *Comprehensive Psychiatry* 21:411–427.

Kleinman, A. 1986. *Social Origins of Depression and Disease: Depression, Neurasthenia, and Pain in Modern China*. New Haven, CT: Yale University Press.

Klerman, G. L. 1978. The Evolution of a Scientific Nosology. In *Schizophrenia: Science and Practice*. J. C. Shershow, ed. Pp. 33–58. Cambridge, MA: Harvard University Press.

Lang, P. J. 1985. The Cognitive Psychophysiology of Emotion: Fear and Anxiety. In *Anxiety and the Anxiety Disorders*. A. H. Tuma and J. D. Maser, eds. Pp. 130–170. Hillsdale, NJ: Erlbaum.

Martin, L. H., H. Gutman, and P. H. Hutton. 1988. *Technologies of the Self: A Seminar with Michel Foucault*. Amherst: University of Massachusetts Press.

McNally, R. J. 1994. *Panic Disorder: A Critical Analysis*. New York: Guilford Press.

Orr, J. 2006. *Panic Diaries: A Genealogy of Panic Disorder*. Durham, NC: Duke University Press.

Pitts, F., and J. McClure. 1967. Lactate Metabolism in Anxiety Neurosis. *New England Journal of Medicine* 277:1329–1336.

Rapee, R., M. Craske, and D. H. Barlow. 1995. Assessment Instrument for Panic Disorder That Includes Fear of Sensation-Producing Activities: The Albany Panic and Phobia Questionnaire. *Anxiety* 1:114–144.

Rosenbaum, J., J. Arana, S. Hyman, L. Labbate, and M. Fava. 2005. *Handbook of Psychiatric Drug Treatment*. Philadelphia: Lippincott.

Scupi, B., B. Benson, L. Brown, and T. Uhde. 1997. Rapid Onset: A Valid Panic Disorder Criterion? *Depression and Anxiety* 5:121–126.

Sheehan, D. V. 1983. *The Anxiety Disease: A Leading Psychiatrist Offers New Hope for Victims of Severe Anxiety*. New York: Scribner's.

Street, L., M. C. Craske, and D. H. Barlow. 1989. Sensations, Cognitions, and the Perception of Cues Associated with Expected and Unexpected Attacks. *Behaviour, Research, and Therapy* 27:189–198.

Taylor, S. 2000. *Understanding and Treating Panic Disorder: Cognitive-Behavioural Approaches.* Chichester, UK: Wiley.

Tuma, A. H., and J. D. Maser, eds. 1985. *Anxiety and the Anxiety Disorders.* Hillsdale, NJ: Erlbaum.

Visker, R. 1995. *Michel Foucault: Genealogy as Critique.* London: Verso.

Weissman, M., and G. Klerman. 1978. Epidemiology of Mental Disorders. *Archives of General Psychiatry* 35:705–712.

Part I

Theoretical Approaches to the
Study of Panic Disorder

Theoretical Perspectives on the Cross-Cultural Study of Panic Disorder

Laurence J. Kirmayer and Caminee Blake

IN RECENT PSYCHIATRIC LITERATURE, panic disorder is usually portrayed as a biologically based disorder resulting from the hypersensitivity of brain systems involved in the anxious response to specific types of threat—especially to the threat of separation from loved ones or to choking or suffocation. At the same time, it is clear from clinical and experimental work that catastrophic cognitions play a crucial role in the genesis and recurrence of panic. Because our thoughts about catastrophe reflect cultural models and concerns, panic disorder provides an interesting opportunity to explore the interaction of bodily and social processes in the cultural shaping of distress.

In this chapter, we explore some ways in which culture may contribute to the pathogenesis, symptomatology, course, and treatment outcome of panic attacks. As with other forms of distress, social interactional processes can contribute to the onset as well as to the recurrence and chronicity of panic. Detailing these interactions involves consideration of both psychosomatic and sociosomatic processes. At the same time, culture provides the larger matrix of knowledge and practice in which our understandings of panic as disorder are framed. Hence, we also consider the issue of the cultural construction of panic in folk psychology and professional nosology. Finally, we explore the role of panic in a larger moral and political economy that identifies regions of the wild, the intolerable, and the "out of control."

The Cognitive Origins of Panic

A substantial body of theory and research argues that specific cognitive processes and cognitive schemas are central to the development and maintenance of panic disorder (Clark and Beck 1988). Schemas, in this context, are sets of dysfunctional beliefs and rules of related content areas that are associated in memory to form higher-order cognitive structures. Some schemas are related to specific types of experience (such as specific bodily sensations, symptoms, or illnesses) while other schemas are related to more global situations or domains. Once a schema is activated, it facilitates the processing of information consistent with that schema and may inhibit the processing of inconsistent or irrelevant information. Central to the cognitive schemas that underlie panic disorder are concerns about vulnerability, loss of control, and sensitivity to anxiety. More specifically, patients with panic disorder have been found to be preoccupied with thoughts of physical catastrophes (death, heart attack, fainting, loss of breath, illness, and seizure), mental catastrophes (going crazy), or behavioral catastrophes (loss of control) (Ottaviani and Beck 1987). In addition, a high proportion of patients with panic disorder fear experiencing public humiliation because of anxious behavior or loss of control.

Consistent with the schema theory of panic disorder, Beck's cognitive model of anxiety suggests that patients with panic disorder experience two levels of disturbed thinking (Beck and Clark 1997). The first level involves patients' negative *automatic thoughts*, that is, thoughts and images that arise spontaneously in specific situations when an individual is anxious. The second level of disturbed thinking involves individuals' dysfunctional assumptions and ways of reasoning, which include general beliefs that individuals hold about themselves and the world that make them prone to interpret specific situations in an excessively negative manner. Dysfunctional assumptions are believed to derive from early learning experiences but may lie dormant until activated by a specific stressful or disturbing event.

Cognitive theory explains the development of panic disorder in terms of two main processes, one involving vicious circles of anxiety, attention, and attribution, and a second consisting of cognitive and behavioral strategies of avoidance.

Individuals who experience panic disorder engage in a narrowing of attention and in a focus on bodily sensations resulting from arousal of the autonomic nervous system, which may be triggered by either external or internal cues. This autonomic arousal is misinterpreted as dangerous, indicating potential threat or disaster. This misinterpretation then serves to intensify and maintain the physiological arousal, leading to an exacerbation of the panic symptoms, thus confirming the person's fears. Once an individual develops a tendency to interpret bodily sensations catastrophically, panic may be triggered through persistent hypervigilance toward the body, that is, scanning for any of the feared sensations. In fact, there is evidence that individuals who experience panic attacks may perceive even trivial bodily changes such as slight increases in heart rate as catastrophic (Craske and Tsao 1999).

Avoidant coping also contributes to the vicious circles that trigger, aggravate, and maintain panic attacks. People use a variety of cognitive and behavioral strategies to prevent the feared events from occurring. Although their fears are unrealistic, the effect of these strategies is to prevent people from disconfirming their negative beliefs. Beck (1988) suggests that a person's cognitive capacity may be so taxed by coping with perceptions of danger that little capacity remains to satisfy other demands. Furthermore, experimental studies suggest that individuals with panic disorder have a memory bias for catastrophic associations, and that this bias can occur in both conscious (explicit) and nonconscious (implicit) memory processes (Khawaja and Oei 1998).

Sensation schemas, or ways of attending to and interpreting bodily sensations, can develop independently of disease and illness schemas (Kirmayer et al. 1994). Panic disorder also reflects broad social influences. Stressful life events around the time of the first panic attack have been found to be primarily interpersonal and social (Craske and Barlow 1993). Stress may raise the level of physiological arousal or enhance cognitive schemas of uncontrollability of and apprehension about bodily sensations. Individuals' beliefs and expectations about their personal competency and power clearly play a role in their perceptions of their ability to keep themselves safe and secure. Certain life experiences may be related to the development of panic disorder, such as receiving warnings from significant others (such as overly protective parents) about the physical or mental dangers of certain bodily sensations, or significant unpredictable and uncontrollable negative life events (such as loss of a parent) (Craske and Barlow 1993).

Fears of personal catastrophe are central to panic. The interpretation of specific sensations or events as evidence of impending catastrophe depends on culture-specific information. The catastrophic consequences may be physical (heart attack), psychological (losing one's mind), or social (public embarrassment due to inappropriate behavior). One and the same event—for example, feeling dizzy—may carry any or all of these implications. In several chapters in this volume, Hinton and colleagues provide many examples of culture-specific types of panic based on interpreting common bodily sensations (or symptoms of emotional distress) as evidence of life-threatening illness or injury.

In panic disorder, fears of catastrophe are frequently linked to worries about a specific type of physical sensation, that is, those that are increased by anxiety and autonomic arousal (such as tinnitus, shortness of breath, palpitations, and cold extremities). Such expectations set up a vicious circle: increasing anxiety increases the physical symptoms, and the increase of physical symptoms of concern in turn leads to a greater conviction that something bad is happening, resulting in even greater anxiety. Hyperventilation often plays a key role in this loop because it may be initiated by anxiety or by sensations of not getting enough air and may lead to many physical symptoms that give further cause for anxiety (Sharpe and Bass 1992).

Through cognitive-evaluative processes, anxiety is influenced by self-schemas that represent behavioral standards for self-efficacy and self-control. People strive to match their behavior to their standards or expectations for what is personally and socially important. We are likely to feel anxious in situations where we think we ought to be in control but are unable to get our behavior to match our standards (Kirmayer 1990). This failure may occur because of anxiety or other factors, but the experience of lack of control then causes more anxiety. If the resultant anxiety leads to further failure, then we have a runaway feedback loop of emotional exacerbation (Storms and McCaul 1976). Table 2.1 displays some of the consequences of attributions of cause and control of behavior for the maintenance of cognitive coherence through specific cognitive mechanisms.

These cognitive mechanisms are all predicated on the need to maintain control and the coherence and consistency of self-schemas. Cultures may differ, however, in the degree to which they demand coherence or tolerate contradiction and ambiguity. This may in turn influence the prevalence and impact of cognitive attributions that contribute to vicious spirals of anxiety. Expectations for coherence and control thus set the stage for anxiety when personal power and control reach their inevitable limits. "The more the body is subject to rational mechanisms of control, the more 'uncertain' it becomes and the more anxious and uncertain we become about those anxious margins, including cancer and AIDS, that elude control" (Williams and Bendelow 1998:120).

Although it has stimulated a productive research program and led to the development of effective clinical interventions, cognitive theory needs to be amended to

Table 2.1   Impact of attributions on cognitive-emotional responses to distress symptoms

Attribution of Cause of Symptom	Attribution of Control of Symptom	
	Self	Other
Self	Cognitive dissonance (Frustration and anger directed toward self)	Reactance or rebellion (Anger toward other)
Other	Emotional exacerbation (Anxiety, panic)	Withdrawal (Helplessness, depression)

SOURCE: Adapted from Kirmayer 1990.

take more seriously the social and interpersonal contexts of panic. The emphasis on cognitive appraisals and beliefs is highly rationalistic (McNally 2001). Although this approach fits well with the emphasis on explanatory models in medical anthropology, there is evidence that reasoning about symptoms does not always follow explicit causal models but may be based on reasoning by analogy from salient prototypes and on bodily learned patterns of responding or procedural knowledge (habits, skills, or know-how) that are difficult to articulate (Kirmayer et al. 1994; Young 1982). Much learning and information processing occurs implicitly, outside awareness, and too rapidly and evanescently to be reliably incorporated into self-representations. Instead, knowledge may be embodied in dispositions to respond and in distributed patterns of interaction that are not well captured by models of rational belief (Turner 2002).

Finally, although cognitive theory focuses on the thoughts of the individual, panic is also an interactional phenomenon that can involve the responses of others in mutually amplifying feedback loops. The feared catastrophe need not be personal, because one can experience intense fear anticipating catastrophe for loved ones. If this fear causes one to respond in a way that is perceived as increasing the loved ones' vulnerability—for example, by making them more anxious or causing oneself to freeze instead of taking protective action—one's fear may become a sort of runaway feedback loop and crescendo of panic. Both anxious concern and disinterested neglect by others may play a role in escalating acute anxiety as well as in evoking the memories and vivid reliving of frightening events that in turn lead to panic. Hence, networks of relationship, closeness, identification, contact, and communication can contribute to individuals' sense of vulnerability and risk of panic, and to the spread of anxiety through a family system or local population.

Strategies of Cross-Cultural Comparison

The cross-cultural study of any human problem assumes that there is a valid basis for comparison across different populations, ethnocultural groups, and communities. At the broadest level, cross-cultural comparison involves defining a common object, issue, or event in a way that allows one to recognize it in diverse cultural contexts. The common object could be a symptom, a behavior, or an experience. The issue could be a specific type of problem in adaptation (such as failure to maintain stable interpersonal relationships). An event-based comparison could look at a generic predicament—for example, the loss of a long-term intimate relationship or the impact of domestic violence—and ask what forms of pathology emerge in such situations. Such comparison presupposes some equivalence in the social contexts that define discrete events. Each form of comparison will give different maps of the forms of distress and lead to different models of psychopathology, with distinct implications for treatment.

In psychiatry, cross-cultural comparisons have tended to center on specific diagnostic entities. Thus, the construct of panic disorder is taken as the anchor point for comparison. Cross-cultural comparison may then be centered on particular core symptoms of panic, on related syndromes having a family resemblance to panic disorder, or on the identification of an underlying biological or psychological marker or mechanism.

The core symptom approach requires that a person have a certain set of symptoms before inquiring about the co-occurrence of other, subsidiary symptoms. This requirement may be problematic because cultural variations in the expression of distress can make any given core symptom more or less prevalent and hence insufficient to identify individuals with other features of the syndrome. For example, many patients with panic disorder report predominately heart-related symptoms and present to a cardiologist (Dammen et al. 1999), some individuals report panic symptoms without fear (Fleet et al. 2000), and others identify their emotional distress as intense anger (Fava et al. 1990). Simply using the term *panic* or *anxiety* to identify a common condition may also be insufficient either because there is no simple translation or because the cognate term has different connotations (Hinton et al. 2002). This limitation can be addressed by using multiple core symptoms or anchor points to define the disorder, by using culturally adapted language, and by systematically inquiring into the whole range of symptoms in every case.

Standardized epidemiological instruments have been used to estimate the prevalence of panic disorder in different countries (Weissman et al. 1997). However, as Kleinman (1988) has insisted, such comparisons run the risk of a category fallacy, that is, of imposing categories drawn from one culture onto another and failing to see what lies "outside the box." Diagnostic interviews and algorithms that skip more detailed inquiry on the basis of a negative response to a few core symptoms can make it impossible to study alternative configurations of syndromes that may better fit local cultural modes of symptom experience and expression (Canino et al. 1997). The limitations of this approach can be mitigated with a methodology that supplements the standard diagnosis with additional inquiry designed to elicit culture-specific symptoms and idioms of distress. It is then possible to determine how well the construct of panic disorder captures prevalent forms of distress. This is the approach taken in work on *ataques de nervios* by Guarnaccia and Lewis-Fernandez (see, for example, Chapter 6).

The use of multiple core symptoms, that is, requiring only a few symptoms from several different categories to make a diagnosis, leads to a polythetic classification, in which cases of a disorder may share no single symptom or essential characteristic. In the absence of any method to identify common underlying pathological mechanisms, such heterogeneity may be a problem for research. The polythetic category approach is justified clinically on the grounds that a common treatment approach may suffice for a wide range of problems related by family resemblance. In fact, medications such as antidepressants or anxiolytics have broad spectrums of action, through multiple mechanisms or final common pathways. Consequently, the mere fact that two conditions both respond positively to the same medication provides little evidence that they share common mechanisms at the level of pathophysiology or psychopathology.

The identification of a common pathogenic mechanism or diathesis provides another way to approach cross-cultural comparison. Following the cognitive theory of panic, we could compare problems that share a process of symptom and anxiety amplification through vicious cycles of attention, catastrophizing, and avoidance. We could call any such pattern of feedback amplification involving attention, interpretation, and behavioral avoidance a form of panic. Alternatively, we could group together syndromes of somatic amplification, emotional exacerbation, and hyperventilation that involve bodily symptoms aggravated by a specific physiological mechanism. Each way of anchoring our definition of a specific disorder will give rise to different sorts of comparison, with implications for how we understand and treat the problem and with consequences for the way in which we explore the sufferer's social world.

Cross-cultural comparisons also run into a more fundamental problem concerning what philosopher Ian Hacking (1995, 1999) has called the "looping effect of human kinds." Briefly, our conceptual categories, the ways we agree to partition the world, have a social reality that governs behavior and experience. Once launched into the world, a diagnostic entity becomes reality by shaping symptom experience, interpretation, and help-seeking. Diagnostic categories then have a life of their own, emerging from psychiatric theory to become social objects that serve as a wider basis of communication, interpersonal interaction, and economic exchange. The economic implications are especially important in a global context in which pharmaceutical companies work hand in hand with psychiatry to define new niches and markets for their products. As a result of this looping effect, the global circulation of psychiatric knowledge and practice, mediated by multinational corporations and international organizations, influences illness experience in ways that confirm existing nosology. Increasingly we find the sorts of human problems that official nosology tells us we should find, and the disappearance of culture-specific forms of distress is a result of both technical blind spots (the category fallacy) that prevent us from looking in the right way, and the actual reshaping of illness experience (the looping effect), which changes the nature of bodily experience (Kirmayer 2002).

Culture, Discourse, and Embodiment

Cultural psychiatry begins with the recognition that culture can influence the causes, symptomatology, course, and outcome of any illness. Table 2.2 lists some of the ways in which culture shapes bodily experience, affect, and emotion; any of these factors may in turn affect the prevalence, form, and impact of panic symptoms (Kirmayer et al. 1995).

Cultural variations in infant and child development may make individuals more or less vulnerable to separation anxiety and to other forms of anxiety that may predispose them to panic. There is evidence from animal research, for example, that experiences in infancy can make animals more or less prone to fear and associated stress responses, including neuroendocrine, immunological, and behavioral aspects (Meaney 2001; Suomi 2003). Children's responses to separation from caregivers have been examined cross-culturally using the *strange situation* (Ainsworth et al. 1978). These studies provide evidence for differences in the prevalence of patterns of anxious responding that can be related to cultural differences in child rearing (Rothbaum et al. 2000).

Culture provides a lexicon for understanding and describing feelings and experiences. Such understanding does not always give priority to discrete emotional states but may reference particular bodily sensations or point to one's position in the social world. As a result, the symptoms of panic may be thought of as primarily bodily events, as indications that something is wrong with the body, and as cognitive or affective concomitants that are understood as secondary reactions or responses to the fact of being ill. Alternatively, in sociosomatic explanations, panic may be linked directly to social concerns.

Basic emotions involve bodily stances and physiological patterns of activation that have adaptive value (Porges 2001). For example, the rate and rhythm

Table 2.2   Some cultural influences on emotion

1. Determines developmental experiences that prime and shape affect systems

2. Regulates style and pattern of emotional expression

3. Provides the contexts for interactional processes and sequences that underlie complex emotions

4. Provides categories and lexicon of emotion

5. Sets limits of tolerance of specific emotions or strong affect

6. Establishes the social meaning of affect and disorder

7. Provides lay theories of how to handle dysphoria and distress

8. Guides individuals and institutions involved in helping and healing problems associated with excessive or abnormal emotional responses

of breathing is integral to the biobehavioral systems that subserve aggression and withdrawal (fight or flight) as well as the systems of affiliation, attachment, and sexual desire. Cultural knowledge may be embodied through specific bodily practices that include implicitly or deliberately learned patterns of respiration (Lyon 1999). Thus culture may influence panic disorder not just through the content of specific cognitive schemas but also through the regulation of relevant bodily processes in social contexts.

More complex notions of emotion refer to culturally scripted or patterned sequences of interaction occurring in specific social contexts. Thus specific arrangements of intimate relationships, family life, and dynamics of power reflect culturally shaped social worlds. The salience of the social world in understandings of emotion may lead to people experiencing panic not exclusively as a bodily event but as a sense of being trapped in a social predicament with no way out.

The influence of culture on illness is sometimes held to be sufficient to give rise to completely distinct forms of psychopathology limited to one cultural context, the so-called *culture-bound syndrome* (CBS). The distinctiveness of a CBS may arise from cultural influences on the mechanisms of disease causation or pathogenesis, or on the shaping of symptoms, illness experience, and the temporal course of the disorder.

A CBS is a correlated, co-occurring set of symptoms with a specific course and outcome. However, many of the terms for what are considered to be culture-bound syndromes in Appendix I of *DSM–IV* and in the classic literature in cultural psychiatry refer to illness explanations or causal attributions rather than to syndromes. For example, *susto*, or "fright-illness" attributes symptoms or problems to the impact of a sudden fright. *Susto* may be invoked to explain conditions ranging from anxiety to infectious disease, and to account for congenital malformations when a pregnant woman is exposed to a frightful shock (Rubel et al. 1984).

Many other supposed CBSs are better understood as *cultural idioms of distress*. This term, introduced by Nichter (1981), refers to the use of a local, conventional mode of expression of distress (which can be verbal, gestural, or expressed through symbolic action) to convey suffering that may have many different origins and locations. For example, intolerable social circumstances of marital or family conflict, poverty, and oppression may be alluded to through talk about "nerves" (Low 1994), excessive heat (Jenkins and Valiente 1994), or other bodily or emotional symptoms. The degree to which an idiom of distress is understood and experienced as actual symptoms or used metaphorically as a conventional idiom may vary among individuals in a specific cultural context, and for the same individual across different settings.

There is a feedback loop between the bodily experiences in which metaphorical expressions originate and the effects of metaphoric language in focusing attention and guiding the interpretation of bodily sensations in ways that may give rise to symptoms (see, for example, Gibbs et al. 1994; Kirmayer 1992, 1994, 2008). Kövecses (2000) suggests a development genealogy of emotion in which there is a progression from bodily experiences mediated by physiological processes to conceptual structures of emotion elaborated in terms of metonyms (for example, anxiety understood as a "shiver of fear" for an English speaker or as a "wind attack" for a Cambodian; see Chapter 3), to metaphorically constructed models, to extensive cognitive models that are linked to explicit recognition of social interactions and their attendant dilemmas. In the models of panic developed by Hinton and colleagues in this volume, these steps in the development of emotions correspond to different perspectives or concurrent levels of meaning.

The construction of panic as disorder involves a specific way of conceptualizing human distress. To some extent the notion of panic disorder reflects the natural covariation of symptoms in experience, but these clinical patterns of symptoms are not simply expressions of physiological perturbations. As the contributions to this volume clearly show, cultural models and interactions with others, both of which are embedded in larger discursive formations, shape patterns of symptoms. Centering our analysis on a given concept of panic predetermines what we will find when we conduct cross-cultural comparisons. To avoid simply replicating conventional wisdom, it is useful to take a step back from the standard definition of panic disorder to consider a wider field of potential meanings.

Panic may be understood as a symptom, emotion, syndrome, disorder, idiom of distress, or novel metaphor. As a symptom, panic is an intense wave of fear with accompanying bodily sensations of autonomic arousal and catastrophic thoughts of impending death or other terrible consequences. The term *panic* is sometimes used to label any intense fear or to indicate that a fear is particularly horrible. Although some core element of the experience of panic may be related to sensations of asphyxiation, in general panic has a wide discursive field and does not refer to as discrete a sensation as dizziness, pain, or shortness of breath (dyspnea). It is not only intensity but especially the sense that fear is escalating without bound or foreseeable end that turns fear into panic. Panic is therefore tied to a particular sense of time or temporality. In fact, convincing oneself that a sensation of panic will end tends to reduce it to merely fear and anxiety. This raises the possibility that culturally different modes of experiencing time can influence the experience of panic. Of course the strategy of reinterpreting the meaning of symptoms to change the temporality of panic is a mainstay of the cognitive treatment of panic disorder.

As a syndrome, panic is associated with a wide range of symptoms, some of which are physiological concomitants of fear based on central mechanisms, peripheral autonomic arousal, or secondary processes such as hyperventilation. Dizziness and disorientation, which are both bodily and psychologically situated experiences, are prominent aspects of panic (Yardley 1997). The syndrome of panic attacks also includes terrifying thoughts, which are experienced as part of the torment of the condition. The links among fear, specific patterns of autonomic activation, hyperventilation, and other physiological changes result in the typical intercorrelations of symptoms over time. However, the cognitive interpretation of sensations and symptoms plays a key role in generating the clusters of symptoms that people report in clinical settings. Because the bodily changes associated with fear are widespread and the sensations are sometimes ambiguous, individuals may focus on many different aspects. This selective attention and subsequent interpretation and labeling are guided by cognitive schemas, which in turn reflect cultural knowledge about the body—its ills and upsets.

Sporadic panic attacks and less intense waves of anxiety are common (Cox and Endler 1991). The release of adrenalin that occurs with a sudden pang of anxiety has its own time course that may not respond immediately to modulation or dampening by the parasympathetic nervous system. This slower time course of autonomic and neuroendocrine responses imposes a period of grappling with intense arousal, a period in which cognitive, behavioral, and interactional responses can shape the persistence or resolution of anxiety. Cultural models that tend to interpret such bodily distress as normal or expectable responses in specific situations will lead people to respond with relative equanimity to the period of ambiguous distress. Indeed, the same sensations that herald (or trigger) panic in one cultural context may have a positive value in another. For example, for the !Kung of the Kalahari, the sensations of fear, trembling, lightheadedness, and even muscular tetany evoked during healing rituals by hyperventilation are evidence of the transformation of consciousness necessary to achieve a desired therapeutic end (Katz 1982).

Isolated or sporadic panic attacks become a disorder when they cause sufficient suffering in the individual to impair day-to-day functioning and motivate help-seeking. The psychiatric labeling of panic as a disorder conveys the notion of a clinically significant disturbance in functioning. This clinical significance is based on two sorts of criteria: evidence of impact of the symptom or syndrome on the individual's functioning in his or her social world, and the presumption that this disability is due to an underlying disruption of healthy functioning of psychophysiological regulatory mechanisms. Because the current state of psychiatric knowledge does not provide a means to measure the underlying disturbance, the ascription of the causal mechanisms of panic to inner disturbances (whether psychological or physiological) remains part of the cultural construction of disorder (Kirmayer and Young 1999).

Another view of panic emphasizes its social origins and its function as a cultural idiom of distress. Panic may occur in epidemic form when specific ideas about bodily vulnerability and the meaning of somatic symptoms and sensations become prevalent and salient. A wide range of symptoms can take part in the vicious circles of emotional exacerbation that contribute to panic. Indeed, any symptom that is exacerbated by anxiety or anxious thoughts may lead to its own amplification by positive feedback. The runaway feedback loops that amplify somatic distress not only may occur in the cognitions, emotions, and bodily experiences of the individual but also may traverse the social world through behavioral and communicative loops that include others. Once panic becomes part of this wider looping effect, it readily becomes a common language for talking about distress in the social world, and as it is codified over time it becomes a cultural idiom of distress. In the colloquial idioms of North America, talk of panic serves to indicate a loss of control. Talk of panic is thus part of a larger cultural ideology of the person that emphasizes self-control, emotional containment, and rational self-direction (Gaines 1992). Where cultural notions of the person differ along with notions of self-control and emotional display, both the cognitions that contribute to vicious circles of anxiety and the idiomatic uses of panic will also differ.

Attributions of agency play an important role in panic. The fundamental paradox of panic is that the person feels that the symptoms are evidence of a process that is out of their control, while efforts to reassert control lead to greater symptomatology (Kirmayer 1990). This out-of-control quality may apply to a specific behavior or physiological process, or to the whole sense of self and social self-presentation. Hence the damage to the person's sense of agency may be focal and limited or more pervasive (as when panic generalizes to agoraphobia and leads to a constricted social world).

The presentation of the experience of panic in terms of symptoms serves to deflect attention from the agency of the sufferer. "A central feature of the indirect communication function of symptoms is that the sufferer is not responsible or accountable for the messages conveyed" (Capps and Ochs 1995:103). This effect leads to the rhetorical use of symptoms as an interpersonally or politically "safe" language through which to draw attention to intolerable or oppressive social circumstances. At the same time, the very urgency of panic allows the sufferer to exert control over others, conferring a measure of power on the weak and oppressed.

Finally, panic may serve as a metaphor for other forms of intense anxiety and concern that grip individuals or collectives (Dunant and Porter 1996). In this use of the term, *panic* is torn loose from its bodily origins and set free in the world to lend rhetorical force to our concerns and reshape the moral landscape. This rhetorical use of panic might be viewed as "just metaphorical" and hence sharply distinguished from the psychiatric construct of panic disorder. However, prevalent metaphors shape our experience of the body and may lead individuals to think of themselves as vulnerable in ways that promote anxiety. There may be a moment in the evolution of a panic attack in which an individual decides whether he or she is really out of control, whether to go with or resist the rising wave of anxiety. This decision is shaped not only by individual strategies of coping but also by a larger stance toward oneself that is conditioned by social forces. This crucial interval is one place where culture can reach down into individual experience and shape its most basic quality. Cultural views of the meanings of fear may lead individuals to attribute their symptoms to forces beyond themselves or to their own loss of control, and hence predispose them to repeated episodes of panic.

Geographies of Fear

The phenomenon of epidemic anxiety or "mass hysteria" provides clear evidence that social and cultural factors can engender panic on a wide scale. Episodes in which many people develop intense anxiety with somatic symptoms and anticipation of ill effects have occurred in many settings. For example, in England, North America, and other industrialized countries, epidemic anxiety has occurred in association with poor environmental conditions in the workplace ("sick building syndrome") or exposure to toxins (Bartholomew and Sirois 2000). In China there have been several epidemics of *koro*, which shares many features with panic but in which the core symptom is a fear that the penis will retract into the body, resulting in death (Tseng et al. 1992). Outside of China and other areas where similar physiological notions are shared, *koro*-like symptoms occur only in sporadic cases, usually in individuals with psychotic disorders. Although individual factors may determine who is most vulnerable in a population and therefore most likely to go on to have persistent or recurrent symptoms, broader social forces must account for the geographic distribution and spread of epidemic anxiety.

These epidemics have several features: (1) they typically occur where a population or group is stressed; (2) they involve culture-specific beliefs that make the presumed threat plausible and credible; (3) they spread from person to person, affecting those who have preexisting vulnerabilities to anxiety and who in some respects identify with or share characteristics with the other cases; and (4) they are typically short-lived and do not result in chronic disorders. The social and medical response likely determines whether the epidemic persists or is quickly dampened.

The transmission of anxiety in epidemics may involve several parallel channels of communication. Interpersonal communication can increase vulnerability to panic and other forms of anxiety by focusing attention on bodily sensations, attributing sensations to abnormal causes, predicting catastrophic consequences, sanctioning avoidance behavior, and undermining efforts to self-soothe or regulate emotion. This communication can occur both explicitly and implicitly, through language but also through gesture and facial expression, and by arranging the environment in ways that influence experience. The facial and bodily expressions of anxiety have direct effects, eliciting a similar emotion from others (Hatfield et al. 1994). This effect can occur even without conscious awareness of the anxious state of the other. This mechanism of empathic mimesis likely has its roots in the adaptive value of rapid communication of danger, and the organization of a corresponding disposition to react with fight or flight.

Anxiety serves to map terrain as safe or dangerous. Panic is closely related to agoraphobia from its inception, indicating that social space is a key trigger and arena for the unfolding of panic. These social spaces or landscapes have both local and global scales. On the local scale we think of urban environments that expose individuals to variable risk for violence as well as to high levels of noxious sensory stimulation requiring constant efforts and filtering and explaining away of the resultant physical sensations. Thus the discourse of women with agoraphobia focuses on their efforts to maintain control over the circumscribed world of home and protect the individual from the unpredictability and threat of a chaotic or hostile outer world. This concern with safety and control may be reflected both in discourse and in the maintenance of architectural boundaries such as the threshold of a home (Capps and Ochs 1995:3).

The creation of places that are no place—disarticulated from a larger social world of familiar comforts and attachments and unable in crucial ways to provide a secure base—is part of the condition of supermodernity (Augé 1995). Among urban dwellers, panic and agoraphobia are commonly associated with such unmoored places as shopping malls, elevators, underground tunnels, subways, and other forms of mass transportation. These spaces of dislocation and displacement may give rise to feelings of disorientation and provoke panic in vulnerable individuals (Yardley 1997).

At the global level, political and economic events that make whole communities view themselves as at risk or besieged may set the stage for epidemic anxiety. This argument was deployed by H.B.M. Murphy (1982) to explain *koro* epidemics in Thailand and Singapore, where the affected ethnic groups felt their collective survival threatened by conflict or competition with others. The eruption of ethnic rivalries into genocidal violence indicates the very real threat to collective identity represented by such anxieties. Communal spaces that were home to diverse people have quickly become fractured and chaotic, presenting sites of overwhelming threat and catastrophe. Although acute threat may give rise to panic, the terror may not be felt until one is removed from the site of conflict and freed from the overriding effort simply to survive, which often brings with it a protective numbing and a narrowing of attention.

Many of the recent epidemics of mass anxiety are associated with the stresses of the workplace, where workers may endure much pressure and harsh working conditions (Bartholomew and Sirois 2000). The distribution of anxiety thus mirrors the political economy of globalization, which is structured according to the strategies of multinational corporations and reflects gender roles. Modernization and industrialization have brought with them a host of concerns that are reflected in common health worries (Furedi 2002). Surveys in New Zealand and Norway have identified four clusters of common health-related concerns linked to modernity: environmental pollution, toxic interventions, tainted food, and exposure to radiation (Petrie et al. 2001). These areas of concern give rise to moral panics with direct affects on health anxiety.

Consider the creation in Nova Scotia of public spaces with "no scent" in response to concerns about environmental sensitivity (Fletcher 2002, 2006). An outbreak among hospital workers in Halifax of medically unexplained symptoms including rashes, dizziness, and breathing problems that was attributed to environmental toxins led to a government investigation and the establishment of a specialized clinic to study and treat environmental illness. Public concern was such that the provincial government enacted legislation to create scent-free areas where people are asked to protect the health of others by not using perfume, deodorant, or other scented products. This unusual level of sensitivity about the environment may be related to wider social concerns about the economic and geographic marginality of the Atlantic provinces, an area that witnessed an economic decline over the last century and that has been exposed to air and water pollution carried up the Atlantic seaboard by the Gulf Stream from the megalopolis of New York–Washington. Nova Scotians thus find themselves suffering from the depredations of urban over-development without enjoying many of its benefits.

Of course it is not simply geography but also social position that marks groups of people as more or less vulnerable to anxiety-provoking threats. Friedman and Paradis (2002) note the higher levels of panic reported by African Americans in epidemiological surveys in the United States. This result may parallel socioeconomic disadvantage, racial discrimination, and the stress of life in places where one experiences a lack of safety on many levels. More subtle social vectors may give rise not to overt epidemics but to endemic distress, characterized by its wide prevalence and persistence. Routinization can lead to the nonrecognition of endemic distress resulting from social problems, or to its incorporation into normalizing discourses that may nevertheless fail to completely neutralize the anxiogenic effects of a precarious existence.

Panic in Context: A Case Vignette

Current psychiatric nosology privileges universal psychological and physiological mechanisms of psychopathology that can be described in a context-free way. Psychiatric diagnosis, which focuses on discrete disorders, wrenches human problems from their larger social context. This leads us to focus in great detail on the particulars of panic while ignoring its common co-occurrence with other problems. These issues are illustrated in the following case vignette.

> Mr. Rodriguez is a twenty-two-year-old Hispanic man who was assessed as part of his treatment in a community outpatient clinic where he was receiving methadone and day treatment for substance abuse. A referral was made for a psychological evaluation because of staff concern about his sudden high levels of anxiety and possible psychotic symptoms.
>
> Mr. Rodriguez was born and raised in Puerto Rico until the age of sixteen, when he immigrated to the mainland United States. He is the youngest of three children and lived with his older brother when he first came to the States. Currently he lives with his girlfriend and their two children. His mother, father, sister, and extended family continue to live in Puerto Rico. Mr. Rodriguez does not have much contact with his father, who separated from Mr. Rodriguez's mother when Mr. Rodriguez was a young child. He is very close to his mother and speaks with her regularly by telephone.
>
> Mr. Rodriguez was described by the staff at the treatment center, who had high expectations for him, as a model client. He had been abstinent from heroin and marijuana use for close to a year and was close to being detoxified from methadone, having been on a one milligram dose for several months without any signs of withdrawal. His counselor had begun to discuss his discharge from the clinic in the coming weeks. Mr. Rodriguez's goals were to find steady employment and resume his education.
>
> Six months prior to the psychological assessment, Mr. Rodriguez had tried to return to school to obtain a high-school equivalency diploma, that is, the General Education Development (GED) certification. Around this time he started to have panic-like symptoms and reported experiencing a lot of anxiety when going to school. He was unable to tolerate being in the classroom and quit after a few weeks. He was disappointed and attributed his failure to the effects of tapering off methadone. He pleaded with his counselors to increase his methadone dosage to help him calm down. They complied with his request and he once again improved. At the time of his first clinical assessment session, however, there was no possibility of a further methadone increase and his insurance coverage for his treatment was coming to an end. His counselor felt he was ready to be transferred to an out-

patient clinic for weekly meetings but was concerned about the return of the client's high level of anxiety. Mr. Rodriguez was phoning his counselor three to four times a day, complaining about feeling that he was going crazy and insisting that he desperately needed help.

During the psychological assessment, Mr. Rodriguez appeared very anxious; he fidgeted in his chair and looked around the room, seemingly desperate for some relief from his distress. Initially he denied that he had any worries and said he felt strongly that all of his anxiety was due to the methadone reduction. However, he had been on the same dosage for many weeks without a problem, so this explanation was eliminated. After several sessions, Mr. Rodriguez began to admit that he was experiencing severe nightmares and that he was afraid to go to sleep at night. He described classic symptoms of panic attacks, with shortness of breath, heart pounding, and the distinct feeling that he was going to die. He also stated that he could not distinguish his dreams from waking experience. In his dreams, demons pursued him and he felt they were angry with him because he was not doing what he was supposed to do. He believed there were people in the community who envied him and did not want to see him progress. He seemed convinced that these individuals had "set bad spirits upon" him as a result of their envy.

Mr. Rodriguez also admitted that he felt extremely guilty that he had not been calling his mother recently. He was concerned about disappointing her and ashamed to let her know that he had quit school. He and his girlfriend had been fighting a lot and she had become increasingly demanding. He wanted to move out but had nowhere else to live and no means to provide for himself economically. He could not turn to his brother because he felt it was due to his brother's influence that he had first became involved with drugs.

Mr. Rodriguez described how "naive" he had been when he first came to the United States. Living and working conditions were not what he had imagined and he was surprised to find that his brother was not doing as well as he had expected. He felt isolated and alone.

Mr. Rodriguez did not understand his episodes of intense anxiety as being due to panic attacks or as related to his many worries. Instead, he thought he was being punished and needed to resist the devil in the form of drug relapse. He felt he was being tested but was not strong enough to survive the test.

This case illustrates the social and cultural embedding of panic attacks. From the start it reminds us that patients rarely come in the pure types defined by psychiatric nosology. Mr. Rodriguez has a dual diagnosis—substance use and panic disorder—and any discussion of one disorder must take into account his intertwined problems (comorbidity) as well as the many-tiered social world he navigates.

Notions of loss of control, of going mad, and other fears central to the cycle of panic have both idiosyncratic personal meanings and specific cultural meanings. Again, the personal draws from cultural constructs even as it contributes to them. For Mr. Rodriguez, the culture of reference is not simply that of some fictive ethnoracial bloc of Hispanics, or even of Puerto Ricans, but of a person from Puerto Rico who has lived in the mainland United States since adolescence, moving constantly across the boundaries of different cultural worlds that maintain a degree of distinctness through geography, politics, and processes of individual and collective self-definition and social exclusion.

In Puerto Rico, the notion of loss of control is reinforced by the cultural idiom of *ataques de nervios* (Guarnaccia 1993; see also Chapter 6). It is also linked to a gender ideology that views being in control as manly and loss of control as feminizing. At a larger level, loss of control is linked to the political history of colonization and subordination to the United States, and in recent times to the invasion of multinational corporations that have appropriated and redefined the Puerto Rican identity. All of these social levels interact with personal experiences to increase the propensity to interpret experiences as out of control, and to sanction such behavior and give it broader cultural meaning.

Mr. Rodriguez's story also highlights the impact of migration as uprooting, as bringing about the loss of familiar structures, routines, and supports. Despite the distance, he is able to maintain frequent contact with his mother, a feature of the new migration in which electronic telecommunication and ease of travel promote transnational identities. This connection does not only translate into social support, however, for it also brings with it anxiety about letting her down. Interestingly, Mr. Rodriguez's panic erupts when he is faced with a school situation that demands social exchange with new people and academic performance.

Mr. Rodriguez's panic was also tied to worries about leaving the treatment center. He sought a "community" in which to develop a sense of belonging, which the center provided. Services at the center, including counseling, were in Spanish; at other clinics in the area, such language-specific services were usually not available.

Mr. Rodriguez's insistence on attributing his symptoms to the effects of decreasing his methadone speak to the centrality of substance use in his own understanding of his vulnerability and coping with distress. He frames his symptoms in terms of a moral test or trial—his recovery from substance use. This way of looking at his problems also contributes to his sense of having been damaged by the process of migration to a land where he experiences racism and marginalization. Finally, Mr. Rodriguez considers that demonic forces may be at work in his illness, adding a dimension of the supernatural that collapses religious, moral, and social concerns in a way that amplifies his fear.

The Work of Culture and the Tenacity of Belief

In the seminal volume *Culture and Depression* (Kleinman and Good 1985), Obeyesekere (1985) presented a cultural critique of the category of depression. He argued that depressed affect need not have pathological implications if it is consonant with cultural beliefs and expectations. He illustrated the oddness of imposing cultural categories on others' experience by arguing that we could look for the prevalence of culture-bound syndromes like *dhat* (symptoms of weakness, fatigue, and anxiety attributed to semen loss) in the West. Since then others have taken him at his word and reported sporadic cases of *dhat, koro,* and *taijin kyofusho* (a social phobia characterized by fear of making others uncomfortable through one's inappropriate social behavior) outside the cultures in which these syndromes were originally described and made salient. But these efforts to count cases miss the point. The cultural embedding of distress is not simply window dressing but is constitutive of specific types of problems. Panic in one context is not quite the same as panic in another, even if the physiological consequences of hyperventilation, adrenaline, or other bodily changes remain the same.

In a later study, Obeyesekere (1991) focused on the psychological dynamics that occur through the interaction of individuals' construction of their selves and larger cultural formations. This dialectic he termed "the work of culture." From this perspective, a diagnosis such as panic, which emerges from a particular social world with its own etymology and cultural construction of emotion, provides a conceptual vocabulary for individuals to use to think through and articulate their own predicaments. As they do this, they contribute to the creation and stabilization of culture, now understood as a dynamic system of discursive practices and institutions.

The idiom of panic provides people with ways of understanding intense feelings of distress, but it also marks off these forms of distress as distinctive and worthy of medical attention. Understanding one's problem as panic may be comforting: patients are often relieved to have a list of panic symptoms read to them, to discover that others have felt "exactly" what they feel, and that there is a medical name for the condition. Naturally this comfort is vastly greater if coupled with a promise of effective treatment.

What work does panic do in the larger culture? Moral panics use anxiety as the mediating process to drive political agendas. The threats of AIDS, mad cow disease, SARS, and avian flu; of strange mutations from the "hot zone" of the world; and of bioterrorism give rise to a thoroughgoing sense of the world as a risky place; but this danger is always located in ways that are politically significant, as originating in the radically *other,* even if it is an other secreted within (Habermas et al. 2003). Paradoxically, the exteriorization of danger may lead us to downplay the significance of this threat for the individual (Squire 1997). Thus the person with HIV/AIDS is enjoined not to panic but to live positively with their affliction, even as the larger society occupies itself with walling off the threat of contagion. The suffering of the individual is subordinated to more general moral panic. This may serve adaptive functions as it lets sufferers escape from their individual plight into a generic "script" of tribulation, but it comes at the cost of ignoring the pains of everyday life. Such externalizing attributions have been used clinically by narrative therapists as a way to move patients beyond the confines of their self-defeating stories (White and Epston 1990). At the same time, moral panics serve to articulate and sustain cultural values. When these values are threatened and a collapse of cultural order and coherence seems imminent, it may be meaningful to speak of a "cultural panic."

The tension between moral or cultural panic as a source of individual anxiety and as a frightening but engrossing generic story into which one can dissolve one's own suffering is regulated by global dynamics, local social interactions, and individual psychology. Whether one finds the generic story comforting or it prompts more remonstrations about the uniqueness of one's own misery depends on the extent to which suffering is adopted as a defining characteristic of an individualized self.

From the perspective of global marketing, moral and cultural panics may be good business in that they may create new needs and intense motivation to acquire goods and services that promise safety, such as organic vegetables, good medicines, security devices, weapons, and the like (Furedi 2002). Although moral panics may block some forms of consumer activity, on balance they surely promote consumption. Indeed, one moral panic begets another as concerns must be expressed ever more stridently in order to have a place on agendas crowded with urgent problems.

Ironically, the political economic account of the origin of cultural panics breeds more anxiety because it reveals the insignificance of individual agency (Furedi 2002). A more complete model would include the dynamics of the spread of knowledge, and the active role of individuals in working with culture to advance their own ends. Following Sperber (1985), we might think of an epidemiology of representations that promote, disguise, and transform experience according to specific interests. Culture is located in specific places and practices, and people are differentially affected by a range of cultural representations depending on their social position. Specific social positions are also actively sought and negotiated by individuals in accord with their psychological needs and opportunities for power. Each position brings with it a set of commitments and concerns, some of which may seem outlandish to others but may be deeply held convictions for others.

Culture determines what beliefs are credible, and how deeply and persistently they are held. The credibility of specific beliefs centers on their fit with larger cultural models and ideologies, their link with various forms of authority, and their grounding in folk epistemologies. The depth at which beliefs are held can be understood in terms of both individual psychology and social dynamics, involving (1) interconnectedness (how many other beliefs and values it is connected to in patterns of mutual reinforcement, consonance, and coherence, or in patterns of conflict, dissonance, and destabilization); (2) affective meaning or salience (how strongly a belief evokes specific emotions, core values, or commitments); (3) unconsciousness (how inaccessible a belief is to everyday awareness because we defend ourselves against looking at it directly); and (4) implicitness (how deeply a belief is buried or hidden in our everyday assumptions). The stability of beliefs for the individual depends both on an internal psychological economy (dissonance reduction, coherence, desirability) and on larger interactions, rhetorical practices, and positions within social contexts and institutions (overarching value systems or participation in discourse). These processes of cultural participation confer on certain ideas and interpretations compelling significance and the power to shape experience.

Beyond these dynamics of belief, cultural worlds shape individual and interpersonal responses to distress through tacit knowledge and practices that may lie outside the realm of explicit models or beliefs about bodily and personal vulnerability. Indeed, individuals may be led to panic by the expectations and responses of others. The meaning of panic is then located not within the brain or the individual person but between people in the local systems of family, community, work, and health care. These local systems are in turn embedded in global systems of exchange that may contribute to the prevalence and form of panic as a direct or indirect consequence of the pursuit of their own political and economic agendas (Kirmayer 2002). Clearly the logic of panic as a form of social suffering cannot be captured by approaches that focus exclusively on its cognitive dimensions.

Conclusion: Implications for Research and Clinical Work

The view of panic as a biologically based response to stimuli viewed as life-threatening encourages an emphasis on pharmacological treatments. This fits with the patients' perceptions that the symptoms come from "out of the blue" and are out of their control. Clinical phenomenology and ethnographic research on the social contexts of panic, however, underscore its close connection to culturally mediated thoughts of catastrophe.

Current cognitive-behavioral approaches to the treatment of panic disorder encourage patients to look at their experiences in an empirical way to see how specific thoughts and interpretations of bodily events lead to increased anxiety and more distressing bodily sensations. Through discovering how the mind engenders anxiety, individuals come to understand the origin of their symptoms and may no longer experience them as coming from out of the blue or as lying entirely outside their control. Pharmacological treatment does not convey the same meanings. Instead, patients may view their symptoms as controllable only through the external means of taking a pill. This may help account for the observation that patients who attribute their improvement to drugs rather than to their own efforts are more prone to relapse (Basoglu et al. 1994).

Panic involves an initial wave of anxiety, which may be exacerbated by efforts to suppress and control the experience. The failure to suppress anxiety, along with the fear that it will persist, leads to more anxiety and hence to the very outcome that the person dreads. Cognitive interventions aim to interrupt this vicious cycle of secondary anxiety. Cognitive therapy bears a striking resemblance in theory as well as practice to elements of Buddhist meditation. Buddhist psychology recognizes the origins of suffering in misinterpretations of experience, especially in the sometimes frantic efforts of the self to stabilize itself and ensure its survival in the face of inevitable flux and change. Insight meditation trains individuals simply to watch experience without judgment or anxious efforts at control (Miller et al. 1995). This stance can diminish the secondary efforts at control that set up the vicious circles that lead to sustained panic. At the same time, the Buddhist perspective has more far-reaching implications: panic is but one form of suffering that arises from the ceaseless exertions of the self to resist change and impermanence. This has its mirror in constructivist views of the self as a narrative center of gravity or a bundle of rhetorical strategies. Learning new narratives of agency can reduce panic if it reduces one's inner struggle and increases one's tolerance of uncertainty.

Exploring the feedback loops that sustain anxiety leads us from the psychophysiology of metaphor to the sociophysiology of interpersonal interaction and, ultimately, to the politics of power and control. A world filled with dangers, aggravated by human greed, malevolence, and caprice, is fertile ground for fears. Indeed, it would be foolish not to worry under such a regime. However, in parallel with the horrors of war and the threats of crime and environmental catastrophe that pose real dangers, the notions of risk and vulnerability are actively manipulated by a wide range of groups and institutions to further their aims, which range from selling newspapers and other commodities to advancing political agendas.

The current emphasis in psychiatry on the intrinsic phenomenology and mechanisms of panic rather than on the circumstances of its emergence fits with the limited focus of biomedicine as a problem-solving endeavor centered on the individualized body. However, the larger contexts in which panic arises need to be considered.

Otherwise, we may find ourselves treating the symptoms rather than the underlying disorder and unwittingly participating in a moral economy in which the social origins of distress are conveniently hidden and obscured.

References

Ainsworth, M.D.S., M. C. Blehar, E. Waters, E., & S. Wall. 1978. *Patterns of Attachment: A Psychological Study of the Strange Situation*. Hillsdale, NJ: Erlbaum.

Augé, M. 1995. *Non-Places: Introduction to an Anthropology of Supermodernity*. London: Verso.

Bartholomew, R. E., and F. Sirois. 2000. Occupational Mass Psychogenic Illness: A Transcultural Perspective. *Transcultural Psychiatry* 37:495–524.

Basoglu, M., I. M. Marks, C. Kilic, C. R. Brewin, and R. P. Swinson. 1994. Alprazolam and Exposure for Panic Disorder with Agoraphobia: Attribution of Improvement to Medication Predicts Subsequent Relapse. *British Journal of Psychiatry* 164:652–659.

Beck, A. T. 1988. Cognitive Approaches to Panic Disorder: Theory and Therapy. In *Panic: Psychological Perspectives*. S. Rachman and J. D. Maser, eds. Pp. 91–109. Hillsdale, NJ: Erlbaum.

Beck, A. T., and D. A. Clark. 1997. An Information Processing Model of Anxiety: Automatic and Strategic Processes. *Behaviour, Research, and Therapy* 35:49–58.

Canino, G., R. Lewis-Fernandez, and M. Bravo. 1997. Methodological Challenges in Cross-Cultural Mental Health Research. *Transcultural Psychiatry* 34:163–184.

Capps, L., and E. Ochs. 1995. *Constructing Panic: The Discourse of Agoraphobia*. Cambridge, MA: Harvard University Press.

Clark, D. M., and A. T. Beck. 1988. Cognitive Approaches. In *Handbook of Anxiety Disorders*. C. Last and M. Hersen, eds. Pp. 362–385. New York: Pergamon Press.

Cox, B. J., and N. S. Endler. 1991. Clinical and Nonclinical Panic Attacks: An Empirical Test of a Panic-Anxiety Continuum. *Journal of Anxiety Disorders* 5:21–34.

Craske, M. G., and D. H. Barlow. 1993. Panic Disorder and Agoraphobia. In *Clinical Handbook of Psychological Disorders*. 2nd ed. D. H. Barlow, ed. Pp. 1–47. New York: Guilford Press.

Craske, M., and J. C. Tsao. 1999. Self-Monitoring with Panic and Anxiety Disorders. *Psychological Assessment* 11:466–479.

Dammen, T., O. Ekeberg, H. Arnesen, and S. Friis. 1999. The Detection of Panic Disorder in Chest Pain Patients. *General Hospital Psychiatry* 21:323–332.

Dunant, S., and R. Porter. 1996. *The Age of Anxiety*. London: Virago.

Fava, N., K. Anderson, and J. F. Rosenbaum. 1990. "Anger Attacks": Possible Variants of Panic and Major Depressive Disorders. *American Journal of Psychiatry* 147:867–870.

Fleet, R. P., J. P. Martel, K. L. Lavoie, G. Dupuis, and B. D. Beitman. 2000. Non-Fearful Panic Disorder: A Variant of Panic in Medical Patients? *Psychosomatics* 41:311–320.

Fletcher, C. M. 2002. Equivocal Illness and Cultural Landscape in Nova Scotia, Canada. Ph.D. dissertation, Department of Anthropology, Université de Montréal.

———. 2006. Environmental Sensitivity: Equivocal Illness in the Context of Place. *Transcultural Psychiatry* 43:86–195.

Friedman, S., and C. Paradis. 2002. Panic Disorder in African-Americans: Symptomatology and Isolated Sleep Paralysis. *Culture, Medicine, and Psychiatry* 26:179–198.

Furedi, F. 2002. *Culture of Fear: Risk-Taking and the Morality of Low Expectation.* London: Continuum.

Gaines, A. D. 1992. From DSM–I to III-R: Voices of Self, Mastery and the Other: A Cultural Constructivist Reading of U.S. Psychiatric Classification. *Social Science and Medicine* 35:3–24.

Gibbs, R. W., Jr., D. Beitel, M. Harrington, and D. Sanders. 1994. Taking a Stand on the Meanings of Stand: Bodily Experience as Motivation for Polysemy. *Journal of Semantics* 11:231–251.

Guarnaccia, P. J. 1993. Ataques de Nervios in Puerto Rico: Culture-Bound Syndrome or Popular Illness? *Medical Anthropology* 15:157–170.

Habermas, J., D. Jacques, and B. Giovanna. 2003. *Philosophy in a Time of Terror: Dialogues with Jürgen Habermas and Jacques Derrida.* Chicago: University of Chicago Press.

Hacking, I. 1995. The Looping Effect of Human Kinds. In *Causal Cognition: A Multidisciplinary Debate.* D. Sperber, D. Premack, and A. J. Premack, eds. Pp. 351–383. Oxford, UK: Oxford University Press.

———. 1999. *The Social Construction of What?* Cambridge, MA: Harvard University Press.

Hatfield, E., J. T. Cacioppo, and R. L. Rapson. 1994. *Emotional Contagion.* Cambridge, UK: Cambridge University Press.

Hinton, D. E., M. Nathan, B. Bird, and L. Park. 2002. Panic Probes and the Identification of Panic: A Historical and Cross-Cultural Perspective. *Culture, Medicine, and Psychiatry* 26:137–153.

Jenkins, J., and M. Valiente. 1994. Bodily Transactions of the Passions: El Calor Among Salvadorean Refugees. In *Embodiment and Experience: The Existential Ground of Culture and Self.* T. Csordas, ed. Pp. 163–182. Cambridge, UK: Cambridge University Press.

Katz, R. 1982. Accepting Boiling Energy: The Experience of !Kia Healing among the !Kung. *Ethos* 10:344–368.

Khawaja, N. G., and T. P. Oei 1998. Catastrophic Cognitions in Panic Disorder with and Without Agoraphobia. *Clinical Psychology Review* 18:341–365.

Kirmayer, L. J. 1990. Resistance, Reactance, and Reluctance to Change: A Cognitive Attributional Approach to Strategic Interventions. *Journal of Cognitive Psychotherapy* 4:83–104.

———. 1992. The Body's Insistence on Meaning: Metaphor as Presentation and Representation in Illness Experience. *Medical Anthropology Quarterly* 6:323–346.

———. 1994. Improvisation and Authority in Illness Meaning. *Culture Medicine and Psychiatry* 18:183–214.

———. 2002. Psychopharmacology in a Globalizing World: The Use of Antidepressants in Japan. *Transcultural Psychiatry* 39:295–312.

———. 2008. Culture and the metaphoric mediation of pain. *Transcultural Psychiatry* 45:318–338.

Kirmayer, L. J., and A. Young. 1999. Culture and Context in the Evolutionary Concept of Mental Disorder. *Journal of Abnormal Psychology* 108:446–452.

Kirmayer, L. J., A. Young, and J. M. Robbins. 1994. Symptom Attribution in Cultural Perspective. *Canadian Journal of Psychiatry* 39:584–595.

Kirmayer, L. J., A. Young, and B. C. Hayton. 1995. The Cultural Context of Anxiety Disorders. *Psychiatric Clinics of North America* 18:503–521.

Kleinman, A. 1988. *Rethinking Psychiatry: From Cultural Category to Personal Experience.* New York: Free Press.

Kleinman, A., and B. J. Good, eds. 1985. *Culture and Depression.* Berkeley: University of California Press.

Kövecses, Z. 2000. *Metaphor and Emotion: Language, Culture, and Body in Human Feeling.* Cambridge, UK: Cambridge University Press.

Low, S. 1994. Embodied Metaphors: Nerves as Lived Experience. In *Embodiment and Experience: The Existential Ground of Culture and Self.* T. Csordas, ed. Pp. 139–162. Cambridge, UK: Cambridge University Press.

Lyon, M. L. 1999. Emotion and Embodiment: The Respiratory Mediation of Somatic and Social Processes. In *Biocultural Approaches to Emotion.* A. L. Hinton, ed. Pp. 182–212. Cambridge, UK: Cambridge University Press.

McNally, R. J. 2001. On the Scientific Status of Cognitive Appraisal Models of Anxiety Disorder. *Behaviour, Research, and Therapy* 39:513–521.

Meaney, M. J. 2001. Maternal Care, Gene Expression, and the Transmission of Individual Differences in Stress Reactivity Across Generations. *Annual Review of Neurosciences* 24:1161–1192.

Miller, J. J., K. Fletcher, and J. Kabat-Zinn. 1995. Three-Year Follow-Up and Clinical Implications of a Mindfulness Meditation-Based Stress Reduction Intervention in the Treatment of Anxiety Disorders. *General Hospital Psychiatry* 17:192–200.

Murphy, H. 1982. *Comparative Psychiatry: The International and Intercultural Distribution of Mental Illness.* New York: Springer-Verlag.

Nichter, M. 1981. Idioms of Distress: Alternatives in the Expression of Psychosocial Distress: A Case Study from India. *Culture, Medicine, and Psychiatry* 5:379–408.

Obeyesekere, G. 1985. Depression, Buddhism, and the Work of Culture in Sri Lanka. In *Culture and Depression.* A. Kleinman and B. J. Good, eds. Pp. 134–152. Berkeley: University of California Press.

———. 1991. *The Work of Culture: Symbolic Transformation in Psychoanalysis and Anthropology.* Chicago: University of Chicago Press.

Ottaviani, R., and A. T. Beck. 1987. Cognitive Aspects of Panic Disorders. *Journal of Anxiety Disorders* 1:15–29.

Petrie, K. J., B. Sivertsen, M. Hysing, E. Broadbent, R. Moss-Morris, H. R. Eriksen, and H. Ursin. 2001. Thoroughly Modern Worries: The Relationship of Worries About Modernity to Reported Symptoms, Health, and Medical Care Utilization. *Journal of Psychosomatic Research* 51:395–401.

Porges, S. W. 2001. The Polyvagal Theory: Phylogenetic Substrates of a Social Nervous System. *International Journal of Psychophysiology* 42:123–146.

Rothbaum, F., J. Weisz, M. Pott, K. Miyake, and G. Morelli. 2000. Attachment and Culture: Security in the United States and Japan. *American Psychologist* 55:1093–1104.

Rubel, A. J., C. W. O'Nell, and R. Collado-Ardón. 1984. *Susto: A Folk Illness.* Berkeley: University of California Press.

Sharpe, M., and C. Bass. 1992. Pathophysiological Mechanisms in Somatization. *International Review of Psychiatry* 4:81–97.

Sperber, D. 1985. Anthropology and Psychology: Towards an Epidemiology of Representations. *Man* 20:73–89.

Squire, C. 1997. AIDS Panic. In *Body Talk: The Material and Discursive Regulation of Sexuality, Madness and Reproduction.* J. Ussher, ed. Pp. 50–69. London: Routledge.

Storms, M. D., and K. D. McCaul. 1976. Attribution Processes and Emotional Exacerbations of Dysfunctional Behavior. In *New Directions in Attribution Research.* J. H. Harvey, W. J. Ickes, and R. F. Kidd, eds. Vol. 1. Pp. 143–164. Hillsdale, NJ: Erlbaum.

Suomi, S. J. 2003. Gene-Environment Interactions and the Neurobiology of Social Conflict. *Annals of the New York Academy of Sciences* 1008:132–139.

Tseng, W.-S., M. Kan-Ming, L. Li-Shuen, C. Guo-Qian, O. Li-Wah, Z. Hong-Bo. 1992. Koro Epidemics in Guangdong China: A Questionnaire Survey. *Journal of Nervous and Mental Disease* 180:117–123.

Turner, S. P. 2002. *Brains/Practices/Relativism: Social Theory after Cognitive Science.* Chicago: University of Chicago Press.

Weissman, M. M., R. C. Bland, G. J. Canino, C. Faravelli, S. Greenwald, H. Hwu, P. Joyce, E. G. Karam, C. Lee, J. Lellouch, J. Lépine, S. Newman, M. Oakley-Browne, M. Rubio-Stipec, J. Wells, P. J. Wickramaratne, H. Wittchen, and E. Yeh. 1997. The Cross-National Epidemiology of Panic Disorder. *Archives of General Psychiatry* 54:305–309.

White, M., and D. Epston. 1990. *Narrative Means to Therapeutic Ends.* New York: Norton.

Williams, S. J., and G. A. Bendelow. 1998. Malignant Bodies: Children's Beliefs about Health, Cancer, and Risk. In *The Body in Everyday Life.* S. Nettelton and J. Watson, eds. Pp. 103–123. London: Routledge.

Yardley, L. 1997. Disorientation in the (Post) Modern World. In *Material Discourses of Health and Illness.* L. Yardley, ed. Pp. 109–131. London: Routledge.

Young, A. 1982. Rational Men and the Explanatory Model Approach. *Culture, Medicine, and Psychiatry* 6:57–71.

A Medical Anthropology of Panic Sensations

Ten Analytic Perspectives

Devon E. Hinton and Byron J. Good

THIS CHAPTER PROVIDES an analysis of panic and panic disorder from the perspective of a *medical anthropology of sensations*. Our overall argument is that sensation is not precultural but is very much embedded in culture. It follows that cross-cultural analysis of panic experiences and panic disorder, dependent as they are on the experience and interpretation of particular sensations, requires an explicit framework for the analysis of sensation. In the following pages we outline such a framework and illustrate its utility for understanding panic and panic disorder from a cultural perspective.

We use the term *sensation* to indicate a variety of somatic forms of experience, from feelings of heat in the body to dizziness to palpitations. The terms *sensation*[1] and *somatic symptom* are often interchangeable; the former, however, emphasizes sensory experience, an emerging bodily experience, while the latter emphasizes the medical interpretation of sensation, the somatic event as a symptom of a certain "disorder." In a panic attack, certain sensations give rise to fearful cognitions. Often a sufferer focuses on—and gives as the presenting complaint to a clinician—a single sensation that occurs in a panic attack, selected from among many sensations felt during the episode. Because somatic experiencing forms a core aspect of panic attacks, a complex understanding of sensations is needed to analyze these attacks adequately.[2]

To research sensation experience, we suggest ten analytic perspectives. Investigating sensation through such a framework prevents the committing of a certain kind of *category error* (Kleinman 1988)—the naive assumption that an illness or symptom in our society has exact equivalents in other societies, that the problem of translation of categories across cultures can be solved by simply finding the correct words or categories in another society. What might be called a *sensation error* (shorthand for a *sensation-type category error*; Hinton et al. 2007) is a similarly naive assumption that a sensation—its causation, semiotic networks, and "local biology" (Lock 1993)—in our culture has equivalents in all others, that translation requires simply identifying local terms for the equivalent sensation, for example, the naive assumption that the experience of dizziness for a Cambodian refugee during a panic attack is the same as that of a native English speaker born in the United States. This assessment carries the implicit assumption that the meaning of the sensation, or the semiotic network (Good 1977, 1994:169–174) associated with it, is equivalent for the two individuals. We argue throughout this chapter that such an equivalence cannot be assumed.

To guard against committing such a category fallacy, we adduce in this chapter ten perspectives from which to examine the sensations that give rise to and that occur in panic attacks. These perspectives delineate key features of sensations in panic, as in how they arise, how they are interpreted and lead to experiences of panic, the prominence of culturally or individually specific sensations in panic, and the structure of meanings associated with those sensations. It is our argument that a serious comparison of panic experience—and of panic disorder—across cultures requires attention to these analytic perspectives. In this chapter we focus largely on Cambodian examples—many pertaining to dizziness—drawn from the first author's experience as a psychiatrist and anthropologist treating and conducting research with Cambodian refugees, primarily in a mental health clinical setting.

1. The Descriptive Perspective:
The Most Prominent Sensations During Panic

According to the fourth edition of the *Diagnostic and Statistical Manual of Mental Disorders* (*DSM–IV*; APA 1994), in order to qualify as having had a panic attack, a person must have experienced at least four of the following symptoms or clusters of symptoms: (1) palpitations, pounding heart, or accelerated heart rate; (2) sweating; (3) trembling or shaking; (4) sensations of shortness of breath or smothering; (5) feeling of choking; (6) chest pain or discomfort; (7) nausea or abdominal discomfort; (8) feeling dizzy, unsteady, lightheaded, or faint; (9) derealization or depersonalization;[3] (10) fear of losing control or going crazy; (11) fear of dying; (12) numbness or tingling sensations; and (13) chills or hot flashes. Of these thirteen criteria, ten consist of sensations (1 through 8, 12, and 13) and three consist of cognitions (9 through 11). Several of these sensation-type criteria lump together multiple sensations; for example, criterion 8 consists of four potentially distinct sensations, and criterion 13 lumps together chills and hot flashes. For this reason, we refer hereafter to each of the thirteen *DSM* criteria as a *symptom category*. (The three cognition-type symptom categories listed in the *DSM–IV* panic attack criteria—items 9 through 11: "fear of losing control or going crazy," "fear of dying," and "derealization and depersonalization"—are best considered *catastrophic cognitions* and are discussed later in the chapter.)

To investigate cross-cultural differences in the types—and salience—of sensations experienced during panic, certain questions must be kept in mind, questions that need to be empirically investigated. Do the severity and frequency of the panic sensations listed in the *DSM–IV* vary across cultures? Are all of the sensations listed in the *DSM–IV* panic attack criteria identifiable in other cultural groups? In other cultural contexts is it valid to lump together several sensations (such as chills and hot flashes) in one symptom category, or should they be individually assessed? Is it sometimes the case that sensations identified in the *DSM–IV* are too broad whereas a more specific complaint is present in the culture in question, as in "heat in the head" rather than "hot flashes"? Do persons experiencing panic in other cultures have sensations not listed in these thirteen symptom categories?

Even when one considers only the sensations listed in the *DSM–IV* criteria, the frequency and severity of those sensations vary across cultures. The following sections explore some reasons for such variation, such as differences in the semantic networks—from associated ethnophysiology to metaphor—of sensations across cultures. One type of *sensation meaning* that influences a sensation's prominence in panic is the sensation's perceived role in the ethnophysiology, that is, its associated catastrophic cognitions. Across cultures, because of catastrophic cognitions specific to each particular locality, certain of the thirteen *DSM–IV* symptom clusters may be more prominent in anxiety and panic. Among English-speaking Americans, palpitations and shortness of breath, both associated with the feared illness category *heart attack* (Taylor 2000), tend to become the focus of panic experience. Khmer refugees often focus on dizziness, a key sign of the onset of a *"khyâl* attack" (*kaoet khyâl*), a condition in which the windlike *khyâl* surges upward in the body toward the head. They often survey the body for evidence of dizziness on standing, because an extremely dangerous form of *khyâl* attack, called *"khyâl* overload" (*khyâl koa*), is thought to be most likely to occur upon standing (Hinton et al. 2001a, 2001b). (In other publications we have used the term *kyol goeu*, but here we use the transliteration system of Heder and Ledgerwood [1996], and we use *"khyâl* overload" rather than *"wind* overload" because it is a more experience-near description.) Nigerians focus on one type of "hot flash," namely, cephalic heat, a key indicator of bodily disorder (Ebigbo 1986); and Puerto Ricans focus on symptoms such as trembling hands, which suggest a disorder of *nervios* and the onset of an *ataque de nervios* (see Guarnaccia et al. 1996; Hinton et al. 2001b, 2006b, in press a).

As previously noted, several of the *DSM–IV*'s thirteen symptom categories combine multiple complaints. A particular person's panic attack or panic attacks typical of members of a specific cultural group may emphasize a more specific symptom than that given in an omnibus *DSM–IV* category—for example, heat in the head rather than the more general *DSM–IV* category of "chills or hot flashes" (among Nigerian panic sufferers); "hand trembling" rather than the *DSM–IV*'s "trembling or shaking" (among Puerto Rican panic sufferers); "true vertigo," that is, a feeling of surrounding objects spinning around oneself, rather than the *DSM–IV*'s "feeling dizzy, unsteady, lightheaded, or faint" (among Cambodian panic sufferers).

Asphyxia complaints are highly represented in the *DSM–IV* panic attack criteria ("shortness of breath or smothering," "feeling of choking," "chest pain or discomfort"), but dizziness complaints are lumped together into one symptom category consisting of "feeling dizzy, unsteady, lightheaded, and faint." As Chapter 5 in this book argues, this bias has resulted from various sources, including the influence of Klein's theory of how panic is generated. Had the *DSM–IV* been developed primarily in an Asian country, one might well imagine that dizziness-related complaints would be parsed into several symptom categories (for example, true vertigo versus lightheadedness versus a feeling of blacking out) and asphyxia complaints lumped into one.

Besides the sensations listed in the thirteen categories of the *DSM–IV* panic attack criteria, other sensations often occur in acute episodes of anxiety (Hiller et al. 1997; Liebowitz et al. 1984; Reich et al. 1988). In some cultural settings, these non-*DSM–IV* symptoms may be a core aspect, or *the* core aspect, of the panic attack. For example, during panic attacks, Khmer often worriedly focus on tinnitus, neck tension, bodily weakness, and blurry vision, none of which are listed in the *DSM–IV* panic attack criteria (Hinton et al. 2000, 2001c, 2006a, 2006b).[4]

As indicated previously, the *DSM–IV* panic attack criteria are insufficient to describe in an accurate way the sensations experienced during panic when viewed from a cross-cultural perspective. The criteria include sensations that often are present in panic, but the panic investigator must also survey the panic sensations within the *DSM–IV* symptom categories, and sensations more specific than those in the symptom categories, such as the "heat in the head" experienced during the panic of a Yoruba-speaking population in Nigeria rather than simply hot flashes. And in many cases, panic sensations that are important in one cultural group, such as tinnitus or neck soreness in the Cambodian refugee population, may not be found in the *DSM* panic attack criteria. Cultural analysis of panic disorder requires identifying sensations that are most prominent in panic attacks, that are most culturally salient, then exploring those sensations through the following analytic perspectives.

2. The Physiological Perspective:
How Local Biology May Generate Specific Panic Sensations

In states of acute anxiety, a person often experiences a strong physiological response, the so-called *fight-or-flight response* (Cannon 1929; Noyes and Hoehn-Saric 1998; Ohman 2000:577), which results in various sensations. Activated by fear, the sympathetic and parasympathetic branches of the autonomic nervous system may produce palpitations, shortness of breath, intestinal upset, cold hands, numb hands, blurry vision, shakiness, muscle tension, buzzing in the ear (tinnitus), or some combination thereof. Rather than assuming physiology to be universal, researchers should consider the possibility that certain differences in panic symptomatology among cultures may result from differences in the autonomic nervous system due to differences in genetics, socialization, and diet.[5]

Each individual's autonomic nervous system may cause certain symptoms during fear states—for one individual, increased muscle tension and acceleration of heart rate; for another, intestinal peristalsis, shortness of breath, and sweating. This phenomenon has been referred to as *autonomic response specificity* (Lacey et al. 1953). Some studies suggest autonomic response specificity across cultures. Among some Asian groups, dizziness seemingly figures prominently during states of distress (see, for example, Kleinman and Kleinman 1994; see also Chapters 7 and 8 in this book). As an experimental correlate to this finding, in response to being seated inside a spinning drum that has vertical stripes, Chinese, when compared to Caucasians, had a far greater tendency to experience motion sickness as measured by nausea, gastric activity (by EGG), and dizziness (Stern et al. 1996). This apparent dizziness predisposition among Asian populations may reflect biological differences, cultural processes, or a dynamic interaction of both.[6]

Panic triggers also may vary across cultures due to physiological differences. The fact that the panic attacks of Cambodian patients are commonly triggered by dizziness inducers such as traveling in a car or entering a complex visual environment may result in part from a biologically determined predisposition to dizziness. Similarly, the frequency of orthostatic panic among Cambodian refugees with posttraumatic stress disorder may have, in part, a biological explanation. Upon standing and feeling dizzy, Cambodians worry about the onset of an episode of *khyâl* overload, a disorder that may cause syncope and death (Hinton et al. 2000, 2001a, 2001b, 2004a, 2006b). These orthostatic panic episodes could be given a purely psychological explanation, that is, that the syndrome of *khyâl* overload leads to an attentional amplification of any dizziness felt upon standing and to catastrophic cognitions about any experienced dizziness sensations. Alternatively, for physiological reasons Cambodians may experience more dizziness sensations upon standing (perhaps due to a less vigorous blood pressure reaction to standing based in ethnic differences in blood pressure adjustment caused by genetics, diet, and so on), followed by catastrophic cognitions about the physiologically caused dizziness sensations, which may lead to panic (Hinton et al. 2004a; Lu et al. 1990; Porth 1990).

3. The Ethnophysiological Perspective: Local Theories of How Physiology Produces Sensations

The term *ethnophysiology* refers to popular ideas about physiology that are more or less shared by members of a society, including *laypersons* and *folk experts*. Certain societies may have a highly complex ethnophysiology elaborated in texts—for example, Ayurvedic medicine in India and traditional Chinese medicine in East Asian societies—and many societies have multiple, interacting traditions. Text-based medical traditions are variably appropriated by different social groups and subcultures within the society in question. The physiological ideas of Cambodian refugee patients in the United States, for example, combine multiple influences—Indian and Chinese sources, as well as Western biomedicine, especially French colonial medicine (see this chapter's section on the historical perspective, and Chapters 5 and 8). Ethnophysiologies have distinctive forms of theorizing, categorizing, and interpreting bodily sensations. A society's popular ethnophysiologies affect self-surveillance, sensation amplification, and ideas about the implications of a particular symptom (Good 1977, 1994; Good 1980; Strathern 1996).

Once an anxiety-type sensation—such as dizziness, cold extremities, palpitations, or tinnitus—is experienced, the local ethnophysiology will have a major impact on how it is interpreted and on the degree of fear it causes. The Cambodian ethnophysiology offers an example of how cultural ideas about how the body functions may produce great fear of anxiety and panic sensations. The Cambodian ethnophysiology is in large part a *pneumatic system*, according to which *khyâl*, a windlike substance, flows in tubes distributed throughout the body, often alongside blood (Hinton et al. 2001a, 2001b, 2001c, 2006a, 2006b).[7] As suggested above, anxiety symptoms are often attributed to a dysregulation of the flow of *khyâl*, and a panic attack is usually referred to as a *khyâl* attack (*kaoet khyâl*). It is thought that in dysregulated states *khyâl* surges upward in the body, causing the various anxiety-type symptoms. It strikes the lungs, impeding breathing; hits the heart, causing palpitations; distends the neck vessels, causing neck pain; swirls the cranial contents, causing dizziness; shoots from the eyes, causing blurry vision; and rushes through the ear canals, causing tinnitus, or ear ringing, referred to as "*khyâl* shooting from the ears" (*khyâl choenh pii troechia*). To treat these various symptoms, Cambodian refugees frequently utilize various *khyâl*-removing measures (see Hinton et al. 2001a, 2001b): "coining," applying medicated pads, and rubbing *khyâl* oil (*preeng khyâl*) onto the skin.

To understand how ethnophysiology affects panic subjectivity, one must examine a culture's conceptualization of the vulnerability of the body to perturbation by emotional states, food intake, or weather (Hinton et al. 2003). One must determine the range of events, from worry to dietary intake to weather shifts, that are thought to cause physiological dysregulations, the ease with which those dysregulations may be induced, and the degree of danger caused by those perturbations. These expectations guide self-surveillance of the body and form a key aspect of the local panic ontology.[8]

An ethnophysiology may produce a sensation just by expectation. If one worries about having—that is, expects to have—a sensation that indicates a serious disturbance of physiology, that sensation may be induced by two processes: attention, that is, by the searching of the body for that particular sensation and focusing on it; and fear-caused activation of the autonomic nervous system, with that activation possibly producing the feared symptom and others (see Figure 3.1). In this way, an ethnophysiology may result in the induction of a sensation, or the same processes may amplify a sensation when it occurs for any reason, and a spiral of panic may soon occur.

4. The Catastrophic Cognitions Perspective

An extensive scientific literature supports the view that catastrophic cognitions about bodily symptoms lead to panic (for a review, see Hinton et al. 2006a), and that the more a person fears somatic symptoms, the more likely it is that he or she will have panic disorder.[9] Fear may focus on any of various somatic sensations—palpitations, cold extremities, stomach bloating, or a feeling of unusual lightness in the body. These research findings clearly have profound implications with respect to variation in rates and subtypes of panic disorder across cultures. If fear about somatic symptoms differs across cultures, then the rate and subtypes of panic disorder should also differ significantly. If catastrophic cognitions about somatic symptoms generate panic attacks, then culture lies at the very center of panic. To carry out research on panic, cultural ideas about the body must be elucidated in a sophisticated fashion.

Fear about a sensation often results when the sensation is thought to indicate the presence of some syndrome or a certain disorder within a local ethnophysiology. Catastrophic cognitions resulting from cultural syndromes and ethnophysiology—for example, a Cambodian worrying that neck tension indicates the imminent rupture of the vessels by *khyâl* and blood (Hinton et al. 2001c, 2006b)—profoundly shape which symptoms trigger panic. Owing to varying cultural syndromes and ethnophysiologies, catastrophic cognitions about sensations would be expected to differ across cultures and subcultures, so the sensations that are most feared and

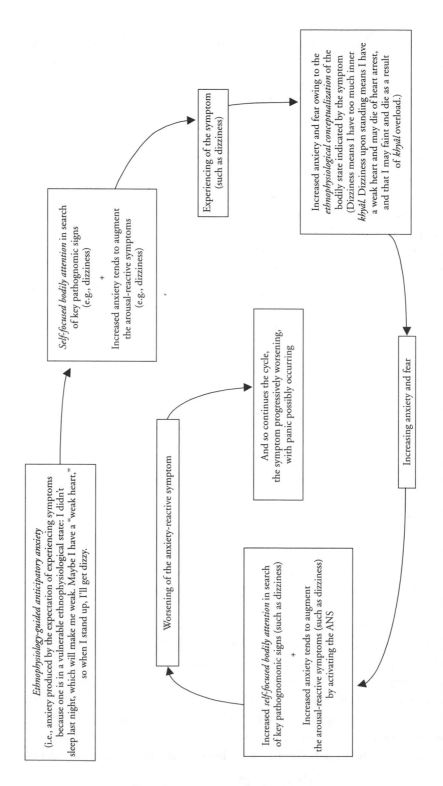

Figure 3.1 Ethnophysiology-guided somatization: A Cambodian example

most likely to give rise to panic would likewise be expected to differ (Hinton et al. 2006b).

Fear of somatic sensations varies across cultures, creating different panic ontologies. Upon experiencing joint pain and muscle soreness, an American may worry about having a chronic disease such as fibromyalgia (Hudson and Pope 1994) or about overstraining the muscles and tendons. But according to the ethnophysiology espoused by Khmer refugee patients, uncomfortable joint sensations indicate the blockage of vessels (*sâsai*) through which *khyâl* and blood flow, with such blockages possibly causing limb paralysis and the upsurge of *khyâl* and blood into the abdomen, chest, neck, and cranium (Hinton et al. 2001a, 2006b). Such catastrophic cognitions about the physiological correlates of joint and muscle discomfort produce fear. That fear may increase joint and muscle discomfort by (a) activation of the autonomic nervous system, which will increase muscle tension, leading to uncomfortable sensations in the muscles and where muscle tendons insert into the bone, for example, at the elbow and knee; and (b) attentional amplification, that is, the narrowing of attention onto the bodily areas of concern—in this case, the joints and muscles—resulting in an increase of their salience in consciousness. A panic spiral may result (Clark 1986; Hinton et al. 2001a, 2001b, 2006b) as fear itself increases the feared symptoms.

The prominence of actual biological diseases in a locality may greatly influence panic ontology if those diseases have somatic symptoms like those induced by anxiety, such as dizziness, palpitations, or shortness of breath. Upon having those somatic symptoms during an anxiety episode, the patient may fear the onset of an episode of that disease. To give one example, malaria is prominent in Southeast Asia, and its symptoms include periodic rigors marked by chills, tinnitus, dizziness, and palpitations. Cambodian refugees often worry that cold extremities and other symptoms indicate the onset of a malaria attack—and it is not uncommon for them to have rigors like those of a malaria episode during states of anxiety. Another example would be an American construing palpitations to indicate the onset of a heart attack. And even when an actual biological disease does not have somatic symptoms like those occurring in anxiety episodes, fear of having that disease may still increase fear of anxiety-type somatic symptoms if a cultural group considers anxiety-type symptoms to indicate the onset of the pathophysiology that generates the dreaded disease, as in Cambodians ascribing joint soreness and hand coldness to the plugging up of the peripheral blood vessels, which may cause permanent limb paralysis, that is, a "stroke"—a disease that is rather common and greatly feared in the Cambodian population. Misattribution of anxiety symptoms to a dreaded disease, that is, to the pathophysiology thought to generate the disease, results in great fear of somatic-type anxiety sensations, so the local biological diseases may shape panic ontology.

As noted in the early section on the descriptive perspective, the *DSM–IV* panic attack criteria include three catastrophic-cognition-type criteria: fear of losing control or going crazy, fear of dying, and derealization and depersonalization. One would expect great cross-cultural variation in the meaning and generation of the first catastrophic-cognition-type criterion, depending on local ideas about the mind, personhood, insanity, and losing control. And clearly, the experience of fear of dying will vary immensely across cultures, depending on what the person fears dying of, that is, on the meaning of the experienced sensations. The catastrophic cognition of derealization and depersonalization does not appear to be present in panic in all other cultural contexts, although a closely related experience, *soul loss*, is often found—for example, in the Cambodian culture.

Cambodian refugees do not seem to experience derealization and depersonalization as part of panic attacks—although after extensive questioning the patient may endorse the complaint. But Cambodians do experience a closely related feeling in panic: a sense of "soul loss" associated with feelings of lightness, of bodily alteration, of strangeness. According to Cambodian understandings, when the "soul" (*prolung*) leaves the body, feelings of lightness, strangeness, or fatigue may result (compare Shweder 1985). Other symptoms heighten soul-loss fears, particularly tinnitus, called "*khyâl* shooting from the ears" (*khyâl choenh troechea*), considered to be a sign of the soul leaving the body. Bodily sensations and mental processes that English-speaking Americans refer to as *derealization* or *depersonalization*—a feeling of strangeness or otherness—would seem to be related to the experience of soul loss that some Cambodians have. The physiological basis of these feelings of strangeness found in derealization and depersonalization and in soul loss may in some cases be anxiety-caused changes in the body, such as vasoconstriction, and anxiety-caused changes in mental processing, such as accelerated thought. These feelings or sensations may be variably interpreted, and no simple translation is possible between abstract categories such as depersonalization and local forms of experience in other societies, such as soul loss.[10]

5. The Perspective of Metaphor

Sensations may be used as metaphors. For example, *shortness of breath* may be used as a metaphor for relationships, as in "You are suffocating me." The meanings associated via metaphor with particular sensations vary by culture. Metaphors influence the meaning of bodily sensations and guide the embodiment of distress (Kirmayer 1984; Lakoff and Kovecses 1987; Scheper-Hughes and Lock 1987).[11] Metaphors may cause a sensation to conjure current life problems; for example, for an English speaker, cold hands may bring to mind a lack of interpersonal warmth, or shortness of breath may conjure thoughts about a relationship. Alternatively, cognizing current problems in certain metaphors may induce sensations; for an English speaker, for example, cognizing a troubled relationship in lack-of-warmth tropes may actually induce a feeling of cold in the body, or thinking "I am suffocating in this relationship" might lead to an actual feeling of shortness of breath.[12]

In any particular culture there occurs a complex *semiosis* (Chandler 2002) of anxiety terms by means of which anxiety comes to acquire specific *dynamic interpretants*.[13] In the Cambodian language, spinning imagery figures prominently in metaphors used to express dysphoria and anxiety. If a Cambodian wants to convey feeling overwhelmed by concerns or obligations, he or she may draw from a rich repertoire of spinning metaphors: "the face spins" (*weul muk*: "to spin," *weul*; "face," *muk*), "my brain spins" (*weul khua*), or *wuat*, which means literally "spinning-like-a-stirred-semisolid," thus conjuring the image of palm sugar being stirred and heated over a fire to coagulate it. And to express anxiety-type distress, Cambodians often use *chrâbook chrâbâl*, a reduplicative, that is, a word composed of two units that are similar but slightly different.[14] *Chrâbâl* means "to mix several ingredients together through a kneading-like action," such as various spices to make a sauce; and *chrâbook* is a rhyming word that has no meaning on its own.

Analysis of panic should specifically attend to metaphors—from phrases or idioms to the etymology of individual words—used to describe anxiety, fear, worry, negative events, and the specific sensations associated with panic. In a given language, anxiety descriptors may use metaphors that suggest that anxiety is particularly associated with a certain symptom. If so, that symptom will tend to be central to anxiety and panic, and that sensation will be more easily induced by anxiety. Also, if a sensation is induced for any reason—such as worry, stress, or physical exertion, as in climbing stairs—that sensation's metaphor-type semantic networks may be activated and thereby cause great distress. And thinking about negative events using metaphors involving a sensation—for example, upon learning of some new problem, thinking "this is a pain in the neck"—may bring about that sensation, and that induced sensation may then trigger or amplify panic.

6. The Perspective of Sound and Kinetic Symbolism

Whenever we objectify our inchoate sensations in words provided by language—a process of *linguistic objectification*—those words will tend to shape our experience of the associated sensations (Berger and Luckmann 1967). As we scan our bodies, if we have in mind certain linguistic labels for sensations, the very nature of those labels and the gestures and postures typically associated with them shape expectation and guide attention. These labels vary greatly by culture, historical period, and social class. A certain word used to express a sensation may have *sound symbolism* (that is, the sound may be iconic of the meaning) and *articulatory iconicism* (that is, the movements made in the vocal tract upon saying the word, such as tongue movements, may be iconic of the meaning) that make it affectively vivid, amplifying the very sensation it describes. Associated gestures and postures may have a similar effect (see, for example, Geurts 2002; Hinton 1999; Hinton et al. 2004b).

In the Western construction of anxiety, shortness of breath is emphasized.[15] In the English language, multiple tropes use shortness of breath to express a dysphoric state (see, for example, DeSalvo 1997:65), such as "no breathing room," "suffocating in this life," "can't breathe in the relationship," and "so busy I can't catch my breath." The close pairing of shortness of breath and anxiety in the English language is etymologically enshrined in the word *anxiety* itself. The word *anxiety*— and closely related words such as *anxious, anguish, anger,* and *angst*—derives from the Greek root *angh,* meaning "to strangle" or "to press tight" (Barlow 1988:9). But *angh* is not just an ideophone (that is, a sound cluster associated with a certain meaning); the root *angh* is an *articulatory kineme* (an analogy to the *phoneme* where *kin* indicates "movement" and *eme* means "meaning"),[16] that is, the movements that occur in the vocal tract upon saying the sound cluster evoke a specific meaning. Upon saying *angh,* the throat closes as the back of the tongue moves backward, blocking off the throat; thus, saying *angh* results in the embodiment of the meaning of the word.

In the Cambodian language, the configuration of anxiety as a kind of vertigo is linguistically objectified through various terms used to describe it. In Khmer, several of the words used to express our concept of anxiety have a specific polysyllabic sound form that has rich sound and kinemic-type symbolism. This sound form, not only through its very sound but also through the mouth movements used to say it, evokes the conventional meaning: a back-and-forth, repetitive occurrence. To express the concept of anxiety, Cambodians utilize any one of four reduplicatives: (1) *chrâbook chrâbâl,* (2) *rosap rosâl,* (3) *krâwâl krâwaay,* or (4) *antea anteeng.* In these expressions, the ideophone, which is also a kineme, configures anxiety as a repetitive motion involving a shift, as in turning from one side to another (Hinton et al. 2004b). Each of these reduplicatives creates a sense of repetitive motion and shift through sound symbolism and mouth motions that produce and amplify a feeling of dizziness (Hinton et al. 2004b).[17]

Just as tongue and mouth motions may indicate the meaning of *anxiety* and *sensation* in a particular cultural context, so too may gestures and body postures, that is, arm and postural kinemics (Beattie 2004; Birdwhistell 1970; Geurts 2002); for example, upon articulating one of the reduplicatives that indicates anxiety, Cambodians will often make one of the following two gestures: (1) pointing the index finger toward the head and making circular motions, or (2) placing one forearm just above the other and then making rotatory motions so that the two forearms revolve around each other. These gestures indicate that "anxiety is a spinning." In contrast, when Puerto Rican patients are feeling anxious, they may place their hands against their chests and speak of feeling "squeezed" (*apretado*) or of "drowning" (*ahogado*) (see Hinton et al. 2001b).

7. The Landscape Perspective: How the Environmental Surround Triggers and Gives Meaning to Sensations

The environmental surround, including both the built and natural environments, may give meaning to sensations in three ways.[18] First, specific aspects of the environment may be invoked as a cause of dysphoric sensations; for example, an agoraphobic may attribute dizziness to the complexity of the visual environment (Hinton et al. 2002a); a sufferer of multiple chemical sensitivity may attribute dizziness to encountering ambient smells; and a Vietnamese refugee may attribute it to "being hit by a poisonous wind" (Hinton et al. 2003). Second, the environmental surround may be used as a descriptor of sensation via metaphor. And third, the environment may serve as a model of pathophysiology, of how sensations result.

The words used to describe sensation often involve landscape imagery. For example, when overwhelmed or anxious, Cambodian refugees will often describe themselves as "dizzy" and will convey their emotional state by using various environmental images—the spinning motions of a water bug (*kânteh lâng*), the rotations of a millstone (*khbaal koen sroew*), the whirling of a dust devil (*khyâl kuach*) in the dry season, the swirling of ash that has been placed in water and stirred to make soap (*weul khbong*), or the rotational motions of liquid palm sugar being stirred over a fire to cause a slow evaporation to form a hard paste (*wuat*) that later will be poured into molds to make discs of palm sugar. Khmer will also compare the sound of tinnitus to the cyclical call of the cicada that is heard during the hot season, most prominently one month before the New Year's celebration, when most family members return to the village (Hinton et al. in press b). Such cultural representations may lead a Cambodian to associate tinnitus with a range of memory and affects. To give an example from the United States, back discomfort and pain resonate with and activate networks of meaning uniting built environment, bodily sensations, and multiple cultural domains: the prominence of column-like elements in our lived environment, from studs to posts to pillars to piers; the use of contemporary stress-related idioms such as "mental collapse," "burdened," "to break down," "stressed out," and "can't stand the stress"; the use of architectural terms to express ideas about morality (such as "upright," "has backbone," "pillar of the community," and "spineless") and about the aesthetics of the body (favoring the upright stance and straight spine, with no rolled-forward shoulders suggesting defeat). These images contrast being upright with being bent over in pain, uniting emotional experience and the columnar aspects of our environment. Thus built environment, posture, back pain, emotion, metaphor, ethics, aesthetics, and physical vigor together form a dynamic and resonating cultural system (Kugelmann 1992; Scheper-Hughes and Lock 1987; Young 1980).

The natural and built environments may give rise to theories of the mind and the body. Rooted in the lived surround (*Umvelt*), these theories seem self-evident and "natural" (Delaney 1991; Feld 1982; Hsu 1999; Kuriyama 1999; Lo 2001; Scheper-Hughes and Lock 1987). Among Laotian speakers experiencing anxiety, the agitated heart is compared to the swinging of a ripe mango on a long stem. Someone suffering from palpitations therefore worries about acute demise, thinking that the "stem of the heart" (*khua hua cay*) will snap, just as would the stem of a mango if hit by a strong wind (Hinton 1999). And Laotians consider abdominal distention to indicate an "upward-hitting *lom*" (with *lom* considered to be a wind-like substance) that may strike the heart and cause it to swing to the point that the heart-stem snaps (Hinton 1999).

8. The Memory Perspective

Any sensation may have certain memory associations. Consequently, experiencing the sensation may trigger those memories, or conversely, thinking about the memory may produce the sensations.

Among Cambodian refugees, dizziness may recall multiple memories, such as malarial episodes marked by severe vertigo; slave labor while starving, including repeatedly bending over to transplant rice or swinging the arms and twisting the torso to thresh rice stalks; falling down due to the dizziness caused by starvation and overwork; being struck in the head by a Khmer Rouge soldier; and events marked by disgust, such as witnessing an execution involving the spilling of blood at a public evisceration. Traumatic events that provoked dizziness through the emotion of terror, such as being threatened with death, cause the trauma to be encoded and evoked by dizziness.

Cultural ideas influence the perception of the degree of bodily damage caused by a trauma. If certain sensations are thought to reflect a disturbance of physiology caused by the trauma, these sensations may evoke memories of that trauma (Kirmayer 2002). According to traditional Khmer belief, a woman should perform minimal work for several months after giving birth and should undergo certain postpartum steaming rituals; if these two injunctions are not followed, the vessels of the body, which are thought to be in a "soft" and vulnerable state, may become permanently disordered and predispose the body to joint soreness and *khyâl* attack, producing such symptoms as dizziness. The Khmer Rouge forced new mothers to undertake hard labor and did not allow them to perform the traditional postpartum rituals. Consequently, whenever a joint pain is felt or dizziness is noticed, a Cambodian woman may think of her postpartum experiences in the Pol Pot time and attribute the symptoms to irreversibly damaged bodily conduits.

As these examples illustrate, "history is written on the body" (Pandolfi 1990). Cambodians need to understand both individual and communal experiences of the Cambodian holocaust in order to understand how trauma moves into the body, how the body remembers, and how the corporal serves as the archive of memory. An adequate analysis of panic must therefore detail the memory associations to sensations that are prominent in panic. Simply to describe a Khmer patient as having a somatic complaint without detailing the testimonial dimension of this complaint, without hearing it as embodied history, is inadequate for understanding the patient's experience.

9. The Sociosomatic Perspective

The social course of sensation, that is, the sensation's role in the *sociosomatic reticulum*—how it affects social relationships, and its origins in a particular social situation—must be taken into consideration (Kleinman 1986; Kleinman and Kleinman 1994). More broadly, the sociosomatic perspective considers the sensation's role, meaning, consequences, and causes in a certain social, political, and economic context. It considers the nature of the *reticulum* that unites somatic complaint to those domains, that is, the term *sociosomatic perspective* is shorthand for the study of the socio-politico-econo-somatic reticulum (see also Chapters 7 through 9 of this book).

One must consider the social course of a sensation complaint. Does it seem to arise from social conflicts, from familial conflicts, from interpersonal abuse? Does it empower certain persons within the family, or serve as a "weapon of the weak" (Scott 1985)? Do the local explanatory frames consider certain disorders as having social origins? Will the sensation be attributed to different processes by various persons within the family? How will the treatments and putative etiology change the social and economic situation of the person? Many other perspectives described in this chapter, such as the perspective of metaphor, delineate the symbolic bridges that link social context to somatic complaint and panic.

In a cultural context, local explanations of illness may take into consideration social causes and may result in immediate treatment by family members. To recall a Cambodian refugee example, anxiety and its symptoms, such as dizziness, are often attributed to a *khyâl* attack, and the *khyâl* attack is often treated by family members through coining, "cupping," and other methods. These *khyâl* attacks are also often attributed to social and economic causes: the body may be depleted and predisposed to *khyâl* attacks due to worrying about not having the money to pay the rent or about a child not going to school, or due to anxiety and distress caused by abuse perpetrated by a spouse or by difficulties with a child who stays out late at night or is gang involved. Cambodians consider *khyâl* attacks and associated symptoms such as dizziness to be key components of the sociosomatic reticulum, and the complaint of *khyâl* attacks and associated somatic complaints will be understood in this way by the family and other persons.

10. The Historical Perspective

In a recent book, Hacking (2002) calls for the study of *historical ontology*, or as Foucault put it, "the historical ontology of ourselves" (quoted by Hacking 2002:2). How have we come through time to constitute ourselves as certain kinds of subjects? In order to attain a processual view of changes in non-Western medical traditions, one must examine the incorporation and embodiment of Western illness categories through time (Hsu 1999:88), the extent to which there occurred a *colonization of ontology*[19] by new idioms of distress, how the adoption of Western illness categories created new constellations of power and knowledge, and how and why certain Western discourses were adopted and produced new, hybrid-type collective representations of disorder.

Sing Lee (1994, 1995, 1999) shows how the Western concept of *neurasthenia* was localized in China, and how it came to have a specific kind of meaning, a meaning constituted in large part by a dynamic interaction of preexisting notions of *weakness* (such as "kidney weakness") and the Western category of neurasthenia (compare Kleinman 1986). The Cambodian notion of *weak heart* is almost certainly of colonial origin. An adequate analysis of the cultural syndrome must examine the interaction of local ideas about weakness and colonial discourses and practices, including the early-twentieth-century French understanding of *heart weakness*, as in *faible de coeur* and *neurasthenie cardiaque*, and of neurasthenia, as in *surmenage mental* and *surmenage physique* (Hinton et al. 2002b).

One might call such a syndrome, produced from a combination of local and colonial syndromes and thus forming a congeries of local and imported ideas, a *hybrid syndrome*. By *hybrid* we seek to emphasize the historically situated syndrome—the historical heart, the *historicized heart*, the heart as an emergent entity—to highlight its composite nature, the way it brings together disparate concepts. It represents a "synthesis of meanings," to use Nietzsche's phrase (1967:80). Genealogy should reveal that shifting synthesis as it transforms itself through time (Foucault 1977)—the heart as emergent and polythetic entity.

In many societies, the lived body, the anxious body, came to be constituted in no small part by the complex interaction through time of local aesthetics, the "great traditions" (such as Ayurveda), and historically specific Western, biomedical-type theories and practices, such as that of the late nineteenth-century British empire.

Only careful research will reveal this "sickness history" (Gaines 1992). To historicize contemporary, non-Western medical systems, the process of indigenization of Western medical systems should be traced, to determine how a certain local poetics of being emerged through time by a complex process of localization (Good and Good 1992; Laderman 1992). So, for instance, how a certain group reacts to a "pounding heart," and how the overactive heart is described (and considered), should be analyzed in relation to notions and syndromes that evolved over time.

In the 1960s, after returning to Cambodia following medical training in France, many Cambodian doctors diagnosed *khyâl* symptoms as due to poor blood flow caused by a "weak heart." To counteract the low calcium thought to produce "spasticity" of the heart and the entire nervous system, they treated patients with pills and injections (French pharmaceuticals) to increase "energy" and strengthen the heart, and with calcium pills and injections (again, French pharmaceuticals) to reduce the spasticity (see Chapter 5 and Hinton et al. 2002b). In this way a new form of the commodification of health (Nichter 1996:265–326) emerged, with energy purchasable in the form of injectable vials, versus the poor man's option of imbibing the juice of a young coconut. Through such means and processes, a colonization of panic ontology, of panic subjectivity, occurred. In this case, palpitations and other sensations took on new dynamic interpretants; the sensations became hybrid entities, incorporating both local and Western meanings.

Given that we live in a so-called postcolonial period, such sickness history might be better described as the study of the emergence of cosmopolitan ontology—of the process of the cosmopolitization of ontology—as applied to specific disorders (Beck 1999; Inda and Rosaldo 2002). Through time there occurs a cosmopolitization of panic ontology and its symptoms.

Concluding Remarks

In a panic attack, certain sensations are prominent. The present chapter has introduced ten analytic lenses through which to examine those sensations. In each culture, in each subculture, and for every individual, a sensation's meaning varies. There is not simply dizziness; when viewed from these various perspectives, differences emerge at the level of individuals, genders, subgroups, and cultures. By attending to sensation via these perspectives, the investigator or clinician can avoid ethnocentric assumptions of equivalence of meaning and better understand a patient's panic attack or symptoms.

In investigating a panic attack, one should determine which sensation is most intense and which sensation is of most concern. In some cases, a sensation may be less severe but cause more concern; for example, the person suffering panic may have severe sweating but be far more concerned about mild shortness of breath. The reason for concern may vary: the sensation may, for example, cause fear of death, evoke current life distress through metaphoric resonances, or recall memories of past traumas. The framework described in this chapter indicates the various processes that may lead to *sensation amplification*, that is, an increase in the emotional and experiential salience of a particular sensation (compare Barsky's term, *somatosensory amplification*: Barsky et al. 1988; Barsky and Wyshak 1990).

The method of sensation analysis outlined in this chapter has both clinical and research importance. If a clinician considers a bodily complaint simply as evidence of somatization arising from anxiety and depression, he or she is providing inadequate care. Adequate ethnography and clinical care require attending to the details of meaning associated with the somatic complaint, as outlined in this chapter—for example, dizziness as generating catastrophic cognitions about the state of bodily functioning, dizziness as the somatization of interpersonal distress according to metaphors in that person's language group, and dizziness as evoking past traumatic events. Attending to the meanings associated with sensations in the ways described in this chapter promotes empathy and provides information that is invaluable for clinical care and for the ethnography of the body. The specific elements described in this chapter suggest a series of questions for empirical research.

In sum, we advocate that research on panic and panic disorder should analyze local panic sensations from the perspectives outlined in this chapter, thus attending to the complex ways that sensations emerge, that is, to the process of sensation semiosis, that is, the sensation's accumulation of meanings—from metaphor to ethnophysiology to social context. Sensations act as multireferential symbols (Myerhoff 1974:194), simultaneously rooted in the biology of the body. Many of the chapters in this book support such an interpretation. We believe that an analytic framework such as this will contribute to the development of a medical anthropology of panic and an anthropology of the sensations.

Notes

1. The term *sensation*, derived from the word *sense*, tends to mean the experience that results from the activation of sensory organs. Elsewhere the first author of this chapter has used the term *polymodal sensations* to describe sensations that result from multiple sensory systems (Hinton et al. in press c), for example, dizziness may result from the vestibular sense (such as turning the head), from visual sensations (such as watching speeding cars), from auditory sensations (such as hearing a jumble of sounds), and so on.

2. Panic attacks that occur in panic disorder may also be analyzed in terms of a medical anthropology of emotion (Shweder 2004). During such a panic attack, the person has an emotion, namely, terror, characterized by fear of insanity or of death from internally generated bodily dysfunction. People with panic disorder have recurrent bouts of a certain type of

fear; they are predisposed to a certain emotional state. As an emotion, panic attacks should be analyzed according to the categories suggested by the anthropology of emotion: environmental determinants, self-appraisal, somatic phenomenology, affective phenomenology, social appraisal, self-management, and communication (Shweder 2004). On the need for a contextualized analysis of emotion terms such as *fear*, see also Kagan (2008).

3. *Derealization* is a feeling that things are "not real," the experiencing of the surrounding world as having a frighteningly surreal quality. *Depersonalization* is the feeling of a frighteningly altered sense of self, as if your body is not yours, as if the thoughts passing through your mind are not your own.

4. In fact, in previous periods in the West, tinnitus was a prominent aspect of panic attacks. Such was the case in Paris in the 1870s, as described by Krishaber (1873).

5. Analogously, Lock (1993) argues that among Japanese women the menopausal experience, referred to as *koneki*, cannot be understood solely from the perspective of cultural schemas; rather, local biology plays an important role. Lock hypothesizes that the lower rate of menopausal hot flashes among Japanese women, compared to that of North American or European women, results (at least in part) from local biology rather than from attentional processes (Lock 1993:372).

6. Multiple dizziness-related metaphors in Chinese culture, representing a hypercognizing of dizziness in metaphoric expression, may increase sensitivity to dizziness; or hypervigilance to dizziness may result from dizziness being considered a key symptom of illness syndromes (such as neurasthenia) or of physiological dysregulations (for example, weakness or increased bodily "wind"). On the other hand, a biological predisposition to motion sickness and dizziness, such as that indicated by the Stern et al. (1996) experiment, may give rise to a dizziness emphasis in metaphoric expression and illness models.

7. This pneumatic system is widespread in Asia and possibly originated in Ayurvedic medicine (see Chapters 7, 8, and 10).

8. For example, in several countries of Southeast Asia, such as Cambodia, Laos, and Vietnam, there is a bridging of mind and body through local theories about how psychology affects physiology and vice versa, hinging on such concepts as bodily energy; this lack of dualism predisposes persons to panic, through the belief that thought processes directly affect bodily state and that bodily state directly affects mental state.

9. Two of the most utilized psychological measures in panic disorder research are the Anxiety Sensitivity Index (ASI; see McNally 1994; Taylor 2000) and the Agoraphobic Cognitions Questionnaire (ACQ; Chambless et al. 1984). The ASI asks a person about fear of different bodily sensations. The ACQ asks the person whether she or he has certain catastrophic cognitions during a panic attack, such as "I must have a brain tumor" or "I am going to have a heart attack." The higher the total score is on either the ASI or the ACQ, the more likely it is that the person will suffer from panic disorder, and if he or she is already suffering from panic disorder, the more severe the disorder is. If these worries are reduced by a therapeutic intervention (such as by a cardiac examination proving that the heart is perfectly normal, so palpitations need not be feared), the panic disorder decreases in severity.

10. In other cultural contexts, other related states may be prominent. As a case in point, a feeling of the "uncanny," or *unheimlich*—literally, "not-at-homeness"—plays a key role in the experience of anxiety (*Angst*) in Germany (see, for example, Freud 2003; Wierzbicka

1999). Such states as derealization and depersonalization in the United States, *unheimlich* in Germany, and soul loss in various locales need to undergo cultural and ethnographic analysis, and their role in the generation of anxiety, panic, and agoraphobia-like states needs to be explored.

11. For example, Scheper-Hughes and Lock (1987) suggest some of the complex meanings of back pain in the United States, meanings influenced by phrases such as *a shirker, spineless,* and *a monkey on his back,* and by the meaning of being "upright" in American culture.

12. Of course the line between putative ethnopsychology and trope is not clear. On a cultural syndrome that must be understood from both the standpoint of metaphor and physiology, see the literature on the Korean syndrome *hwa byung*, a form of acute distress centering on abdominal complaints in which the person experiences heat rising upward from the belly (Lin 1983; Pang 1990).

13. When we refer to *dynamic interpretants* (Nattiez 1987, 1988; see also Chandler 2002; Muller and Brent 2000), we mean the full spectrum of ideas and images evoked by a particular word in the mind of the person who hears the word, that is, in the mind of the *interpreter of the sign*—hence Peirce's neologism, *interpretant* (on Peirce's conception of the "*interpretant*," see the references cited earlier in this note). To give an example, if the word *red* is spoken, any of a number of dynamic interpretants might come to mind, such as lipstick, blood, or apples; and if it happens to be near Valentine's day, perhaps saying *red* will evoke a red rose and all the associated feelings. The dynamic interpretants of a term will vary by culture and personal experience; for instance, if you recently experienced a car accident, the red of blood may be evoked as well as the entire trauma scene.

14. As in the English terms *wishy washy, dilly dally,* and *flip-flop.*

15. This emphasis on shortness of breath may rise in part from the prominence in the Western ontology of *breath, spiritus, pneuma*—considered an animating breath in both religious experience and theories of physiology (for a review, see Hinton 1999). One of the most famous images of Western embodiments of anxiety also involves shortness of breath: from Greco-Roman times to the nineteenth century, the periodic suffocating of the hysteric when vapors from the uterus, or the uterus itself, rose upward to block inhalation by pressing on the lungs and wind pipe (Veith 1993). In current theories of panic (particularly that of Klein; see Chapter 5 in this book), shortness of breath plays a key role.

16. On this term, see Birdwhistell 1970; Hinton et al. 2004b.

17. These reduplicative ideophones, which are also reduplicative kinemes, have the following abstract form, where *syl* means syllable, *c* means a consonant, and *v* means a vowel: syl1c1v1c2 syl1c1v2c3.

18. Scheper-Hughes and Lock (1987) write of the "embodied world"; Hsu (1999:78–79) calls this the "body ecologic"; this might also be called the "lived-landscape body," or "*Umwelt* body"(on Heidegger's notion of *Umwelt*, see Cumming 2001).

19. Habermas uses the term *colonization of the life-world* to describe "the shaping of the experiential world or our moral lives by instrumental rationality, highly routinized procedures, by both technical and technological management" (Good 1994:85; see also Braaten 1991). In using the term *colonization of ontology,* or *ontology colonization,* we wish to emphasize how aspects of ontology become shaped by colonial idioms of distress, personhood, self, physiology, aesthetics, and health. The new ontology may become a key part of *symbolic reproduction* (on Habermas's notion of symbolic reproduction, see Braaten 1991).

References

American Psychiatric Association (APA). 1994. *Diagnostic and Statistical Manual of Mental Disorders.* 4th ed. [*DSM–IV.*] Washington, DC: American Psychiatric Association.

Barlow, D. H. 1988. *Anxiety and Its Disorders: The Nature and Treatment of Anxiety and Panic.* New York: Guilford Press.

Barsky, A., and G. Wyshak. 1990. Hypochondriasis and Somatosensory Amplification. *British Journal of Psychiatry* 157:404–409.

Barsky, A., J. Goodson, R. Lane, and P. Cleary. 1988. The Amplification of Somatic Symptoms. *Psychosomatic Medicine* 50:510–519.

Beattie, G. 2004. *Visible Thoughts: The New Psychology of Body Language.* London: Routledge.

Beck, U. 1999. *World Risk Society.* Cambridge, UK: Blackwell.

Berger, P., and T. Luckmann. 1967. *The Social Construction of Reality: A Treatise in the Sociology of Knowledge.* Harmondsworth, UK: Penguin.

Birdwhistell, R. 1970. *Kinesics and Context: Essays on Body Motion.* Philadelphia: University of Pennsylvania Press.

Braaten, J. 1991. *Habermas's Critical Theory of Society.* New York: State University of New York.

Cannon, W. B. 1929. *Bodily Change in Pain, Hunger, Fear, and Rage.* New York: Appleton.

Chambless, D., G. Caputo, P. Bright, and R. Gallagher. 1984. Assessment of Fear of Fear in Agoraphobics: The Body Sensations Questionnaire and the Agoraphobic Cognitions Questionnaire. *Journal of Consulting Clinical Psychology* 52:1090–1097.

Chandler, D. 2002. *Semiotics: The Basics.* London: Routledge.

Clark, D. 1986. A Cognitive Approach to Panic. *Behaviour Research and Therapy* 24:461–470.

Cumming, R. D. 2001. *Phenomenology and Deconstruction.* Chicago: University of Chicago Press.

Delaney, C. 1991. *The Seed and the Soil: Gender and Cosmology in Turkish Village Society.* Berkeley: University of California Press.

DeSalvo, L. 1997. *Breathless: An Asthma Journal.* Boston: Beacon Press.

Ebigbo, P. 1986. A Cross-Sectional Study of Somatic Complaints of Nigerian Females Using the Enugu Somatization Scale. *Culture, Medicine, and Psychiatry* 10:167–186.

Feld, S. 1982. *Sound and Sentiment: Birds, Weeping, Poetics, and Song in Kaluli Expression.* Philadelphia: University of Pennsylvania Press.

Foucault, M. 1977. *Language, Counter-Memory, Practice.* Ithaca, NY: Cornell University Press.

Freud, S. 2003. *The Uncanny.* New York: Penguin Books.

Gaines, A. D. 1992. Medical/Psychiatric Knowledge in France and the United States: Culture and Sickness in History and Biology. In *Ethnopsychiatry: The Cultural Construction of Professional and Folk Psychiatries.* A. D. Gaines, ed. Pp. 171–201. Albany: State University of New York.

Geurts, K. 2002. *Culture and the Senses: Bodily Ways of Knowing in an African Community.* Berkeley: University of California Press.

Good, B. J. 1977. The Heart of What's the Matter: The Semantics of Illness in Iran. *Culture, Medicine, and Psychiatry* 1:25–58.

————. 1994. *Medicine, Rationality, and Experience: An Anthropological Perspective.* Cambridge, UK: Cambridge University Press.

Good, B. J., and M. J. Good. 1992. The Comparative Study of Greco-Islamic Medicine: The Integration of Medical Knowledge into Local Symbolic Contexts. In *Paths to Asian Medical Systems.* C. Leslie and A. Young, eds. Pp. 257–272. Berkeley: University of California Press.

Good, M. J. 1980. Of Blood and Babies: The Relationship of Popular Islamic Physiology to Fertility. *Social Science and Medicine* 14b:147–156.

Guarnaccia, P., M. Rivera, F. Franco, and C. Neighbors. 1996. The Experiences of Ataque de Nervios: Towards an Anthropology of Emotions in Puerto Rico. *Culture, Medicine, and Psychiatry* 20:343–346.

Hacking, I. 2002. *Historical Ontology.* Cambridge, MA: Harvard University Press.

Heder, S., and J. Ledgerwood, eds. 1996. *Propaganda, Politics, and Violence in Cambodia.* New York: Sharpe.

Hiller, W., A. Janca, and K. Burke. 1997. Association Between Tinnitus and Somatoform Disorders. *Journal of Psychosomatic Research* 43:613–624.

Hinton, D. E. 1999. Musical Healing and Cultural Syndromes in Isan: Landscape, Conceptual Metaphor, and Embodiment. Ph.D. dissertation, Department of Anthropology, Harvard University.

Hinton, D. E., P. Ba, S. Peou, and K. Um. 2000. Panic Disorder Among Cambodian Refugees Attending a Psychiatric Clinic: Prevalence and Subtypes. *General Hospital Psychiatry* 22:437–444.

Hinton, D. E., P. Ba, and K. Um. 2001a. *Kyol Goeu* ("Wind Overload") Part I: *Kyol Goeu* and Orthostatic Panic Among Khmer Refugees. *Transcultural Psychiatry* 38:403–432.

————. 2001b. *Kyol Goeu* ("Wind Overload") Part II: Prevalence, Characteristics, and Mechanisms of *Kyol Goeu* ("Wind Overload") and Near-*Kyol Goeu* Episodes of Khmer Patients Attending a Psychiatric Clinic. *Transcultural Psychiatry* 38:433–460.

————. 2001c. A Unique Panic-Disorder Presentation Among Khmer Refugees: The Sore Neck Syndrome. *Culture, Medicine, and Psychiatry* 25:297–316.

Hinton, D. E., M. Nathan, B. Bird, and L. Park. 2002a. Panic Probes and the Identification of Panic: A Historical and Cross-Cultural Perspective. *Culture, Medicine, and Psychiatry* 26:137–153.

Hinton, D. E., S. D. Hinton, K. Um, A. Chea, and S. Sak. 2002b. The Khmer "Weak Heart" Syndrome: Fear of Death from Palpitations. *Transcultural Psychiatry* 39:323–344.

Hinton D. E., T. Pham, H. Chau, M. Tran, and S. D. Hinton. 2003. "Hit by the Wind" and Temperature-Shift Panic Among Vietnamese Refugees. *Transcultural Psychiatry* 40:342–376.

Hinton, D. E., V. So, M. H. Pollack, R. K. Pitman, and S. P. Orr. 2004a. The Psychophysiology of Orthostatic Panic in Cambodian Refugees Attending a Psychiatric Clinic. *Journal of Psychopathology and Behavioral Assessment* 26:1–13.

Hinton, D. E., V. Pich, D. Chhean, and M. H. Pollack. 2004b. Olfactory Panic Among Cambodian Refugees: A Contextual Approach. *Transcultural Psychiatry* 41:155–199.

Hinton, D. E., D. Chhean, V. Pich, K. Um, J. Fama, and M. H. Pollack. 2006a. Neck-Focused Panic Attacks Among Cambodian Refugees: A Logistic and Linear Regression Analysis. *Journal of Anxiety Disorders* 20:119–138.

Hinton, D. E., V. Pich, S. Safren, M. H. Pollack, and R. J. McNally. 2006b. Anxiety Sensitivity Among Cambodian Refugees with Panic Disorder: A Factor Analytic Investigation. *Journal of Anxiety Disorders* 20:281–295.

Hinton, D. E., L. Nguyen, and M. H. Pollack. 2007. Orthostatic Panic as a Key Vietnamese Reaction to Traumatic Events: The Case of September 11th. *Medical Anthropology Quarterly* 21:81–107.

Hinton, D. E., R. Chong, M. H. Pollack, D. H. Barlow, and R. J. McNally. In press a. Ataque de Nervios: Relationship to Anxiety Sensitivity and Dissociation Predisposition. *Depression and Anxiety*.

Hinton, D. E., S. D. Hinton, R. Loeum, and M. H. Pollack. In press b. The "Multiplex Model" of How Somatic Symptoms Are Generated and How They Generate Distress: Application to Tinnitus Among Traumatized Cambodian Refugees. *Transcultural Psychiatry*.

Hinton, D. E., D. Howes, and L. J. Kirmayer. In press c. Towards a Medical Anthropology of Sensations: Definitions and Research Agendas. *Transcultural Psychiatry*.

Hsu, E. 1999. *The Transmission of Chinese Medicine*. Cambridge, UK: Cambridge University Press.

Hudson, J., and H. Pope. 1994. The Concept of Affective Spectrum: Relationship to Fibromyalgia and Other Syndromes of Chronic Fatigue and Chronic Muscle Pain. *Balliere's Clinical Rheumatology* 8:839–856.

Inda, J. X., and R. Rosaldo, eds. 2002. *The Anthropology of Globalization: A Reader*. Cambridge, UK: Blackwell.

Kagan, J. 2008. *What Is Emotion? History, Measures, and Meanings*. New Haven, CT: Yale University Press.

Kirmayer, L. J. 1984. Culture, Affect, and Somatization. *Transcultural Pyschiatric Research Review* 21:159–188.

———. 2002. The Refugee's Predicament. *Evolution Psychiatrique* 67:724–742.

Kleinman, A. 1986. *Social Origins of Distress and Disease: Depression, Neurasthenia, and Pain in Modern China*. New Haven, CT: Yale University Press.

———. 1988. *Rethinking Psychiatry: From Cultural Category to Personal Experience*. New York: Free Press.

Kleinman A., and J. Kleinman. 1994. How Bodies Remember: Social Memory and Bodily Experience of Criticism, Resistance, and Delegitimation Following China's Cultural Revolution. *New Literary History* 25:707–723.

Krishaber, M. 1873. *De la névropathie cérébro-cardiaque*. Paris: Librairie de l'Académie de Médecine de Paris.

Kugelmann, R. 1992. *Stress: The Nature and History of Engineered Grief*. Westport: Praeger.

Kuriyama, S. 1999. *The Expressiveness of the Body and the Divergence of Greek and Chinese Medicine*. New York: Zone Books.

Lacey, J., D. Batemen, and R. Vanlehn. 1953. Autonomic Response Specificity. *Psychosomatic Medicine* 1:8–21.

Laderman, C. 1992. A Welcoming Soil: Islamic Humoralism on the Malay Peninsula. In *Paths to Asian Medical Systems*. C. Leslie and A. Young, eds. Pp. 272–289. Berkeley: University of California Press.

Lakoff, G., and Z. Kovecses. 1987. The Cognitive Model of Anger Inherent in American English. In *Cultural Models in Language and Thought*. D. Holland and N. Quinn, eds. Pp. 195–222. Cambridge, UK: Cambridge University Press.

Lee, S. 1994. Neurasthenia and Chinese Psychiatry in the 1990s. *Journal of Psychosomatic Research* 38:487–491.

———. 1995. Rethinking Neurasthenia: The Illness Concepts of Shenjing Shuairuo Among Chinese Undergraduates in Hong Kong. *Culture, Medicine, and Psychiatry* 19:91–111.

———. 1999. Diagnosis Postponed: Shenjing Shuairuo and the Transformation of Psychiatry in Post-Mao China. *Culture, Medicine, and Psychiatry* 23:349–380.

Liebowitz, M., A. Fyer, and J. Gorman. 1984. Lactate Provocation of Panic Attacks. *Archives of General Psychiatry* 41:764–770.

Lin, K. M. 1983. Hwa-Byung: A Korean Culture-Bound Syndrome. *American Journal of Psychiatry* 140:105–107.

Lo, V. 2001. The Influence of Nurturing Life Culture on the Development of Western Han Acumoxa Therapy. In *Innovation in Chinese Medicine*. E. Lu, ed. Pp. 19–51. Cambridge, UK: Cambridge University Press.

Lock, M. 1993. *Encounters with Aging: Mythologies of Menopause in Japan and North America*. Berkeley: University of California Press.

Lu, A., B. Metzger, and B. Therrien. 1990. Ethnic Differences in Physiological Responses Associated with the Valsalva Maneuver. *Research, Nursing, and Health* 13:9–15.

McNally, R. J. 1994. *Panic Disorder: A Critical Analysis*. New York: Guilford Press.

Muller, J., and J. Brent, eds. 2000. *Peirce, Semiotics, and Psychoanalysis*. Baltimore: Johns Hopkins University Press.

Myerhoff, B. G. 1974. *Peyote Hunt: The Sacred Journey of the Huichol Indians*. Ithaca, NY: Cornell University Press.

Nattiez, J. 1987. *Musicologie générale et semiologie*. Montréal: Christian Bourgois.

———. 1988. *De la semiologie à la musique*. Montréal: Université du Québec à Montréal.

Nichter, M. 1996. *Anthropology and International Health: Asian Case Examples*. Sidney, Australia: Gordon and Breach.

Nietzsche, F. 1967. *On the Genealogy of Morals and Ecce Homo*. New York: Vintage Books.

Noyes, R., and R. Hoehn-Saric. 1998. *The Anxiety Disorders*. Cambridge, UK: Cambridge University Press.

Ohman, A. 2000. Fear and Anxiety: Evolutionary, Cognitive, and Clinical Perspectives. In *Handbook of Emotions*. M. Lewis and J. Haviland-Jones, eds. Pp. 573–594. New York: Guilford Press.

Pandolfi, M. 1990. Boundaries Inside the Body: Women's Suffering in Southern Peasant Italy. *Culture, Medicine, and Psychiatry* 14:255–273.

Pang, K. 1990. Hwa Byung: The Construction of a Korean Popular Illness Among Korean Elderly Immigrant Women in the United States. *Culture, Medicine, and Psychiatry* 14:495–512.

Porth, C. 1990. Re: Ethnic Differences in Physiological Responses Associated with Valsalva Maneuver. *Research, Nursing, and Health* 13:445–447.

Reich, J., R. Noyes, and W. Yates. 1988. Anxiety Symptoms Distinguishing Social Phobia from Panic and Generalized Anxiety. *Journal of Nervous and Anxiety Disorders* 176:510–513.

Scheper-Hughes, N., and M. Lock. 1987. The Mindful Body: A Prolegomenon to Future Work in Medical Anthropology. *Medical Anthropology Quarterly* 1:6–41.

Scott, J. C. 1985. *Weapons of the Weak: Everyday Forms of Resistance*. New Haven, CT: Yale University Press.

Shweder, R. 1985. Menstrual Pollution, Soul Loss, and the Comparative Study of Emotion. In *Culture and Depression: Studies in the Anthropology and Cross-Cultural Psychiatry of Affect and Disorder*. A. Kleinman and B. J. Good, eds. Pp. 182–216. Berkeley: University of California Press.

————. 2004. Deconstructing the Emotions for the Sake of Comparative Research. In *Feelings and Emotions: The Amsterdam Symposium*. A. Manstead, N. Frijda, and A. Fischer, eds. Pp. 81–98. Cambridge, UK: Cambridge University Press.

Stern, R., S. Hu, M. Uijtdehaage, L. Xu, and K. Koch. 1996. Asian Hypersusceptibility to Motion Sickness. *Human Heredity* 46:7–13.

Strathern, A. 1996. *Body Thoughts*. Ann Arbor: University of Michigan Press.

Taylor, S. 2000. *Understanding and Treating Panic Disorder: Cognitive-Behavioral Approaches*. West Sussex, UK: Wiley.

Veith, I. 1993. *Hysteria: The History of a Disease*. London: Jason Aronson.

Wierzbicka, A. 1999. *Emotions Across Languages and Cultures: Diversity and Universals*. Cambridge, UK: Cambridge University Press.

Young, A. 1980. The Discourse on Stress and the Reproduction of Conventional Knowledge. *Social Science and Medicine* 14:133–146.

Part II

Historical Perspectives on Western Panic

4

The Irritable Heart Syndrome in the American Civil War

Robert Kugelmann

———————————————————————————————●

THE INVENTION OF THE STETHOSCOPE posed new possibilities for perceptions of the body, particularly of the heart, which became the contested site for two quite different concepts. On the one hand, the heart in the West has been seen as the center of emotion and character and, especially in wartime, as an echo of the *thumos* pounding away in the chest of the warriors at Troy. Thumos, neither a physical organ nor a mental entity, was the center of irascible passions, such as courage and anger, but like a horse, tamable. On the other hand, the heart has been conceived as a muscle that pumps blood, an engine subject to overwork and overstrain, to tearing, backflow, and rupture (see Romanyshyn 1982:100–141). *Irritable heart*, a medical condition that emerged as a diagnosis during the Civil War and that with every war thereafter has been revived, with new names, diagnoses, and treatments, has served as a mediating concept between these two contrasting conceptions of the heart.

Physicians during the American Civil War claimed to observe this disorder for the first time, and it is important first to determine the character of that novelty. To do so, I consider the medical and social contexts within which irritable heart received recognition and a name. I am not interested in finding out what irritable heart "really" is according to present cosmopolitan medical criteria. Rather, I locate it within its own world and within the practices and discourse of the mid-nineteenth century during, to boot, a war. Irritable heart belonged to a set of concepts and concerns about excess, fatigue, masculinity, disease, and courage. I analyze events and actions and sensations—the signs and symptoms described and interpreted by soldiers and their physicians of the time. I then consider the enduring relevance of this nineteenth-century condition, even as it indicates the distance between who those soldiers were and who we find ourselves to be. In this spirit, I ask about irritable heart not as a medical term but as an existential possibility.

Describing and Explaining Irritable Heart

When the physician Edward H. Clarke (1820–1877) listed the accomplishments of nineteenth-century American medicine, he paid particular attention to the stethoscope, writing that Laennec's invention had "revolutionized the study and indirectly the therapeutics of affections of the chest" (1971[1871]:33). He then turned to irritable heart. Three American physicians—Alfred Stillé (1813–1900), Henry Hartshorne (1823–1897), and Jacob Mendez Da Costa (1833–1900)—had described this "condition of the heart observed among soldiers as the result of prolonged and violent exertion" (Clarke 1971[1871]:34) during the Civil War. The discovery of the irritable heart with the aid of a stethoscope indicates the modernity of the condition. Other U.S. physicians, including Joshua B. Treadwell, (1840–1885) and British physicians, such as Benjamin Ward Richardson (1828–1896), Clifford Allbutt (1836–1925), and Samuel Wilks (1824–1911), found similar disorders among peacetime patients, as did Da Costa. In these accounts, the fatiguing conditions of an industrializing society were prominent. Irritable heart, a functional disorder, could degenerate into an organic disease of the heart. The rigors of modern warfare and industrial discipline affected not only the mind but also, and more ominously, the body, itself interpreted in terms of the machinery that defined this new age, through the sign of the tell-tale heart.

The discovery of irritable heart did not come out of the blue. The medical community already viewed the body in specific ways in the 1860s. Duden (1993:69) draws attention to two related epistemological contexts that will guide my interpretation: "On the one hand, the training of the eye and imagination by the scientific thought collective and, on the other, the contextualization of the specialist's viewpoint within the everyday perspective of his time." Several aspects of the medical thought collective are especially relevant: the development of equipment, especially the stethoscope and the education of the physician's ear to hear the heart's sounds through it (Da Costa played a leading role in forwarding this skill in his book *Medical Diagnosis*, 1901 [1864]), and the practice of pathology. These developments entailed interrogation by means of an eye informed by the anatomist in order to discover the disease. What I argue is that irritable heart as a diagnosis would have been impossible without the stethoscope and the autopsy. Reiser (1978:38) concludes that the stethoscope transformed medical practice: "Auscultation helped to create the objective physician, who could move away from involvement with the patient's experiences and sensations, to a more detached relation." From now on, symptoms were to be interpreted as anatomical and physiological dysfunctions. The cadaver provided the object for medical interpretation.

The relevant "everyday perspective of his time" here was ethical: What were the consequences of intemperate activity? Immoral behavior was excessive behavior, a teaching that extended back to the ancient world. This ethical conception found expression, for example, a generation before the American Civil War, in an essay by Peter Mere Latham (1789–1875), a leading English physician. He asked whether it was possible that the passions of the mind or "disorders called nervous [could] lay the foundation of organic diseases of the heart" (1829:529). It was an understanding of long standing that the passions are felt as changes in the heart and in the blood around the heart. To this concept Latham brought the new medical gaze. Whereas popular belief held that violent passions could cause heart disease, and although for years Latham had held that very view, he had come to doubt it: only "from causes long and uninterruptedly applied" (1829:530) can the heart become dilated. That conclusion, to his mind, excluded emotional upsets and nervous disorders from the causes of pathological changes in the heart. Instead, he attributed such changes to certain constitutional temperaments or to "the constant and excessive stimulus of excessive liquors" (1829:532). Latham asked, "Is it not possible that the common language of mankind, making the *heart metaphorically expressive of all moral emotions*, may upon this point have done some secret prejudice to the observation and better judgment of physicians?" (1829:529, italics in original). The new medical thought collective produced a "new heart" that made the "old heart" merely metaphorical. Narratives of paroxysm of rage causing palpitations and death gave way as physicians listened no longer to patients' words but rather to the heart sounds coming through the hollow tube. A dissociation of the medical heart and the everyday heart of popular belief appeared not as a new certitude but as a vexing problem.

First Appearance of Irritable Heart
After Combat and Defeat in Virginia

In April 1862, the Army of the Potomac, under General George B. McClellan, invaded Virginia, marching from the sea toward Richmond. In a series of battles, Robert E. Lee's Confederate troops repulsed the Federals, who slowly withdrew in retreat. The shock of the loss shook Northern confidence. Casualties were high, the wounded were sometimes abandoned in the haste of retreat, and sickness took its toll.

> The health of McClellan's army, already affected by the heavy rains and humid heat among the Chickahominy swamps in May and June, deteriorated further after the army's arrival at Harrison's Landing in July. Nearly a fourth of the unwounded men

were sick. Scores of new cases of malaria, dysentery, and typhoid were reported every day. . . . With the sickliest season of the year (August-September) coming on, the administration decided over McClellan's protest to withdraw his army from the Peninsula. [McPherson 1988:488]

Conditions did not improve, and the subsequent battles of Antietam and Fredericksburg produced heavy casualties. Some of the sick became patients of Stillé, Hartshorne, and Da Costa.

An exhortation to undertake scientific study in medicine preceded Alfred Stillé's first description of irritable heart. Philadelphia could lose its preeminence in American medicine, Stillé had asserted, because of indifference to experimental and clinical research in an epoch "during which physics have been applied to medicine, and auscultation, percussion, and their kindred methods of investigation, microscopical, chemical and physiological, have laid the phenomena of life and of disease open to the senses" (1863:11). Stillé described chronic conditions he had seen in soldiers, including "palpitation of the heart." The soldiers themselves attributed the palpitations to their knapsacks—"either directly by its contusive blows upon the back in marching, or indirectly by its producing a free perspiration of the part, which afterwards became chilled on the removal of the knapsack when the wind was blowing, or else by getting the back wet with rain or in wading streams" (Stillé 1863:18)—or to "prolonged or very rapid marching" (Stillé 1863:18–19). Stillé surmised that the real cause was "a state of extreme exhaustion, especially when produced by prolonged and violent muscular efforts" (1863:19). The condition was not associated with murmurs or hypertrophy. Stillé thought it was "an effect of muscular debility of the heart alone, or of that organ along with the rest of the muscular system" (1863:19), especially because it responded to rest and good food. He concluded that in general the health of the army was very good, and "that it has failed to accomplish all that was justly expected of it is plainly owing not to the muscle and bone which compose, but to the brains which direct it" (1863:18–20).

Stillé would no doubt have insisted that "muscular debility" was meant literally, but the figure of speech suggests that the meaning of *muscular* went beyond the literal. If these men were the "muscle and bone," what were the "burdens" of which they complained? To what extent were their complaints protests against their conditions, expressed in the only acceptable language available? To what extent were they correct in their complaints that they labored under unreasonable burdens? A similar indirection occurred when Stillé spoke of "extreme exhaustion" and "prolonged and violent muscular efforts." He was referring to attacks and retreats, the excitement and terror of battle. The statement refers to war by both understatement and metonymy: exhaustion and effort are but a part of the totality of battle, and they are terms that minimize affective aspects of that totality. Such indirect speech used the new medical discourse to speak of the stresses of war.

Hartshorne (1864) described "cardiac muscular exhaustion" in June 1863 in terms similar to Stillé's. Cardiac muscular exhaustion was not associated with in-flammations of the heart, with pericarditis, with dilatation or hypertrophy of the heart, or with valvular disease. He also differentiated "soldiers' heart exhaustion" from palpitations "or functional disturbance of the heart's action from sympathy with irritated stomach, from nervousness, abuse of tobacco" (1864:89). Its symp-toms included a rapid but feeble pulse when the patient was resting, an abnormally increased heart rate with even the "*slightest* exertion," (1864:90) and dyspnea. The men looked healthy, although often of late their nutrition had not been good. The pulse, the percussion of the chest, and the use of the stethoscope ascertained that these men did not suffer from detectable organic changes of the heart. Hartshorne did not think these were cases of "ordinary sympathetic or nervous palpitation" (1864:91), because the heart action was "less heaving in impulse, more constant in character, and much more susceptible of increase by the slightest exertion" (1864:91). The causes of cardiac muscular exhaustion were "long-continued over-exertion, . . . deficiency of rest, and often, of nourishment" (1864:91).

Most of the soldiers Hartshorne saw had been in the Peninsula Campaign, during which "the soldiers suffered from great and prolonged over-exertion with the most unfavorable conditions possible—privation of rest, deficient food, bad water, and malaria. The heart, being called upon to supply the demands of the overtasked body, must, in such a case, become weakened" (1864:91). Hartshorne did not mention combat itself or the retreats, or the moments of panic and ter-ror for the troops, such as those that Dean (1997) documents. That Hartshorne did not mention the terrors of war and that psychologically minded readers more than a century later expect to find them discussed indicates the different interpre-tive networks in which Hartshorne wrote. For him, "the 'trotting heart' of our soldiers" differed from "sympathetic or nervous palpitation" (1864:91). Even here, Hartshorne's emphasis was on the immoderate use of tobacco, alcohol, coffee, and masturbation; he mentioned "nervousness" only once. As did Stillé, Hartshorne presented selected aspects of the military experiences of these soldiers, although other aspects were certainly presented in the press at the time and in the letters and journals of the combatants. A lack of physical and ethical moderation played the key role in Hartshorne's account.

This new medical phenomenon first appeared, then, as a culturally specific embodiment of the wearying Peninsula Campaign, which brought home the grim realities of the Civil War to both soldier and civilian alike.

Da Costa and Irritable Heart

Da Costa first referred to "irritable heart" in *Medical Diagnosis* (1901 [1864]) and then in a report (Da Costa 1867) published for the U.S. Sanitary Commission. His full presentation appeared later (Da Costa 1871), followed by an extension of his findings to the civilian population, claiming that such diseases "are very common, and, I think, becoming more so" (Da Costa 1874). Da Costa was a renowned diagnostician whose *Medical Diagnosis* received favorable notice as an important contribution to this developing area (see, for example, H. H. 1864). Da Costa's system of diagnosis was based, as far as possible, on pathology, that is, on the localization of disease within the anatomically defined body. Da Costa was developing the "medical gaze" (Foucault 1973), a "symbolic form" (Ernst Cassirer's term, as used by Good 1994) of perceiving the body. Unlike earlier symbolic forms, in this one the literal level of discourse referred exclusively to material, as opposed to mental and emotional, categories. The boundaries between mind and body were, however, not strictly defined (Rosenberg 1992) and the two tended to fuse, especially in indirect speech.

A case history cited in Da Costa (1871:20) clearly illustrates his conception of irritable heart:

> William C., private, 140th N.Y. Vol., twenty-one years of age, single, and a farmer before he volunteered. He enlisted August 27th, 1862, had diarrhea for about three months. . . . [W]hile on a march from Harper's Ferry to Fredericksburg, [William] had his attention drawn to his heart by attacks of palpitation, pain in the cardiac region, and difficulty breathing at night. He remained, however, on duty, though not of very hard kind, until December 24th, 1862, when in consequence of a severe cold which resulted in loss of voice, he was ordered from the front.

Harper's Ferry and the surrounding hills had been in Union hands in the fall of 1862, when they were successfully besieged by the Confederates, led by General Thomas J. "Stonewall" Jackson. Moreover, marching to Fredericksburg meant retreating north to engage in the disastrous battle there on December 13, 1862. McPherson (1988:573–574) describes that battle as "one of [the Union army's] worst defeats of the war. . . . Fredericksburg brought home the horrors of war to northerners more vividly, perhaps, than had any previous battle."

Hard marching with heavy packs over rough terrain was the norm in the Civil War. Dean (1997:48) observes that "following the war, Union veterans frequently claimed 'sunstroke' and 'hard marching' as the basis for military disability pensions—and these claims were often granted." In this retreat north, William C. was marching after a three-month bout of diarrhea, a common ailment of soldiers of the time (Dean 1997:51).

William C. was transferred from one hospital to another until June 1863, when he arrived at Turner's Lane Hospital, where Da Costa saw him.

> Appearance that of fair health; gums rather spongy, says that they bled easily while in the field, and he thinks he had a slight attack of scurvy; . . . respiration 24 in the minute; pulse 122; impulse of the heart extended and very jerky . . . . He is still aphonic, probably from catarrhal laryngitis; was etherized before I saw him, but without effect on voice. He has had lately two nocturnal discharges a week, which has been the case with him for years, excepting when in the field and suffering from diarrhea, when he was free from them. Has occasionally spells of dizziness. [Da Costa 1871:20]

A variety of drugs were used, with little result. "November 16 he returned from a furlough, apparently in excellent health, but with an impulse of 98, and still suffering from palpitations, especially at night." In May 1864, when he was to join the veteran reserve corps, "he still had some cardiac pain and occasional palpitations. These, however, scarcely occurred excepting on strong exertion" (Da Costa 1871:20). Da Costa's prescription of digitalis aimed at improving the action of the heart.

In naming this condition "irritable" heart, Da Costa used a term that had been used in medicine for about a century and indicated the alleged cause of the disease. Disturbed innervation of the heart arises, said Da Costa, from a number of causes, especially exertion in an exhausted man. Many cases of irritable heart were preceded by fever or diarrhea, double-time marches, and poor nutrition. These conditions were seen as pressing the heart into overaction by disordering its innervations:

> It appears most probable that the special nerve centers near the base of the heart which preside over the normal rhythmical movements of the organ are stimulated, and in considering the close connection of these ganglia with the sympathetic, we have the explanation of how their function may have been stimulated, or kept so, by irritation reflected to them from the abdominal ganglia or elsewhere. [Da Costa 1871:40]

Thus the irritation might have begun elsewhere, but it was reflected to the heart via the nervous system. In Da Costa's words, irritable heart resulted from a "hyper-aesthesia of the sensory nerve-fibres," especially from a "disturbance of the sympathetic elements of the cardiac plexus" (1874:11–12).

In short, irritable heart was a *cardiac neurosis*, caused by a functional disturbance of the nervous system. In support of this interpretation, Da Costa referred to the work of Charles Handfield Jones (1819–1890), a British physician who contributed to histology and to the theory of functional diseases of the nervous system. Jones presented the neurological theory behind the diagnoses of functional nervous diseases, in particular the reflex spread of irritation to the heart. He wrote that "nervous tissue . . . becomes more excitable and mobile in proportion as its power becomes weaker" (Jones 1868:44). Jones discussed cardiac neurosis, of which angina pectoris was the chief example but which also included a condition he called *cardiac hyperaesthesia*, which strongly resembles Da Costa's irritable heart. (See also Jones 1870 for a brief discussion of irritable heart.)

Thus, for Da Costa "the mass of cardiac disorder is not organic, but functional. And of these again a very large proportion belong to the group which I have designated 'irritable heart'" (1867:381). But why had this condition not been described earlier? Da Costa wondered. He concluded that "accurate knowledge of diseases of the heart is the knowledge of our times" (1871:18). In other words, changes in medical perception, in particular the invention of the stethoscope and the application of physics to the tissues of the body, constituted epistemological conditions for the possibility of perceiving irritable heart.

As a functional disorder, which Da Costa described as "attacks" and "seizures," the symptoms *were* the disease. Most prominently, these symptoms included palpitations (likened by one soldier "the fluttering of a chicken, when taken by the legs"), cardiac pain of varying degrees, a rapid heart rate ("varying from 100 to 140"), shortness of breath, and "oppression on exertion" (Da Costa 1871:22–23, 25). There were also "nervous" symptoms, including "headache, giddiness," "jerking during sleep and disturbed rest," and unpleasant dreams (Da Costa 1871:22–25). "One soldier spoke often of dreaming that he was falling off high buildings" (Da Costa 1871:25). For all this, Da Costa never stated that irritable heart was a moral or mental disease. His main concern was how this disorder arose from exhaustion and overwork and how it could lead to organic changes in the heart if unattended. Why did he not elaborate on potential psychological causes of irritable heart? Why did he not say explicitly what he said implicitly, that these soldiers, exhausted and sick, had been terrified as well, and that perhaps their concentration on their physical symptoms deflected attention from their fears?

In his 1871 article that addresses irritable heart in soldiers, Da Costa did not emphasize emotional causes. He did not question the motivation of soldiers complaining of irritable heart, but claimed that the symptoms were not easily feigned (Da Costa 1871:37). In fact, he made note of one soldier:

A man who had been in sixteen fights, and for two years had not been off duty a day, though gradually more and more troubled with palpitation, and much distressed while carrying his knapsack on long marches—how such a man, who was often obliged to halt and sit down until the spell had passed off, but who loved the excitement of campaigning so much that he would not leave his regiment—we can well understand how it was that, giving his heart no chance for recovery, he should have presented all the signs of the most marked hypertrophy. [Da Costa 1871:32]

As this case illustrates, exertion beyond the limits of what is physically possible out of zeal and ambition and courage constituted the ground of his irritable heart, rather than fear or cowardice causing the disease.

Constant and heavy duty on the picket line [troops sent out as sentinels] or during active movements in the face of the enemy would develop the cardiac symptoms; or slight[ly] before, these increased and became marked after forced marches . . . ; or during arduous and exciting fighting and marching (Case 119, who noticed it first after fighting and marching for three days, sleeping on his arms, and being greatly depressed in spirits during Gen. McClellan's retreat in front of Richmond). [Da Costa 1871:38]

This functional disease of overexertion was audible and palpable: "When the hand is applied to the praecordial region, it may note the quick impulse happening in a regular manner, or it takes cognizance of the irregularity of the rhythm of the irritable organ. Further, it may at times perceive the two sounds of the heart; feel them as it were" (Da Costa 1871:26). To interpret these heart sounds and feelings properly, one needed to know who the man was and where he had been. The interpretive framework for the diagnosis included anatomy and the stories of hard marches, draining diseases, and prolonged and disheartening battles. The sound and feel of such a heart were indices of a nervous dysfunction and an icon of fatigue.

Da Costa later drew on civilian cases to broaden the picture and simplify his account of the cause of irritable heart, which was to "strain," meaning any state of "over-action, over-exertion, or over-work," whether a sudden or shocking demand put on the heart, or any persistent and excessive condition that exhausts the person and the heart. No other preexisting condition was needed. Moreover, strain included "extraordinary mental emotion or shock":

Some years since a blooming girl of eighteen was brought to my office by her mother, to consult me with reference to palpitations and shortness of breath on exertion, which had developed themselves suddenly. I found a well-marked aortic lesion. She never had had rheumatism, had been, indeed, in perfect health until a certain day, and had been remarkable for the ease and endurance with which she rode and walked long distances. But one night—it was in the midst of the troublesome times in the border States during the civil war—while she and her mother were alone in the house, which stood some distance from any neighbor's, and the father was known to be far away with the army, two men entered the dwelling, and, notwithstanding the entreaty of the mother, slowly ascended the wide staircase. The girl was beside herself with agitation and alarm—the mother, resolute, told them not to advance or she would fire. The warning was unheeded; the flash of the pistol followed. The fire desperately wounded one of the invaders; the other fled. But from that fatal night the girl was a wreck; the palpitations never left; and after a few years, I am sorry to record, the cardiac trouble led to death. [Da Costa 1874:4–5]

Generalizing from his cases, Da Costa thus implicated an emotional etiology for irritable heart.

We can understand how even mental emotion, acting through the nervous system on the nerves of the heart, may produce real trouble, and how the worry of life, and strain on the feelings, when long kept up, may give rise to conditions which, in figurative language, we call "heart-weary," and "heart-sick," and which, not as a figure of speech, but in truth, may be the beginning of actual cardiac malady. [Da Costa 1874:12]

In addition, the causes of irritable heart included anything that produces over-exertion of the heart, including "irregularity or excess in eating or in drinking, sexual disorders, long matrimonial engagements, the abuse of tea, of coffee, of tobacco" (Da Costa 1874:9).

Thus any source of nervous irritability, which is involuntary because it is a reflex, produced irritable heart. It was not a matter of the will or of the intellect, hence it was not a mental disease. A muscle that pumps, with valves that keep blood circulating, was the medical conception of the heart. Like any piece of nineteenth-century machinery, it could take only so much strain. Yet despite Da Costa's scientific stance, he preserved in his figurative use of such ideas as heart-weary and heart-sick a substantial link to earlier conceptions and still-popular beliefs.

Given this view of the problem, Da Costa recommended rest and medication, chiefly digitalis, as treatment. Rest was paramount, and Da Costa concluded his discussion of irritable heart with a warning:

The public . . . err[s] through ignorance, and it is our place to show them that the heart will not, any more than the brain, endure incessant and exhausting labor and excitement; that there are heart-weary as well as brain-weary persons; to point out how some occupations predispose to the disorder more than others, and how, there-fore, the dictates, of science, humanity, and true economy, alike demand that they be less continuously pursued; . . . and how it may be the heart that bears the brunt of the irregularity and abuse, and not the organs which would appear the ones most likely to suffer. [Da Costa 1874:28]

What civilian life had in common with the war, then, was excessive activity. There was something about the way life was conducted that was dangerous for the heart. In Da Costa's view, irritable heart is part of a causal chain that can lead from the excesses of military campaigns or from overwork in industry and commerce to organic diseases of the heart, particularly valvular disease.

Interpreting Irritable Heart

Irritable heart as a condition depended on a number of epoch-specific factors. The most salient factors had to do with exertion, with fatigue and rest, and with the medical and other cultural meanings of the heart. One of the questions that must be addressed is why Civil War accounts did not give primacy of place to what seemed increasingly obvious to later physicians looking at similar complaints, namely, that the symptoms arise in situations when effort and fatigue "induce fear" (Wood 1941). The answer to this question will shed light on the perception of the body and of males in the 1860s.

Exertion, Fatigue, and Rest

Irritable heart was a condition caused by overexertion. Fatigue, both as a consequence of the demands placed on workers to conform to the machine and the clock, and as "a metaphor for the modern form of psychological suffering, for inertia, loss of will, and depletion" (Rabinbach 1990:20), appeared in the accounts of irritable heart. Fatigue, as Rabinbach shows, limited the participation of human beings in mechanized and industrialized society. The soldier with irritable heart was a man with insufficient stamina, often in his own eyes. Fatigue was no longer a natural limit but a defect of hearts understood in engineering terms.

An irritable heart, when listened to by the new techniques, was clearly an overworked organ. Worry about the ill effects of overwork was common in the medical literature at the time. Excessive exertion in pursuit of athletic and business ends produced strain, especially on the heart and the brain. Medical anxiety over the effects of economic and social upheaval was common: "In the present day of excitement and over-exertion of both body and mind, a word in season cannot be out of place. There is a fierce struggle going on. Competition is everywhere. We work as though the capacity of the human system were inexhaustible" (The Danger of Excess in Physical Exertion 1861:165). The terms *overwork*, *wear and tear*, and *life at high pressure* were all used to point to the upheaval of industrialization and urbanization in the nineteenth century. Engineering and economic metaphors in medicine depicted the counterproductive effects of the disembedding of the economy (Polanyi 1957). For Da Costa (1874:28), "it may be the heart that bears the brunt of the irregularity and abuse" of the accelerating pace of life—*accelerating* being a figure of speech for the social and economic upheavals of the late nineteenth century. For Da Costa and others following the Civil War, the observation of William James in his essay "The Moral Equivalent of War" may be apropos. James (1987[1910]:1290) wrote that the "martial virtues . . . [of] patriotic pride and ambition in their military form are, after all, only specifications of a more general competitive passion." Although civilian life may not have held the same terrors that war did, there was nevertheless something warlike in the way life was being led, and in the minds of Da Costa and other physicians of the time, it produced the same kinds of functional disorders as war did. It was "this strange disease of modern life," in the words of Matthew Arnold (1907:279), that made life in industrializing countries so warlike in the eyes of medical men (see also Herschbach 1997).

The mechanics of exertion and fatigue as they affect the anatomically imaged body influenced Da Costa and other physicians. Soldiers often attributed their condition to heavy packs, long marches, debilitation from diarrhea and chills, inadequate rations, lack of sleep, and the hardships of combat. Union physicians noted, as did their British colleagues, that the main complaint was the heavy knapsack. In particular, British military medical man Arthur B. R. Myers (1870:87) concluded that constrictive clothing and equipment obstructed circulation and led to heart disease.

The physicians tended to think, however, that Myers's interpretation misplaced the true culprit, which was strain on the material of the tissues and their nervous supply. Da Costa believed that soldiers' complaints about their equipment had to be taken with a grain of salt. The knapsack was for the soldier "a kind of *bête noir*, which he likes to hold responsible for his mishaps." Da Costa compared, unfavorably, the modern soldier with his Roman counterpart: "It is no longer, as with the Romans, a boast of the overwhelming loads they carry" (1871:38). A similar observation was made by Clifford Allbutt (1836–1925), a British physician who contributed much to the development of medicine as a scientific discipline. In his article entitled "Overstrain of the Heart and Aorta," Allbutt (1873) described irritability of the heart among laborers, noting that overstrain was more common when work was done continually, "in spite of fatigue, of diminished health, and imperfect feeding." He added that "work done *con amore* is less exhausting than the drearier kinds of toil" (Allbutt 1873:291). Allbutt's suggestion is important because it indicates that overwork and exhaustion, as causative agents of irritable heart, were not understood in the nineteenth century as simply mechanical factors. Rather, the physicalistic language connoted something additional. For Da Costa, as for Allbutt, irritability of the heart may owe something to work done without *amore*, that is, passion, or with discouragement or in disillusionment, with "being greatly depressed in spirits" (1871:38) during retreats.

A soldier's report confirms this link between the physical heart and depleted spirit or vitality. Wilbur Fisk (1839–1914) wrote to a newspaper back home in Vermont of the chronic diarrhea he and others contracted "in the swamps of the Chickahominy [in 1862], and which saps the foundations of one's strength. . . . I had marched many a weary mile when I had not sufficient strength to step on" (Rosenblatt and Rosenblatt 1992:44). At the end of the summer in 1863, Fisk wrote:

> No particular malady affects the men, but a sort of general debility, a relaxation of the whole system that has long held out against severe and protracted hardships. The surgeon's call is lately well attended. The long train of sick, lame and halt that find their way to the surgeon's tent every morning, shows conclusively that something is needed to repair the physical vigor of a great many who have been heretofore proof against the severest privations and hardships. . . . It is no more than the truth to say that the bravest and best of us would be almost as willing to see the Constitution of the United States destroyed as to see his own. [Rosenblatt and Rosenblatt 1992:126–127]

"Vigor" and "constitutions" were depleted and tired. Even the "bravest and the best" had reached their limits. Fisk's report suggests that the sick role was one acceptable avenue for protest in the face of grueling conditions. The complaint about the backpacks, although genuine by all reports, was a shorthand way of complaining about the burdens of war, with the pack serving as an icon for them.

The link between physical and mental characteristics in mid-nineteenth-century thought is further demonstrated in the 1867 U.S. Sanitary Commission report on the health problems faced by the Federal army. Roberts Bartholow (1831–1904), a former American army surgeon, summarized the conditions that affected "physical endurance of men [and] . . . their power of resistance to disease" (1867:3). Bartholow was well qualified for this task, having served in the army since 1855 and as author of *A Manual of Instructions for Enlisting and Discharging Soldiers* (1991[1863]), "the standard authority for many years" (Packard 1964). Bartholow's conception of fitness and durability was a composite of mental, moral, and physical traits that were differentially distributed across the five "races" of U.S. troops ("American [referring to 'the composite race now inhabiting the continent, and not . . . the aborigines'], Celtic, Teutonic, Negro, and the mixed Spanish-American of New Mexico" [1867:4]), rank ordered in terms of their fitness and endurance.

> The mental characteristics that fit the American for the military service consist of a spirit of enterprise and an intellectual hardiness which render him superior to fatigue; an easy bearing under defeat, and a buoyant self-confidence which misfortunes do not easily depress. The national vanity and love of popularity may have much to do in the formation and development of these military qualities. . . .

> The physical qualities which fit the American for military service consist, not so much in muscular development and height as in the toughness of his muscular fibre and the freedom of his tissue from interstitial fat, whereby active and prolonged movements are much facilitated. In active service he fails more frequently from defects in his digestive apparatus and from a phthisical tendency, than from a lack of power due to imperfect physical development. [Bartholow 1867:4]

The Irish and the German, who stood below the American, suffered primarily from moral defects. The Negro ranked below the German, even though he had the "physical qualities pertaining to the highest type of soldier." Nevertheless, "the Negro soldier is, unquestionably, less enduring than the white soldier; less active, vigilant, and enterprising, and more given to malingering. The Mulatto is feebler than the Negro" (1867:5). Ranking last were the racially mixed Spanish-Americans of New Mexico, who in addition to having weak constitutions had "syphilitic cachexia, impaired vision, deformities of the hands and feet, and diseases of the urinary organs," and were "cowardly, unreliable, and difficult to control, in consequence of a very mercurial temperament" (1867:5).

Endurance and resistance were thus not simply either physical or psychological qualities; they were physical-psychological-moral characteristics. Bodily traits mirrored those of character in Bartholow's account. Moreover, the subject of the discourse was not, specifically speaking, the empirical individual; it was the individual as a type. Bartholow's analysis reflected a hierarchical social order.

A review of a book published for the U.S. Sanitary Commission seconded Bartholow's assessment (J.H.H. 1869). The reviewer used Bartholow's views to account for the fact that black American troops died at a much higher rate from disease than from combat, in comparison with white troops. Poor sanitation caused disease among whites, but poor racial characteristics did so among blacks. Edward S. Dunster (1834–1888), a U.S. army surgeon who had served in the Peninsula campaign, noted that a much smaller percentage of officers than of enlisted men died of disease, because the officers had better nutrition, housing, sanitation, and morale (Dunster 1867:183). However, in considering the relatively higher death rate due to disease among the black troops, Dunster wrote, "What the causes of this greater susceptibility of the negro to disease are . . . , to use the words of General Fry, 'that they were rather psychological than physical, and arose from lack of heart, hope, and mental activity, and that a higher moral and intellectual culture would diminish the defect'" (1867:184). The reviewer of the *Memoir* concurred (J.H.H. 1869:177). Moral and physical racial traits accounted for the differences (compare Russell 1867:332). This analysis illustrates that *effort* and *endurance* were terms highly charged with moral and racial connotations.

The relationships among race, character, and disease help account for three aspects of irritable heart. First, only excessive and violent conditions could produce such a disorder in these soldiers. Conditions would have to be such that the men could not have been suspected of faintness of heart or cowardice. Second, these conditions are a measure of the concern that irritable heart could lead to organic changes in the heart. Given the moral characteristics of a good soldier, as implicated in Bartholow's descriptions, a man would push his merely physical body beyond its limits in zeal and dedication. Third, the occurrence of so many cases of this new ailment indicates social and political anxiety generated by Northern defeats so close to the capital in late 1862. Physical, moral, and political conditions were extreme—that is one sense of the disorder.

Related to the importance of character and race was youth. Much of the anxiety expressed by medical men about the ill effects of strenuous exercise on the heart focused on young men. Da Costa (1871:40) concluded that young, inexperienced, and ill-trained soldiers made up the preponderance of cases of irritable heart. In this Handfield Jones (1870) concurred, drawing on his own experience in mountain climbing. In discussion after the publication of Allbutt's paper on overstrain of the heart, comments centered on young men permanently debilitated after excessive athletic competition (Clinical Society of London 1873). Irritable heart was, to a degree, a gender- and age-specific disorder—that of young men. Their failure of nerve threatened the future of the race, the nation, and the economy (see Kugelmann 1992).

In the mid-nineteenth century, the nervous power that innervates our organs was understood to be in limited supply. The fatigue that resulted from inadequate nerve force came to be seen in the late nineteenth century as pathogenic, with fatigue replacing idleness as a primary cause of disease. At the same time that the science and technology of energy promised unlimited production, diseases of exhaustion and overwork surfaced. Notable among them, in the post–Civil War period, was neurasthenia, a disease of nerve weakness caused by depletion of nerve force. A major contributor to the treatment of neurasthenia and of other diseases of overwork was Silas Weir Mitchell, who worked in Turner's Lane Hospital with Da Costa during the Civil War. The famous Mitchell cure of "Dr. Diet and Dr. Quiet" emphasized bed rest as a means to restore depleted vitality. So Da Costa's prescription of rest for those suffering from irritable heart fit well with prevailing conceptions of the body, the self, and their relationships to society.

Heart as Pump and Heart as Courage
Irritable heart was unquestionably a heart disorder. The question is, what was the heart in the mid-nineteenth century? It was a hybrid heart—that is, it was both the nineteenth-century physiological conception of the anatomical body, as well as the earlier, and still vernacular, conception of the heart as the organ of passion

and courage. The heart was a hybrid symbol signifying a mechanical part of the mind-body structure that constituted the person and, simultaneously, signifying the person, especially with respect to moral character. The heart was a hybrid because the older meanings of the heart were not simply repudiated. Instead, at times newer meanings were used to explain the older ones; but more important, features of the newer meanings were interpreted according to the older meanings. Thus, weak heart action explained lack of sympathy or lack of competitiveness.

Stearns (1994) discusses that the understanding of the heart changed from the older, humoral perception of the eighteenth century to the mechanistic physiology of the nineteenth century. "Prior to the nineteenth century, dominant beliefs, medical and popular alike, attached anger, joy, and sadness to bodily functions. Hearts, for example, could shake, tremble, expand, grow cold. . . . In the body-machine, emotions were harder to pin down" (Stearns 1994:66–67). In the body-machine of the mid-nineteenth century, the heart was a pump and the emphasis was on its structure and strength, especially of the valves. Da Costa (1901 [1864]:369) noted that the heart "exhibits, when in action, a wonderfully perfect mechanism and regularity of movement." It was a muscle that worked.

The heart often worked too hard. Herbert Spencer recounted that his own heart action, never strong, became enfeebled as a result of overwork, in particular from overexertion while on a hiking holiday in Switzerland in 1853. He wrote that "there was no mental cause" (Spencer 1904, vol. 1:501), but the heart has limited power, and in straining himself he had enfeebled his heart. The explanation for this fatigue was couched in part in terms of the nervous innervations of the heart, as we have seen. It also had a mechanical explanation in that the valves of the heart were what gave out under exertion, hence the concerns among physicians about the potential ill effects of athletic competition and strenuous physical labor.

The new heart of the nineteenth century was in part a product of changing medical technology. The older heart was not available to the physician insofar as he could only listen to it with the stethoscope and probe it with related techniques that silenced the patient (Reiser 1978) and mapped the sounds heard onto the image of an anatomical cadaver. The action of the heart thus heard tells only indirectly tales of fear and courage and love. Its primary grammar and syntax are the muscles and valves.

Something of the older perceptions of the heart as the seat of emotions and feelings lingered not only in the figures of speech that preserved them but also in irritable heart itself. In discussing palpitations, Da Costa acknowledged that "nervous excitement" could produce them: "Every one knows that there is a feeling of slight constriction about the chest, with a hurried breathing, and a strange sensation as if the heart were leaping from its place. . . . The popular notion, that the heart is the seat of the emotions, is based on these striking evidences of its disturbed action" (1901 [1864]:387). Then as now, however, the seat of the emotions was the nervous system, not the heart. This displacement allowed for the conceptualization of irritable heart as a functional heart disease, which physician and soldier alike could describe with only indirect reference to the passions or courage or morale.

The older perceptions occurred in figurative accounts of the heart. J. B. Treadwell, a physician involved with the medical examination of Civil War veterans applying for disability assistance, found considerable evidence of the ill effects of overwork and strain. His account also contains overtones of the older heart. For example, an irritable heart "seems to have been deprived of all governing power, and upon the slightest provocation becomes tumultuous and irregular in its action" (Treadwell 1872:180). This description suggests that the heart has lost self-control. Treadwell wrote that "a strong muscle is, as it were—if I may be allowed the expression—self-reliant, self-sufficient, and consequently self-controlled, and being called upon to perform certain work, does it easily, steadily and quietly, without violent or spasmodic effort, simply because it is sufficiently powerful to overcome resistance opposed to it" (1872:180). This is a hybrid heart insofar as Treadwell interpreted the healthy heart as being that of a strong and virtuous man. His metaphors were explicit, but they were traditional, alluding to the stout- and fainthearted.

A key difference between the perception of the heart as the center of courage and the perception of the heart as a pump turns on the extent to which these perceptions considered men to have or to be hearts. It has not been that long in Western cultures that the body and its parts have been deemed private property (Hyde 1997); certainly slavery considered the other's body to be someone else's property. To the extent that I am my body, *heart* signifies *me* in a variety of ways, including the moral. The question remains, however, what did the soldiers complaining of irritable heart understand their hearts to be? What was the vernacular heart?

An example of the cultural image of the heart in the time of the battle of Fredericksburg occurred in an editorial in the *New York Times*, on the occasion of General Ambrose E. Burnside taking responsibility for losing the battle. The *Times* noted that Burnside's letter was a model of "manliness and true courage," and that his "simple-hearted nobility" could calm the fears that "touch the keenest sensibilities of the public heart." When the public heart is troubled, men are "excited and aroused" to assign blame. But Burnside did well with his letter, and his men did well, for they were "his brave legions [who] climbed the hills to the death which crowned them" (A Good Example 1862). Courage, manliness, nobility, and the passions of fear and anger were all seen to dwell in the heart.

This hybrid heart made possible but also problematic the relationship between irregular action of the heart and courage. In the work of another Victorian physician, Benjamin Ward Richardson, the hybrid heart appeared as the *broken heart*. Richardson took this vernacular term and redefined it as a disease "due to failure of the nervous supply of the heart, and induced by excessive nervous activity." He appealed to those readers "who know even nothing of anatomy and physiology" (1876:124–125) to compare their own experiences of exertion with his explanation of heart action. Richardson bridged almost seamlessly the everyday experience of his readers with his scientific view of the body. He did so by reinterpreting the meaning of *broken heart* as a result of loss of power supply from the nerves:

> The reader is not, however, bound to accept under this term an actual rupture or bursting of the heart. . . . Most commonly the heart is rather to be considered as broken in power, by reason of the disorganization of structure or action, than as ruptured simply in one part: and death may be considered as due rather to the gradual wearing out of a motion that is essential to life. [1876:124]

The men subject to broken heart were "valiants" as youths; their "vital bank is good," but they "live a life that is altogether artificial, and in violent opposition to nature—who sacrifice their powers to overwork of mind as well as body, and who neither in sleeping nor waking give a respite to the labouring heart" (Richardson 1876:128). Vigorous men striving to advance themselves economically wrecked their health by the excess of their passionate competitiveness. Richardson appealed to common experience and common symbols of middle-class life and translated them into an anatomical explanation.

> We say of some men they are "lion-hearted"; of others, they are "faint-hearted." How true are these definitions! Physical courage depends on strength of heart, and men vary, from their babyhood, in their courage according to such strength. . . . The nervous boys have weak, the valiant boys strong, hearts. The first may become, in time, by far the most powerful, morally, and the most reflective; but the latter are the men who supply the chivalry and industry of the world. [Richardson 1876:126]

Richardson's *broken heart* resembles the irritable heart. When "the regulating influence exerted upon [the heart] by the nervous system is imperfect" (Richardson 1876:134), the heart is broken, by grief, overwork, or sudden strain. So the soldiers suffering from irritable heart could be said to have been suffering from faintheartedness, broken hearts, or un-self-reliant hearts.

One does not, however, read such depictions in Civil War literature on the topic. Irritable heart was not seen as a metaphor. The physicality of the disorder had its guarantee in one word: courage. Derived from the Latin *cor* (heart), courage was identified with the heart. The Union physicians did not doubt the courage of the men they treated for irritable heart. Their emphasis was on the overwhelmingly material causes of the disease: diarrhea, hard marching, poor nutrition, and sanitary conditions. It is worth considering, then, the place of courage in the context of the time. Hess (1997:95–96) depicts it as follows:

> Courage itself, enshrined by American culture as a supremely valuable ideal of action and thought, was an immensely potent factor in keeping Northern soldiers on the battlefield. They had been nurtured in a cultural environment that encouraged allegiance to a standard of public conduct few could have guessed would be applied in a conflict against fellow Americans, and they tried to live up to that standard. The ideal of courage, which meant to the Northern soldier "heroic action undertaken without fear," was intertwined with a range of other values such as manliness, religion, duty, and honor.

The setbacks of 1862 for Federal troops in Virginia put this sense of valor to the test. Hess summarized the situation of many:

> Ambrose Burnside ordered his men to repeatedly assault Lee's veterans, who were positioned behind a stone wall, which left this field of battle littered with bodies and soaked with blood. Walter Carter of the 22d Massachusetts survived it and managed to hold on to his faith: "My sense of right and love of country and its glorious cause would impel me forward to death, even if my poor weak nature hung back and human feelings gained control over me." [1997:99]

This passage gives the existential context for irritable heart. In the face of terror and death, Carter fought his own "poor weak nature" even as he fought the enemy. This passage sheds further light on the passage cited earlier from Stillé—that the army "has failed to accomplish all that was justly expected of it is plainly owing not to the muscle and bone which compose, but to the brains [the generals] which direct it"—insofar as "the muscle" meant also the moral muscle of the soldier as Hess describes him.

Courage was essential to "the social expectations of manliness in the face of modern war" (Blight 1992:63), and the horrors and deprivations of the war sorely tested it. During the failed Peninsula Campaign in 1862, the letters of soldier Charles Harvey Brewster

> chronicled his desperate struggle with dysentery and "terrible exposure" while sleeping nightly in the mud. At one point he declares himself so sick that he will have to resign and go home; to fall back now to some makeshift hospital, he believed, would surely mean a hideous and ignoble death. Courage in this instance, Brewster learned, merely meant endurance and a little luck. He could "give up" and seek a furlough, he reasoned, but he feared that the "brave ones that staid [sic] at home

would call me a coward and all that so I must stay here until after the fight at any rate." [Blight 1992:64]

Linderman (1987) argues that courage has a history, and the Civil War marked the end of one epoch of courage. Early in the war, soldiers idealized fearless courage, an ideal that the war attenuated and that faded into mythology by the end of World War I. Courage also signified action, heroic action, "as an extension of the will" (Linderman 1987:17) of the individual. It is not, to be sure, that fear was not there; in the teeth of the cultural ideal of manhood, however, the terrors of battle were suffered privately. The war, writes Linderman, proved disillusioning to that ideal of fearless courage.

Yet the ideal made a difference. Even while hospitalized, soldiers were expected, and they expected themselves, to show bravery in the face of wounds and pain, and their ideal was fearlessness. Twentieth-century psychotherapeutic practices had not yet invited the soldiers to speak about their fears in an effort to exorcize them and the functional ailments that unacknowledged fears are said to produce. In the Civil War, or at least in its early years, signs of fear were repugnant. In a scene that contrasts sharply with Da Costa's examinations, Linderman (1987:22) describes an instance of pulse-taking on the battlefield:

> A teamster—"a dreadful, dirty, snuffy, spectacled old Irishman," certainly no gentleman and not even a solider—one day insisted on taking the pulses of William [Dame, a volunteer in a Confederate artillery battery] and his friends. He then announced that one soldier was excited, another was frightened, that a third "would do all right" in combat, and so on. Some of the judged were pleased, others hated the Irishman for his verdicts, but no one dared either to refuse to submit to the test or to question its results.

So an elevated pulse could have been read as a sign of fear and, in the context of the time, cowardice.

This Da Costa did not do. One must suppose that in examining and treating sufferers of irritable heart, Da Costa treated the men as brave, and that the soldiers with such hearts struggled with doubts about themselves. What would it have taken, in such a situation, for physician and patient to begin to speak of fears, terrors, and panic? The closest Da Costa came to addressing such topics were his remarks about the disordered innervation of the heart. Even there, the defect was of the nerves, not the nerve, of the soldier.

What distinguished Da Costa's medical examination of soldiers from that of the Irish teamster who tested soldiers' mettle by taking their pulse? Why did Da Costa not feel fear in the pulse as the Irishman had? In a sense, of course he did, as he acknowledged in his 1874 lecture. However, the anatomical sense of the pulse, coupled with the cultural ideals of courage and manhood, cancelled the pulse's moral significance. The anatomical action of the heart may be felt and heard, and many things quicken the heartbeat. Da Costa did hear the sounds that the Irishman diagnosed as fear:

> The sounds grow in loudness in any functional disturbance of the heart. When the organ is palpitating violently under strong nervous excitement, they may become short and sharp, and sometimes so loud and ringing as to be audible to the by-standers. They are often permanently louder than in health, and are shorter and more clearly defined when the walls of the heart are thinned. . . . When the walls of the heart are thick, the first sound over the hypertrophied portion is apt to be dull and prolonged. [Da Costa 1901[1864]:375]

Da Costa could hear fear, but he was listening for the sounds of a weakened muscle and the sounds of defective valves. This new language of the heart, heard with Laennec's instrument, together with the ideal of manly courage and the fears of young manhood, constituted irritable heart.

The new language of the heart was manifested in Da Costa's evidence that functional changes of the heart could become permanently inscribed in the heart and its valves as the condition degenerated into organic disease. This concern was a great one among Da Costa and other physicians of the time and was most eloquently expressed by Richardson, who saw the figurative *broken heart* realized in ruptured valves. Because this particular heart—the heart as a pump, a muscle, an engine designed for work—was at stake, irritable heart was a dangerous condition. But this was not the whole story.

Further evidence that *irritable heart* was a hybrid symbol of the heart comes from an account of another Civil War–era physician, Sanford B. Hunt, who claimed that the term *functional disease of the heart* was a misnomer. For Hunt, this heart disease was caused by a variety of other diseases and by the privations of military life: "It was enough that the man had been sick for six or eight months, that a full year north would be required to restore him, and that a second season south would make him the easy victim of pernicious intermittent [fever]" (quoted in Barnes et al. 1991[1870–1888]:864). The term *functional disease of the heart* was for Hunt a term of convenience, but telling convenience. One might say that an even more convenient description would have been *functional disease of the soldier*. The use of *heart* emphasized the severity of the condition, and the compelling necessity of consulting examination boards to decide, and quickly, what to do with a particular man. The heart's action was disturbed, Hunt had no doubt; but much else was also amiss with these debilitated men. The diagnosis of functional disease of the heart—and so of irritable heart—said, in effect, that the heart is the man.

Later Interpretations of Irritable Heart

I will only briefly consider the further fate of irritable heart. Soldier's heart, a World War I diagnosis, presented a symptom picture similar to that of irritable heart. The older diagnosis, the earlier fears that a functional heart disease might become organic, and the recommendations for rest were deemed nonessential. James Mackenzie (1853–1925), the Scottish cardiologist, concluded in 1916, according to Howell (1985:39), that "the cases were overwhelmingly non-cardiac, the most likely etiology being the strain and exhaustion of life in the trenches superimposed on some 'toxic influence' caused by infection." In World War II, with renewed attention to the same symptom picture, the meaning of the condition changed again. In a widely cited study, Paul Wood concluded that irritable heart, soldier's heart, the effort syndrome, and neurocirculatory asthenia had nothing to do with the heart. The condition was instead anxiety neurosis, "an emotional reactive pattern peculiar to psychopathic personalities and to subjects of almost any form of psychoneurosis" (Wood 1941:849). Wood noted, moreover, that women and people from "the emotional races" were more susceptible to this "Da Costa syndrome" (1941:768).

Dunbar's (1946) review of medical literature on the relationship between the heart and emotions complicated the picture. Dunbar referred to the work of Karl Fahrenkamp, who stressed the unity of the psychological and the somatic in heart disorders of this type. Fahrenkamp showed the dilemma of the patient with something like irritable heart (or neurocirculatory asthenia):

> A patient's insistence on his own diagnosis of "nervousness" raises the suspicion of dissimulation; it expresses his hope for confirmation of this self-diagnosis, i.e., the expectation that nothing organic may be found. The neurotic with cardiac complaints, on the other hand, expects confirmation of an organic condition, thus denying his neurotic condition. [Dunbar 1946:213–214]

Finally, Dunbar cited Gustav von Bergmann, who claimed that we cannot separate the "nervous or organic, or functional or organic" (Dunbar 1946:214) components of these conditions. Dunbar searched for a way to conceptualize "heart neurosis" without falling into the culturally defined dichotomies. This incipient deconstruction still awaits its birth.

Although today irritable heart is occasionally diagnosed in a sense that is close to Da Costa's, it is usually labeled something else. The Vietnam War occasioned evaluating the symptom picture in terms of posttraumatic stress disorder (PTSD). A characteristic of PTSD is physiological hyperreactivity: "The two PTSD patterns are generally described by higher than control basal rate and (1) a dramatic overshoot of heart rate with a slow return to a baseline . . . , or (2) a more normal increase in heart rate but a sluggish return to a baseline rate" (Perry 1994). In the continuing trend to interpret irritable heart as a psychiatric condition, it has been classified as a panic disorder or as agoraphobia with panic attacks. In one case study, a woman was initially diagnosed as having an irritable heart:

> At least three times a month Mrs. Williamson notices palpitations and becomes frightened that these palpitations signal a heart attack. . . . Initially Mrs. Williamson was treated with a variety of beta blockers for an "irritable heart." . . . She does experience frequent (about twice weekly) panic attacks. . . . Mrs. Williamson has agoraphobia with panic disorder. [Management Plan for Panic Disorder and Agoraphobia, 2007]

Irritable heart has also been interpreted in the other, strictly physiological, direction as mitral valve prolapse or as orthostatic intolerance. Mitral valve prolapse syndrome occurs regularly with panic disorder, according to the fourth edition of the *Diagnostic and Statistical Manual of Mental Disorders* (APA 1994).

A recent review of war syndromes concludes that no conclusive diagnosis can be made on the basis of Civil War accounts of irritable heart (Hyams et al. 1996). Although Da Costa's descriptions of irritable heart resemble descriptions of the effort syndrome, shell shock, agent orange exposure, and Gulf War syndrome in being attributed to physiological causes (unlike nostalgia, battle fatigue, and PTSD, which have been attributed to psychological causes), "no single, previously uncharacterized illness or underlying cause that is unrelated to psychological stress is apparent from the available reports" (Hyams et al. 1996:403). Despite the constancy of life-threatening circumstances, the role of infectious diseases, diarrhea, and poor nutrition cannot be ruled out in evaluating the medical significance of Da Costa's diagnosis of irritable heart. If there is a consensus, it is that the terrors and exhaustion of battle figure significantly in the occurrence of irritable heart.

Conclusion: Excess and Matters of the Heart

If we view irritable heart as an *existential attunement*, to use a Heideggerian term—that is, as a mode of being-in-the-world—and not as a diagnosis; if we view irritable heart as a medicalized name for an existential possibility that occurred during the American Civil War, what could we say? Da Costa's patients faced squarely the imminent possibility of their own deaths in an experience of the uncanny. I propose that irritable heart, whatever else it signifies, points to an existential attunement of *anxious fatigue*. In calling it *anxious fatigue*, I bring together an analysis of fatigue (Levinas 1978) and anxiety (Heidegger 1962). For Levinas, "the pain of effort or fatigue is wholly made of this being condemned to the present. . . . To be weary is to be weary of being" (1978:35). Fatigue is not a state but a way of existing in which one is unable to relinquish temporarily the burdens of one's existence. As in insomnia, one is condemned to be there ("being there" translates Heidegger's term for human existence, *Dasein*).

According to Da Costa's accounts, fatigue was the context for irritable heart. In addition to fatigue, the soldiers experienced a largely unanticipated brutal, intractable war. In 1862 and 1863, they did not know what the outcome of the conflict would be, especially given the defeats the Union suffered in Virginia, where many of these men fought. They faced the uncanny, the *unheimlich*, the not-being-at-home, which one encounters in an attunement of anxiety, according to Heidegger. These soldiers met the possibility of their own death and the death of their nation, their world. In facing their situation from a position of anxious fatigue, they became conscious of their hearts—an awareness culturally appropriate and medically conspicuous. As Barlow (2000) indicates, attentional biases and hypervigilance play formative roles in anxiety such that increased awareness to heartbeat can be the result. Heidegger suggests that "anxiety is often conditioned by 'physiological' factors" (1962:234), which, according to the case records Da Costa and the other physicians provided, included poor nutrition and illness in addition to the hard marching and other rigors of military life. From this existential point of view, irritable heart is a metaphor in a culturally appropriate discourse for the revelation of the radical contingency of one's own existence in the face of a world and a life that are falling apart.

Irritable heart is scarcely now imaginable. The cultural categories that produced it seem remote. In one respect, Civil War physicians had a perceptual style that was more reminiscent of the *Iliad* than of the medical gaze. Irritable heart was a culture-bound condition that occurred at the limits of the endurable—physically, psychologically, and morally. It occurred during wartime at the limits of endurance and resistance to disease, and it reflected not only physical stamina but character as well. Irritable heart occurred at the limit of the anatomical. As a functional disease, it occupied a space between the physical, defined by the medical gaze, on the one hand, and the psychological and moral, defined by race, character, and temperament, on the other. This category of the functional—a holding place of the anomalous between the duality of the mental and the physical—took shape as the anatomical image of the body displaced earlier humoral and symbolic readings of the flesh. Irritable heart, then, as a functional disease, held a place in two interpretive fields and in two perceptions of self and society. It was simultaneously the heart of courage in a man and the pump in the machine.

Irritable heart signified, moreover, that war had changed. Individual action will always count for something, but war had changed. William James, evoking the Civil War, wrote that "when whole nations are the armies, and the science of destruction vies in intellectual refinement with the sciences of production, I see that war becomes absurd and impossible from its own monstrosity" (1987[1910]:1289). He affirmed that military valor was noble, that the ability to endure and triumph under conditions of "pain and fear" (1987[1910]:1287) marks the best of the human spirit. The contradiction between valor and modern warfare seem to have been precisely the existential condition that produced irritable heart. Whatever the probable medical diagnoses are, then or now, irritable heart signified this contradiction.

Irritable heart signified a heart disease. In the face of diseases that wasted them, battles that shocked them, defeats that discouraged them, and marches that pushed them, many soldiers felt heartsick. Out of respect and discretion, Da Costa did not accuse them of being afraid or of panicking. These young soldiers had "the right stuff," the right character, background, and patriotism. In their lives at that moment, the heart of courage at the limits of endurance became a disordered pump.

References

Allbutt, C. 1873. Overstrain of the Heart and Aorta. *Medical Times and Gazette* 1:291.

American Psychiatric Association (APA). 1994. *Diagnostic and Statistical Manual of Mental Disorders.* 4th ed. [*DSM–IV.*] Washington, DC: American Psychiatric Association.

Arnold, M. 1907. The Scholar-Gypsy. In *Poetical Works of Matthew Arnold.* Pp. 273–80. London: Macmillan.

Barlow, D. H. 2000. Unraveling the Mysteries of Anxiety and Its Disorders from the Perspective of Emotion Theory. *American Psychologist* 55:1247–1263.

Barnes, J. K., G. Otis, and D. L. Huntington. 1991[1870–1888]. *The Medical and Surgical History of the Civil War.* Wilmington, NC: Broadfoot.

Bartholow, R. 1991[1863]. *A Manual of Instructions for Enlisting and Discharging Soldiers: With Special Reference to the Medical Examination of Recruits, and the Detection of Disqualifying and Feigned Diseases.* San Francisco: Norman.

———. 1867. The Various Influences Affecting the Physical Endurance, the Power of Resisting Disease, Etc., of the Men Composing the Volunteer Armies of the United States. In *Contributions Relating to the Causation and Prevention of Disease, and to Camp Diseases; Together with a Report of the Diseases, Etc., Among the Prisoners at Andersonville, Ga.* A. Flint, ed. Pp. 3–41. New York: Hurd and Houghton.

Blight, D. W. 1992. No Desperate Hero: Manhood and Freedom in a Union Soldier's Experience. In *Divided Houses: Gender and the Civil War.* C. Clinton and N. Silber, eds. Pp. 55–75. Oxford, UK: Oxford University Press.

Clarke, E. H. 1971[1871]. Practical Medicine. In *A Century of American Medicine 1776–1876.* E. H. Clarke, ed. Pp. 3–72. New York: Burt Franklin.

Clinical Society of London. 1873, March 15. *Clinical Society and Gazette*, i, 291.

Da Costa, J. M. 1867. Observation on the Diseases of the Heart Noticed Among Soldiers, Particularly the Organic Diseases. In *Contributions Relating to the Causation and Prevention of Disease, and to Camp Diseases; Together with a Report of the Diseases, Etc., Among the Prisoners at Andersonville, Ga.* A. Flint, ed. Pp. 360–383. New York: Hurd and Houghton for the U.S. Sanitary Commission.

———. 1871. On Irritable Heart: A Clinical Study of a Form of Functional Cardiac Disorder and Its Consequences. *American Journal of the Medical Sciences* 61:17–52.

———. 1874. On Strain and Over-Action of the Heart. *Smithsonian Miscellaneous Collections* 15:1–28.

————. 1901[1864]. *Medical Diagnosis, with Special Reference to Practical Medicine: A Guide to the Knowledge and Discrimination of Diseases.* 9th ed. Philadelphia: Lippincott.

Danger of Excess in Physical Exertion, The. 1861. *Lancet* 2:165.

Dean, E. T. 1997. *Shook over Hell: Post-Traumatic Stress, Vietnam, and the Civil War.* Cambridge, MA: Harvard University Press.

Duden, B. 1993. *Disembodying Women: Perspectives on Pregnancy and the Unborn.* Cambridge, MA: Harvard University Press.

Dunbar, H. F. 1946. *Emotions and Bodily Changes: A Survey of Literature on Psychosomatic Interrelationships 1910–1945.* New York: Columbia University Press.

Dunster, E. 1867. The Comparative Mortality in Armies from Wounds and Diseases. In *Contributions Relating to the Causation and Prevention of Disease, and to Camp Diseases; Together with a Report of the Diseases, Etc., Among the Prisoners at Andersonville, Ga.* A. Flint, ed. Pp. 169–192. New York: Hurd and Houghton.

Foucault, M. 1973. *The Birth of the Clinic: An Archaeology of Medical Perception.* New York: Random House.

Good, B. J. 1994. *Medicine, Rationality, and Experience: An Anthropological Perspective.* Cambridge, UK: Cambridge University Press.

Good Example, A. 1862. *New York Times*, December 23:4.

H. H. 1864. Review of *Medical Diagnosis, with Special Reference to Practical Medicine. American Journal of the Medical Sciences* 48:423–440.

Hartshorne, H. 1864. On Heart Disease in the Army. *American Journal of the Medical Sciences* 48:89–92.

Heidegger, M. 1962. *Being and Time.* New York: Harper & Row.

Herschbach, L. M. 1997. Fragmentation and Reunion: Medicine, Memory and Body in the American Civil War. Ph.D. dissertation, Department of History, Harvard University.

Hess, E. J. 1997. *The Union Soldier in Battle: Enduring the Ordeal of Combat.* Lawrence: University of Kansas Press.

Howell, J. D. 1985. "Soldier's Heart": The Redefinition of Heart Disease and Specialty Formation in Early Twentieth-Century Great Britain. *Medical History Supplement* 5:34–52.

Hyams, K. C., F. S. Wignall, and R. Roswell. 1996. War Syndromes and Their Evaluation: From the U.S. Civil War to the Persian Gulf War. *Annals of Internal Medicine* 125:398–405.

Hyde, A. 1997. *Bodies of Law.* Princeton, NJ: Princeton University Press.

J.H.H. 1869. Review of *Contributions Relating to the Causation and Prevention of Diseases, and to Camp Diseases; Together with a Report of the Diseases, Etc., Among the Prisoners at Andersonville, Ga.* Published for the U.S. Sanitary Commission. *American Journal of the Medical Sciences* 58:173–181.

James, W. 1987[1910]. The Moral Equivalent of War. In *William James: Writings 1902–1910.* B. Kuklick, ed. Pp. 1281–1293. New York: Library of America.

Jones, C. H. 1868. *Clinical Observations on Functional Nervous Disorders.* Philadelphia: Henry C. Lea.

————. 1870. *Studies on Functional Nervous Disorders.* London: Churchill.

Kugelmann, R. 1992. *Stress: The Nature and History of Engineered Grief.* Westport, CT: Praeger.

Latham, P. M. 1829. Pathological Essays on Some Diseases of the Heart. *London Medical Gazette* 3:529–533.

Levinas, E. 1978. *Existence and Existents.* Dordrecht, NL: Kluwer.

Linderman, G. F. 1987. *Embattled Courage: The Experience of Combat in the American Civil War.* New York: Free Press.

Management plan for panic disorder and agoraphobia. 2007. In *Clinical Research Unit for Anxiety and Depression.* Electronic document, http://www.crufad.com/site2007/clinicianinfo/clinicianagoraphobia.html, accessed September 17, 2008.

McPherson, J. M. 1988. *Battle Cry of Freedom: The Civil War Era.* Oxford, UK: Oxford University Press.

Myers, A.B.R. 1870. *On the Etiology and Prevalence of Diseases of the Heart Among Soldiers.* London: Churchill. Available at http://books.google.com/books?id=thgDAAAAQAAJ&pg=PA1&lpg=PA1&dq=%22On+the+Etiology+and+Prevalence+of+Diseases%22&source=web&ots=FrAW_ltwuB&sig=3X9cUFOqdc49xgZ9HQUQFlHD8e4&hl=en&sa=X&oi=book_result&resnum=1&ct=result#PPA92,M1.

Packard, F. R. 1964. Bartholow, Roberts. In *Dictionary of American Biography.* Pp. 2–3, Vol. 1, Part 2. New York: Scribner's.

Perry, B. D. 1994. Neurobiological Sequelae of Childhood Trauma: Post-Traumatic Stress Disorders in Children. In *Catecholamine Function in Post-Traumatic Stress Disorders: Emerging Concepts.* M. Murburg, ed. Pp. 253–276. Washington, DC: American Psychiatric Press.

Polanyi, K. 1957. *The Great Transformation.* Boston: Beacon Press.

Rabinbach, A. 1990. *The Human Motor: Energy, Fatigue, and the Origins of Modernity.* Berkeley: University of California Press.

Reiser, S. J. 1978. *Medicine and the Reign of Technology.* Cambridge, UK: Cambridge University Press.

Richardson, B. W. 1876. *Diseases of Modern Life.* New York: Appleton.

Romanyshyn, R. 1982. *Psychological Life: From Science to Metaphor.* Austin: University of Texas Press.

Rosenberg, C. E. 1992. *Explaining Epidemics and Other Studies in the History of Medicine.* Cambridge, UK: Cambridge University Press.

Rosenblatt, E., and R. Rosenblatt, eds. 1992. *Hard Marching Every Day: The Civil War Letters of Private Wilbur Fisk, 1861–1865.* Lawrence: University of Kansas Press.

Russell, I. 1867. Pneumonia as It Appeared Among the Colored Troops at Benton Barracks, Mo., During the Winter of 1864. In *Contributions Relating to the Causation and Prevention of Disease, and to Camp Diseases; Together with a Report of the Diseases, Etc., among the Prisoners at Andersonville, Ga.* A. Flint, ed. Pp. 319–335. New York: Hurd and Houghton.

Spencer, H. 1904. *An Autobiography.* 2 vols. New York: Appleton.

Stearns, P. 1994. *American Cool: Constructing a Twentieth-Century Emotional Style.* New York: New York University Press.

Stillé, A. 1863. *Address Before the Philadelphia County Medical Society.* Philadelphia: Collins.

Treadwell, J. B. 1872. Observations Upon Over-Work and Strain of the Heart. *Boston Medical and Surgical Journal* 10:157–160, 179–184.

Wood, P. 1941. Da Costa's Syndrome (or Effort Syndrome). *British Medical Journal* 1:767–772; 805–811; 845–851.

Twentieth-Century Theories of Panic in the United States

From Cardiac Vulnerability to Catastrophic Cognitions

Devon E. Hinton and Susan D. Hinton

ALTHOUGH PANIC DISORDER (PD) emerged as a nosological category in American psychiatry only in the 1980s, experiences of acute anxiety or panic that cause suffering and disability are hardly new to Americans or to American psychiatrists. Contemporary theories of PD and anxiety have grown out of a history of concepts in American popular and medical culture. PD is not a known, fixed entity but a particular conceptualization of acute anxiety that has evolved historically within psychiatric writing and research, particularly in North America—a set of ideas that continues to evolve. Cross-cultural studies of panic cannot assume a fixed disorder as the basis for comparison. In this chapter we perform a genealogy of our current conceptualization of the cause of PD panic attacks,[1] tracing epistemic shifts linked to other shifts in society in the representation of panic's causation. By examining theories of panic in twentieth-century America, we put the panicker "back into the historical domain of practices and processes in which he has been constantly transformed" (Foucault 2005:525).

As each new theory of what causes acute anxiety and panic became viewed as "scientific," as "fact," its answers to basic questions (What causes panic? Are anxiety- and panic-type symptoms such as dizziness and palpitations dangerous? If so, which ones? What causes those symptoms? What can be done?) were popularized, and therefore profoundly influenced ideas about bodily vulnerability and created certain modes of self-surveillance. As medical theorists introduced new "frames of meaning" (Giddens 1984:285) and presented new panic theories, the panic experience itself changed as the result of a complex dialectic between the *panicker's experience* and the *theoretician's understanding of the panicker's experience*—a process that has been described as *biolooping* (Hacking 1999), as *classificatory looping* (Hacking 1999),[2] and as a *double hermeneutic* (Giddens 1984:374). In addition, as described in previous chapters, if a person fears having a certain symptom, the symptom will tend to be induced not only by attentional processes but also by the very biology of fear (which might be considered a form of biolooping): fear about having palpitations will cause palpitations by activation of the autonomic nervous system. Through these various processes, panic, as scientifically conceptualized, became "real," that is, a part of the historically specific ontology.

The observer changed the observed as scientific terms entered popular consciousness (Giddens 1984:374); that is, the adopted terms and associated theories changed the very structure of panic ontology in a seeming self-fulfilling prophecy (Giddens 1987).[3] Scientific theories of panic causation were variably assimilated into lay discourse and variably influenced *techniques of the self*.[4] Assimilated etiological theory led to a unique constitution of the panic experience, to a particular type of panic subjectivity. Each etiological theory about the acute onset of panic symptoms led to the empowerment of certain groups as diagnosticians, researchers, and providers of cure, resulting in a certain constellation of power and knowledge (Foucault 1980). We now examine the shifts in theories of panic's cause and cure throughout the twentieth century.

Heart-Focused Fear and Its Syndromes in the Nineteenth and Early Twentieth Centuries

As revealed in the previous chapter of this volume, certain heart syndromes prominent in the nineteenth century and the first half of the twentieth century are part of the conceptual history of what are now described as PD panic attacks (Barlow 1988, 2002; Hinton et al. 2002a; Katschnig 1999; Micale and Lerner 2001; Young 1995). These cardiac syndromes were based on a premise of cardiac vulnerability. The heart became the site of increased monitoring and concern. The collective imagination was haunted by worries that the heart might become weakened, hypertrophied, dilated, and inelastic; that it might be damaged by palpitations produced by emotion, exercise, and exhaustion.

As the United States industrialized in the first half of the twentieth century, the heart, the body's motor, became the center of medical investigations of acute anxiety and, more generally, of the hygiene of the body. In parallel, actual motors gave rise to new modes of experience and a new industrial regime. The Model T Ford's engine, for example, made possible the mass production of automobiles, which gave rise to a new experience of the city and country landscapes; and large engines served as the animators of industrialization. The heart, configured as the central motor of the body, thus came under careful scrutiny, with special attention paid to all the effects and signs of its apparent breakdown. It was the site of care (*Sorge*) and concern (*Besorgen*),[5] a zone of surveillance, as reflected in hundreds of articles and multiple books, and in new methods of physical examination and treatment. Medical studies and pronouncements increased the sense of the vulnerability of the heart, creating cardiac hypervigilance and concern.

War-Related Cardiac Syndromes: Da Costa's Syndrome, Effort Syndrome, and Neurocirculatory Asthenia

During armed conflicts in the nineteenth century and the first half of the twentieth century, various panic-like syndromes emerged that were defined as focused on the heart—in the Civil War, *irritable heart*, also called *Da Costa's syndrome* or *soldier's heart;* in World War I, *effort syndrome;* and in World War II, *neurocirculatory asthenia.* Some recent academic articles and books refer to these wartime heart syndromes as PD equivalents (Barlow 2002; Katschnig 1999); others refer to them as the presentation of posttraumatic stress disorder (PTSD; see Engel 2004; Noyes and Hoehn-Saric 1998:236; Saigh and Bremner 1999:1). In fact, both interpretations would seem to be correct; these heart syndromes combined characteristics of both PD (such as fears of cardiac arrest) and PTSD (such as trauma recall causing palpitations and palpitations causing recall of traumatic events).[6]

In the Civil War, the physician Da Costa found irritable heart to be common among battle-exposed soldiers. A key sign of the disorder was the elicitation of palpitations and other symptoms by mild exercise or just standing up—an indication of exhaustion and irritability of the heart muscle (Da Costa 1871). According to Da Costa, the irritable heart was "strained" and "weak" and at great risk of developing hypertrophy and permanent dilatation, conditions that could cause death.

In World War I, more than seventy thousand troops were discharged from the British army because of "heart disease," the second most common cause after wounds. Lewis (1917, 1919, 1940) examined a large number of these patients and determined that almost none suffered from structural heart disease, but most suffered instead from a "functional disorder" he named *effort syndrome.*[7] The cardinal feature of the disorder was the induction of symptoms—such as fatigue, chest pain, fainting, giddiness, headache, sweating, palpitations, and breathlessness—either by mild exertion or by simply standing up. Lewis (1917; see also Skerritt 1983) likened these soldiers to a person pushed in exercise to the point of near collapse, with any additional effort—even that of standing up from a lying or sitting position—producing palpitations, giddiness, and sometimes fainting. Effort syndrome seemingly represented a panic syndrome in which exertion-induced panic was extremely common (compare Taylor 2000); upon effort, the sufferer surveyed the body for any symptom and read effort-induced symptoms as a sign of the depletion of inner energy supplies, of a body and heart about to collapse. So great was the fear of exertion that it was often said that the person with effort syndrome had an *effort phobia*.

After World War I some researchers suggested renaming *effort syndrome* and calling it instead *neurocirculatory asthenia*. They suggested this name change because the term *effort syndrome*—and even more so other commonly used terms like *irritable heart, weak heart,* and *soldier's heart*—heightened fears of having a serious and permanent physical condition, a disorder of the heart. After being given one of these diagnostic labels, patients worried about having a weak and vulnerable heart that might be strained by effort; afflicted by these fears, they often became incapacitated. The new term, which contained the word *asthenia*, meaning weakness, was considered less likely to produce what we now call *catastrophic cognitions* in the person so diagnosed. Until after World War II, neurocirculatory asthenia remained the main presentation of what today would be called PD—and was an important presentation of PTSD.

From World War I to World War II, multiple studies were done to determine the physiological characteristics of persons with effort syndrome and neurocirculatory asthenia. Dizziness upon standing remained a central aspect; it was thought to indicate dysfunction of the autonomic nervous system and possibly of the heart muscle itself (Friedman 1947; Jones 1948:422–423; Whishaw 1939). The military made extensive use of both the Crampton Test, which assessed the change in heart rate and blood pressure upon standing, and the Schneider Index, a key component of which was the Crampton Test (McFarland and Huddleson 1936; Taylor and Brown 1944).[8] It would seem likely that orthostatically induced panic—that is, panic triggered by dizziness upon standing—was common at that time.[9]

Cardiac Concerns Among Civilian Populations: Popular Self-Help Literature

In the early twentieth century, cardiac concerns were increasingly prominent not only among the military but also among civilian populations. We now examine a book from the 1930s that illustrates how medical literature intended for laypersons created fears about the heart and made the heart an area of hypervigilant care and an always-at-risk inner engine.

In 1934, a physician named Calvin Smith published *That Heart of Yours* (1934), a book aimed at a popular audience. Mirroring the opinion voiced by other contemporary authors (such as Deutsch and Kauf 1927), Smith asserted that overstraining the heart—such as by experiencing strong emotion or by engaging in excessive exercise or mental work—could cause permanent dilation of the organ.

As symptoms indicating the possible presence of a serious cardiac condition and the need to consult a physician, Smith (1934:69) mentioned fatigue, chest pressure, fainting, palpitations, "cardiac asthma,"[10] a feeling of gas pressing on the heart, and shortness of breath.

"Physical strain is likely to induce serious damage in an adolescent heart," wrote Smith (1934:34), and overexercise might actually rip the valves of the heart, creating permanent disability.[11] Overexercise would cause the adolescent to develop an *athletic heart*, a heart that was dilated as a result of overstrain. To illustrate the danger of overstraining the heart, Smith (1934:34–35) presented an analogy: if a rubber band is stretched repeatedly, it loses elasticity and becomes permanently elongated; so too the fibers of the heart, if repeatedly strained, lose elasticity, leading to dilatation of the heart.[12] To warn against the dangers of overexercise, Smith advocated inscribing the following dictum, called the *Heart Creed*, in all gymnasiums, in all training quarters, and on all athletic fields: "Effort must cease when it brings on heart hurry, shortness of breath, chest oppression, chest pain, or physical fatigue" (1934:35).

Smith conflated economic imagery and physiological imagery, considering heart effort to be a kind of capital that must not be overspent, especially in one's youth:

> There are times when youth overreaches itself in stretching out to grasp the pleasures of the moment. Young people do not realize that there is a limit to the spending of enthusiasm and energy. The continual seeking for entertainment and diversion throughout the days and into the nights, with no relaxation and but little actual rest, will eventually exhaust the heart's reserve force and threaten its future efficiency. When a youth comprehends that by thoughtless squandering of physical reserve he not only jeopardizes the future of his heart but also his prospects in business, he will watch his expenditures and conserve his physical assets, in order that he may take his place in the world of affairs. [Smith 1934:33]

Smith's book also created hypervigilance about diet and digestion, both of which could reportedly damage the heart: "The eating of rich incompatible foods, the overeating of any food at irregular hours, the eating of simple food when weary or physically engaged, all tax digestion. And the heart pays the tax" (1934:66). Poor digestion produced heart-damaging toxins and a gas-producing fermentation that distended the stomach to the point that it pressed upon the heart. Simply having a feeling of "gas pressing on the heart" was sufficient reason for consulting a physician (Smith 1934:61, 72).

Smith (1934:17–18, 66) presented a pathophysiological model of how poor blood flow from an impaired heart might bring about indigestion and heart damage, resulting in a vicious cycle of worsening. The vicious cycle might begin with heart "disorder" and lead to indigestion, or it might begin with indigestion and lead to heart damage. Smith's pathophysiological model of the cycle beginning with a disordered heart (see Figure 5.1) may be summarized as follows:

1. A disordered heart, which may result from even a slight cause, such as fatigue, results in less blood perfusing the stomach.[13]

2. Poor blood flow to the stomach brings about impaired production of digestive juices.

3. Limited digestion results in food becoming a "fermenting mass" that produces intestinal gas, distending the stomach.

4. Stomach distention causes (a) gastric discomfort, (b) mechanical blockage of heart motion, (c) blockage of the diaphragm action required for normal breathing,[14] and (d) activation of the vagal nerve through a hypothesized "reflex," leading to palpitations and heart-rate acceleration (through a reduction in vagal tone).

5. The irregular and inefficient motions of the heart lead to decreased perfusion of the stomach and heart, resulting in worsened digestion and heart injury, even cardiac collapse and death.

6. The heart becomes weakened and damaged, leading to even poorer blood supply to the stomach, restarting and perpetuating a vicious cycle of worsening.

Because of the production of toxins and the other pathological processes just outlined, a bout of indigestion was to be greatly feared: "The 'acute' phase [of indigestion] promptly subsides. The indigestion is only a matter of a few hours; but the associated heart damage likely persists for weeks, maybe for months" (Smith 1934:46). As Smith noted, "an attack of 'acute indigestion' is in reality a severe and violent heart prostration. . . . To onlookers, it is an attack of 'acute indigestion'; to the heart, it is a revolution that shakes the very foundation of its stability" (1934:46–47).

Smith's book demonstrates how medical discourses in the 1930s produced cardiac (and gastric) hypervigilance. Many things, from emotion to exercise, might strain the heart; a "weakened" heart might cause indigestion and impaired circulation, thereby bringing about further cardiac damage in a vicious cycle of worsening; or simply having indigestion might lead to an initial damaging of the heart that resulted in such a vicious cycle of worsening.

The End of the Episteme of the Vulnerable Heart

As we have seen, an elaborate cardiac ethnophysiology existed well into the first half of the twentieth century, resulting in hypervigilance to cardiac symptoms, in catastrophic cognitions about the heart, in self-surveillance for evidence of symptoms of even minor cardiac dysfunction, and in the medicalization of PD panic attacks as generated by a disordered heart. Only in the 1940s and 1950s would researchers

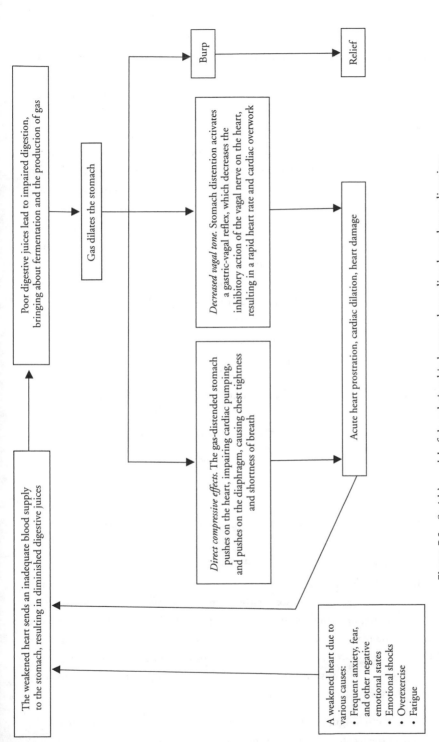

Figure 5.1 Smith's model of the relationship between heart disorder and poor digestion: A vicious cycle of worsening

determine that this vulnerable heart model was physiologically incorrect—that the heart was not injured by exercise, that palpitations caused by emotions did not damage the heart. A shift occurred: an anxious patient complaining of palpitations and other panic symptoms came to be presumed to have cardiac-focused anxiety rather than actual cardiac pathology (see Barlow 1988, 2002).

Prior to 1950, anxiety was frequently attributed to a dangerous heart disorder, and the panicker was compared to a person pushed through overexercise to exhaustion, an exhaustion that might deplete and damage the heart (as in Lewis's effort syndrome). In the 1950s, new views emerged. Anxiety came to be interpreted as due to mental imaginings, which might produce harmless palpitations, and the panicker was analogized to a person suddenly frightened by some event, which caused harmless palpitations. The image of dangerous nervous exhaustion and heart disorder gave way to the image of the neurotic, of a person easily frightened, whose condition posed no risk to the heart (see, for example, Conillera 1954).

In the 1950s and 1960s, new biological models emerged that hypothesized noncardiac causes of panic, such as low calcium and an oversensitive brain-based carbon dioxide detector. But cardiac concern remained prominent among laypersons, as evidenced by the continued frequency of cardiac-focused panic, which resulted from heart attack concerns and the salience of heart-related symbolism and metaphors. (For one review of the cardiac-focused panic literature, see Eifert 1992.)

The Emergence of a Noncardiac Theory of Panic: Low Calcium and Spasticity

In the 1950s and 1960s, two theories of panic emerged that emphasized the role of low calcium.

The Low Calcium Hypothesis and the Birth of Spasmophilie: French Panic in the 1950s

In the 1950s, two Frenchmen described a syndrome of "spasticity" and claimed it was due to low blood levels of calcium (Justin-Besançon and Klotz 1950; see also Klotz 1958). They gave the disorder the name *spasmophilie* or *tétanie chronique* (chronic tetany). *Spasmophilie* was characterized by anxiety attacks, and in France it became the new face of PD (Cathebras 1995; Fraschina 1979; Horenstein 1986; Sidoun et al. 1989; see also Gaines 1992 for a cultural contextualization of *spasmophilie*). *Spasmophilie* was diagnosable by various seemingly scientific means, particularly by the presence of the following:

- The Chvostek sign, in which, when the cheek is tapped so as to deliver a slight blow to the facial nerve, the corner of the lip spasms.

- The emergence or worsening of the Chvostek sign after hyperventilation.

- The emergence or worsening, following hyperventilation, of the Trousseau sign, which consists of a hand contraction after a blood-pressure cuff is inflated at the level of the biceps.

- Excessive muscular contractions, either spontaneous or after hyperventilation or other means of induction, upon examination by the electromyograph (EMG).[15]

All these procedures investigate for the presence of spasm, and the term *spasmophilie*, which contains the root *spasmo*, indicates that spasm is the disorder's key feature.

To correct the disorder's key deficit, French physicians treated *spasmophilie* patients with various calcium supplements (Cathebras 1995; Fraschina 1979; Horenstein 1986; Sidoun et al. 1989). Dating back to the publication of Krishaber's (1873) classic work, one finds *faiblesse irritable* (irritable weakness) to be a key construction of French anxiety states, and the disorder *spasmophilie* gave it a new set of pathophysiological mechanisms. As in Krishaber's first iteration of an irritable weakness paradigm, the reflex (in the case of *spasmophilie*, the Chvostek sign) played a key part in the model of the disorder, and in the anatomical and physiological theories of the time. The medical gaze had now become more penetrating, by contemplating the body from the level of symptom to the calcium ions in the blood, seeing the body through the optic not of anatomophysiology but rather of chemo-anatomophysiology. The diagnosis of *spasmophilie* and the treatment of PD-like panic attacks with calcium were exported to French colonies (such as Cambodia), where they underwent indigenization and became a key aspect of local anxiety and panic syndromes (see Hinton et al. 2002a).

The Lactate Hypothesis and Low-Calcium-Caused Spasticity: Panic in the United States in the 1960s and 1970s

Beginning in World War I, investigators tried to discover a metabolic reason for the poor exercise tolerance of effort syndrome patients. They discovered an abnormally rapid rise of lactate during exercise. (In fact, this abnormal increase resulted from poor physical conditioning; that is, if you compared panic and nonpanic patients with equivalent levels of fitness, no differences in lactate levels would be found [Broocks et al. 1997].) In an extremely influential article, Pitts and McClure (1967; see also Pitts 1971) demonstrated that lactate caused panic among persons with effort syndrome. When they injected those patients with lactate, panic resulted, with headache, dizziness, faintness, weakness, and chest tightness. No doubt influenced by the work of Klotz and other *spasmophilie* researchers, Pitts and McClure

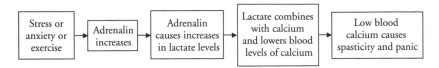

Figure 5.2   Pitts and McClure's model of how low calcium occurred and caused panic

noted the similarity of the symptoms of anxiety neurosis to those of pretetanic hypocalcemia (that is, a state of hyperreactivity, nearly tetanic in severity, seen in persons with low levels of calcium), a state of spastic overreactivity. During lactate infusion, all of the study's subjects had paresthesia, such as numbing and tingling of the skin, which is also found in hypocalcemia. Pitts and McClure hypothesized that lactate combined with calcium, lowering calcium levels. To test the hypothesis, they infused calcium along with lactate to see whether it would block the panic reaction. It did.

On the basis of these experiments, and conjoined with the fact that adrenalin was known to increase lactate, Pitts and McClure put forth the following theory of panic (see also Figure 5.2):

- *Triggers of panic.* Stress, anxiety, or exercise might trigger panic.
- *Panic pathophysiology.* Stress, anxiety, or exercise increases adrenaline, which starts a causal sequence that ultimately results in a drop in calcium, producing spasticity and panic.
- *Predisposition to panic.* A person is predisposed to having panic episodes if he or she has (1) excessive production of adrenaline during stress, anxiety, or exercise; (2) excessive production of lactate in response to a set amount of adrenalin; or (3) chronically low calcium.

Ultimately the lactate theory of panic was disproven, but not until the 1980s (Fyer et al. 1984; Liebowitz et al. 1986). In France, Pitts and McClure's lactate theory reinforced ideas about *spasmophilie* and the efficacy of calcium as treatment.[16]

The Emergence of the Diagnostic and Statistical Manual: The Continued Biologization of Panic

As indicated in the introduction to this volume, the *Diagnostic and Statistical Manual* (*DSM*) presents an extremely narrow definition of PD that fits only a very small part of the spectrum of what would actually constitute *panic disorder* in the broad sense of the word. Here we further discuss the development of the *DSM*, including theories and experiments that guided its development (see also Chapter 1).

Acute Attacks of Anxiety Symptoms in 'DSM–I': Organ-Focused Anxiety Subtypes and Fear of Anxiety-Caused Heart Dysfunction

In the *DSM–I*, published in 1952, what we now call PD was diagnosed most commonly as an *anxiety reaction* (defined as a general state of fear, frequently associated with somatic symptomatology) or as one of the *psychophysiologic autonomic and visceral disorders*. The latter category comprised several subtypes, each classified by its predominant symptom—*psychophysiologic cardiovascular reaction, psychophysiologic gastrointestinal reaction*, and *psychophysiologic nervous system reaction* (general fatigue being the most prominent complaint). These subtypes took the place of such former designations as *cardiac neurosis* and *gastric neurosis*—terms that in turn had replaced *cardiac neurasthenia* and *gastric neurasthenia*. The *DSM–I* discussion of psychophysiologic disorders stated that "such long continued visceral states [such as palpitations] may eventually lead to structural damage" (APA 1952:29). This statement reveals the persistence of a catastrophic view of the effects of emotion and of emotion-related symptoms (such as palpitations). Later versions of the manual no longer mentioned that prolonged anxiety states might damage the bodily organs. PD would increasingly be viewed as a purely biological disorder, a periodic spasm of the autonomic nervous system, brought about by biological rather than psychological causes, with the spasm causing no damage to the body.

The Inclusion of Panic Disorder in 'DSM–III': The Key Role Played by the Suffocation-Alarm View of Panic

The diagnosis of PD first appeared in *DSM–III* (APA 1980), largely due to Klein's research, which greatly shaped the *DSM–III*'s conceptualization of the disorder. Wishing to draw a distinction between *anxiety states* and *paroxysm of fear*, which he considered to differ in respect to biology and phenomenology, Klein referred to *paroxysms of fear* as "panic" (Klein and Fink 1962). When Klein first began to study patients with what he called panic attacks, most psychiatrists continued to conceptualize panic sufferers in a Freudian manner—that is, to consider panic attacks as caused by the sudden eruption of repressed energy, and agoraphobia as resulting from the avoidance of locations that symbolized temptations. Most psychiatrists treated the sufferer of these ailments with intensive psychotherapy, focusing on the exploration of unconscious sexual and aggressive impulses (Klein and Fink 1962).[17]

Klein (1964) postulated two mechanisms for the production of panic attacks: (1) early life experiences of loss that deranged areas of the brain that are responsible for separation anxiety, causing a predisposition to periodic spasms of fear; and (2) hormonal shifts, such as menopausal changes, that through an effect on specific brain structures might trigger panic. According to this model, separation anxiety and hormonal fluctuations shifted the threshold for neuronal firing downward, resulting in periodic spontaneous electrical events in certain brain areas. Klein considered PD panic attacks as coming out of the blue, as a sort of episodic seizure of the autonomic nervous system. Only one type of panic trigger—certain exterior locations—was allowed in Klein's conceptualization. If panic attacks occurred outside the home, the person might develop agoraphobia as a result of pairing the fear of the panic attack with an external situation—a conditioning to the cue of specific outside spaces.

Soon after Klein's theory gained prominence, laboratory studies solidified the conceptualization of panic as a distinct psychopathological entity linked to specific brain structures. As described earlier, exercise often triggered panic in sufferers of panic attacks, giving rise to one of the PD names: *effort syndrome* (see Barlow 1988). Pitts and McClure (1967; see also Barlow 1988) hypothesized that the actual trigger might be endogenous lactate, a substance known to increase with exercise. When it was discovered that panic attacks could indeed be brought about by the administration of lactate, the conceptualization of panic as a specific biology-caused entity gained greater acceptance (Baker 1989; Barlow 1988).

Starting in 1989, Klein published a series of influential articles that attempted to integrate all available experimental and pharmacological data into a unitary theory of panic that resulted from the hypersensitivity to carbon dioxide and lactate in the suffocation-alarm system part of the brain (for a review of Klein's panic theory, see Rachman 1998:97). According to Klein, this alarm system might be triggered not only by an actual increase of carbon dioxide or lactate (which increases when oxygen levels drop in the body), but also by the encountering of cues associated with suffocation: a closed-in space, being in a crowd, or air that seems stale. Klein argued that shortness of breath was the key feature of panic, whereas palpitations took center stage in a state of fear caused by an external threat, as in an imminent attack by an assailant; he also argued that the prominence of shortness of breath in panic reflected the specific biological cause of the disorder: an oversensitivity to carbon dioxide and lactate, and a deranged suffocation-alarm system, leading to frequent triggering of the suffocation alarm and a seizure-like paroxysm of shortness of breath and autonomic arousal.

In this theory, based on the hypothesis that a suffocation-alarm center exists in the brain and on the process of conditioning (that is, on the association of fear to places in which panic occurred in the past), Klein sought to explain both the origins of panic attacks and the phenomenon of agoraphobia. Hence, although earlier researchers such as Carl Westphal (1988), who first described agoraphobia in 1871, minimized the dizziness aspect of agoraphobia in order to prove more global neuropathic origins (Hinton et al. 2002b), Klein wished to prioritize shortness of breath in order to support a biological and conditioning view of the disorder.[18]

Klein's theory resulted in shortness of breath and related symptoms (such as chest tightness) being emphasized in the Western conceptualization of PD. Reflecting this bias, three of the thirteen symptom categories in the *DSM–IV* panic attack criteria (APA 1994) are concerned with shortness of breath: sensations of shortness of breath or smothering, feelings of choking, and chest pain or discomfort. Klein's theory also contributed to the *biologization* of panic disorder as the medical gaze sought panic's origin in the inner recesses of the brain, in a suffocation-alarm brain center. As a result of Klein's theory, the medical problematization of panic placed shortness of breath and the correlated brain area at the center of the disorder.

The Emergence of a Psychological Theory of Panic
In the introduction to this volume (Chapter 1), Good and Hinton critique the *DSM–III* and *DSM–IV* and describe the emergence of the catastrophic cognitions theory of panic causation, a theory that has increasingly challenged a purely biological explanation of panic.

Conclusion
In this chapter we have analyzed theories of PD panic attacks in the nineteenth and twentieth century in Western Europe and the United States, following the frequent transformation of the *medical gaze* (Foucault 1990; Jones and Porter 1994) that has constructed panic. We have delineated historical shifts in theories about the essential nature of PD. Each PD theory hypothesized variations in the following elements:

- *Symptom profiles.* The main symptom has been presumed to be dizziness (Westphal's theory at the end of the nineteenth century), palpitations (as in effort syndrome), shortness of breath (Klein's theory), or a symptom about which the person has extensive catastrophic cognitions (Clark's catastrophic cognitions theory).
- *Sensitivities or triggers.* Exertion, causing a dangerous draining of heart strength (as in effort syndrome); high carbon dioxide or lactate levels in the brain, or suffocation cues (Klein's model); or experiencing the catastrophically cognized somatic sensation (catastrophic cognitions theory).
- *Causal mechanisms.* Eye weakness (as in Westphal's theory), heart frailty (as in effort syndrome), low calcium levels (*spasmophilie*), hypersensitive carbon dioxide and lactate detectors in the brain's suffocation-alarm center (Klein's theory), or excessive catastrophic cognitions (Clark's theory).

Only recently have PD researchers actually investigated the cognitions of PD patients—that is, what PD patients think just before and during a panic attack.

From that research has emerged the next and most recent theory of PD, the theory of catastrophic cognitions, which is described in the introduction and throughout this volume. As outlined in the introduction, this volume's editors consider the multiplex theory of panic, which hypothesizes PD-type panic to result from multiple simultaneous processes—from catastrophic cognitions to trauma associations to metaphoric resonances—to be an even more adequate explanation. The current chapter, as well as the other historical chapter and the ethnographic chapters of this book, illustrate the validity of the multiplex model as applied to PD-type panic attacks. Further theories of panic will no doubt emerge as researchers scrutinize the historical record, do detailed ethnography, conduct biological investigations, and investigate psychological processes.

Notes

1. On Foucault's archaeology and genealogy, see Gutting (1989) and Visker (1995).

2. Hacking (1999) coins the term *interactive kinds* to indicate classifications that constantly shift through time because of their cultural and sociological embeddedness. He advocates *dynamic nominalism,* that is, studying the effects of labeling in a particular cultural and sociological context. *Classificatory looping* is how the classification of something as *x* alters the relationship between the person labeled *x* and the social and institutional context, alters how *x* is scrutinized by the scientific practitioners of the day, and alters how the person labeled *x* views him- or herself, thereby bringing about various complex looping effects. Hacking utilizes the term *biolooping* to indicate how the mind influences physiology, which is an important way by which shifts in the labeling of a person bring about effects; labeling brings about not only mental effects but also physiological ones, creating another level of looping. Interactive kinds display both the classificatory and the psychophysiological kind of looping.

3. On how a psychiatric diagnosis, once established, self-perpetuates through cognitive biases, see also the edited volume by Caplan and Cosgrove (2004).

4. On Foucault's notion of *subjectivation, subjectivity,* and *modes of subjectivation,* see Revel (2002).

5. On Heidegger's use of the terms *Sorge* and *Besorgen,* see Polt (1999).

6. One form of trauma-related disorder, *shell shock,* has been extensively described (Binneveld 1997; Micale and Lerner 2001; Young 1995), but the history of the heart syndromes has been neglected. (For an excellent, brief historical discussion, see Barlow, 2002; see also Oglesby 1987; Skerritt 1983.) In the trauma literature, in respect to the Civil War, irritable heart is often described as being an earlier form of PTSD; however, these same authors, when discussing World War I, assert that shell shock is that period's equivalent of PTSD, yet they ignore effort syndrome. This is a surprising omission, because irritable heart and effort syndrome were very similar syndromes, and in World War I more than seventy thousand British troops seemingly suffered from effort syndrome.

7. *Functional* means the heart is damaged even though there are no visible changes in the heart upon using available means of examination such as viewing cross-sections of the tissue under a microscope; this is in contrast to a disorder in which an actual lesion

can be located, such as when seeing damaged heart valves during an autopsy or hearing a valve defect during auscultation. It is assumed that the damage occurring in a functional disorder exists in some domain still beyond the area of visualization—for example, in the neurochemical synapse.

8. Researchers at that time thought that in a person with neurocirculatory asthenia an unusually great heart-rate acceleration and blood-pressure drop upon standing resulted from a disordered autonomic nervous system.

9. In the contemporary United States, orthostatic dizziness is commonly found in chronic fatigue syndrome and Gulf War syndrome. In chronic fatigue syndrome, orthostatic dizziness is thought to be caused by a disordered autonomic nervous system that is incapable of adequately maintaining blood pressure upon standing (Rowe and Calkins 1998; Schondorf and Freeman 1999). Gulf War veterans with comorbid chronic fatigue syndrome and PTSD have been shown to have not only orthostatic dizziness complaints but also impaired blood-pressure response to standing (Peckerman et al. 2003). On the relationship of Gulf War syndrome to effort syndrome, and on the prominence of orthostatic dizziness in both, see *The Irritable Heart: The Medical Mystery of the Gulf War* (Wheelwright 2001).

10. Smith (1934:69) considers nocturnal awakenings in a state of panic to be a dire cardiac indicator, sometimes called *cardiac asthma*. In fact, nocturnal panic—that is, awakening in a state of terror in the absence of nightmare—is commonly found in PD patients and does not indicate any cardiac pathology (McNally 1994).

11. "Overindulgence in tennis, swimming and wrestling, beyond that point where fatigue sounds the warning note to desist, may so stress the heart that the valve leaflets fail to approximate and a functional murmur results" (Smith 1934:34).

12. Smith also writes of "heart fatigue" (1934:93), "hurting the heart" (1934:37), "breaking the heart" (1934:45) through excessive exercise or through extremes of emotion and "emotional load" (1934:45), "heart prostration" (1934:93), and the "loads" (1934:7) placed on the heart by various activities.

13. Smith asserts that if one consumes food when in a fatigued state, when the heart is "tired," then even less blood can be pumped to the stomach and indigestion worsens.

14. The idea that distention of the stomach might seriously impair breathing and cardiac function was quite prevalent. According to Schott (1914:130), a professor of medicine, "distention of the stomach should be avoided since a full stomach may press the diaphragm up against the heart and lungs and thereby cause marked shortness of breath and palpitations."

15. The EMG is an instrument that registers the electrical activity produced by muscle contraction.

16. Although the theme of irritable weakness, of spasticity, was part of American discourses about panic for much of the twentieth century, it then greatly decreased in importance. Recently, however, spasticity has once more become a prominent collective representation of panic states in the United States. The theme of irritable weakness reemerged at the turn of the twentieth century in the form of certain PD syndromes, for example, *multiple chemical sensitivity*, in which a person frequently experiences panic attacks in response to odors, that is, has odor-triggered panic attacks (Hinton et al. 2004); or in the formulation of a new personality type, the *highly sensitive person*, who is prone to overreactivity to various stimuli (Aron 1996).

17. As briefly described in the introduction to this volume (Chapter 1), Freud theorized that panic resulted from repressed sexual desire, being an explosion of that repressed energy.

18. Modern researchers have increasingly realized the strong association of dizziness with a tendency to experience agoraphobia (Balaban and Jacob 2001). Khmer patients almost always attribute dizziness in public places to *spin-inducers*, that is, for example, a noise that attracts attention (and so causes a rapid rotation of the head) or the sight of many people milling around (Hinton et al. 2004). Increasingly, researchers have become interested in how such mechanisms—for example, looking at spinning objects—may trigger episodes of agoraphobia (Balaban and Jacob 2001).

References

American Psychiatric Association (APA). 1952. *Diagnostic and Statistical Manual of Mental Disorders.* 1st ed. [*DSM–I.*] Washington, DC: American Psychiatric Association.
———. 1980. *Diagnostic and Statistical Manual of Mental Disorders.* 3rd ed. [*DSM–III.*] Washington, DC: American Psychiatric Association.
———. 1994. *Diagnostic and Statistical Manual of Mental Disorders.* 4th ed. [*DSM–IV.*] Washington, DC: American Psychiatric Association.
Aron, E. N. 1996. *The Highly Sensitive Person: How to Thrive When the World Overwhelms You.* New York: Broadway.
Baker, R. 1989. Introduction: Where Does "Panic Disorder" Come From? In *Panic Disorder: Theory, Research, and Therapy.* R. Baker, ed. Pp. 1–12. Hoboken, NJ: Wiley.
Balaban, C., and R. Jacob 2001. Background and History of the Interface Between Anxiety and Vertigo. *Journal of Anxiety Disorders* 15:27–51.
Barlow, D. H. 1988. *Anxiety and Its Disorders: The Nature and Treatment of Anxiety and Panic.* New York: Guilford Press.
———. 2002. *Anxiety and Its Disorders: The Nature and Treatment of Anxiety and Panic.* 2nd ed. New York: Guilford Press.
Binneveld, H. 1997. *From Shellshock to Combat Stress.* Amsterdam: Amsterdam University Press.
Broocks, A., T. F. Meyer, B. Bandelow, A. George, U. Bartmann, E. Rüther, and U. Hillmer-Vogel. 1997. Exercise Avoidance and Impaired Endurance Capacity in Patients with Panic Disorder. *Neuropsychobiology* 36:182–187.
Caplan, P., and L. Cosgrove, eds. 2004. *Bias in Psychiatric Diagnosis.* Lanham, MD: Aronson.
Cathebras, P. 1995. Neurasthenia, Spasmophilie, and Chronic Fatigue Syndromes in France. *Transcultural Psychiatry* 31:259–270.
Conillera, J. S. 1954. Syndrome d'asthenie neuro-circulatoire. *Bulletin international des services desanté des armées de terre, de mer, et de l'air* 27:567–591.
Da Costa, J. M. 1871. On Irritable Heart: A Clinical Study of a Form of Functional Cardiac Disorder and Its Consequences. *American Journal of the Medical Sciences* 61:17–52.
Deutsch, F., and E. Kauf. 1927. *Heart and Athletics.* St. Louis, MO: Mosby.
Eifert, G. H. .1992. Cardiophobia: A Paradigmatic Behavioral Model of Heart-Focused Anxiety and Non-Anginal Chest Pain. *Behaviour, Research, and Therapy* 30:329–345.
Engel, C. 2004. Post-War Syndromes: Illustrating the Impact of the Social Psyche on Notions of Risk, Responsibility, and Remedy. *Journal of the American Academy of Psychoanalysis and Dynamic Psychiatry* 32:321–334.

Foucault, M. 1980. *Power/Knowledge: Selected Interviews and Other Writings, 1972–1977.* London: Harvester Press.

——. 1990. *The Birth of the Clinic: An Archaeology of Medical Perception.* London: Routledge.

——. 2005. *The Hermeneutics of the Subject: Lectures at the Collège de France, 1981–1982.* New York: Palgrave.

Fraschina, B. 1979. Revue critique du concept de spasmophilie. *Acta psychiatrica belgique* 79:391–403.

Friedman, M. 1947. *Functional Cardiovascular Disease.* Baltimore: Williams and Wilkins.

Fyer, A., J. Gorman, M. Liebowitz, M. Levitt, E. Danielson, J. Martinez, and D. Klein. 1984. Sodium Lactate Infusion, Panic Attacks, and Ionized Calcium. *Biological Psychiatry* 19:1437–1447.

Gaines, A. D. 1992. Medical/Psychiatric Knowledge in France and the United States: Culture and Sickness in History and Biology. In *Ethnospsychiatry: The Cultural Construction of Professional and Folk Psychiatries.* A. D. Gaines, ed. Pp. 171–201. Albany: State University of New York.

Giddens, A. 1984. *The Constitution of Society.* Berkeley: University of California Press.

——. 1987. *Social Theory and Modern Sociology.* Stanford, CA: Stanford University Press.

Gutting, G. 1989. *Michael Foucault's Archaeology of Scientific Reason.* Cambridge: Cambridge University Press.

Hacking, I. 1999. *The Social Construction of What?* Cambridge, MA: Harvard University of Press.

Hinton, D. E., S. D. Hinton, K. Um, A. Chea, and S. Sak. 2002a. The Khmer "Weak Heart" Syndrome: Fear of Death from Palpitations. *Transcultural Psychiatry* 39:323–344.

Hinton, D. E., M. Nathan, B. Bird, and L. Park. 2002b. Panic Probes and the Identification of Panic: A Historical and Cross-Cultural Perspective. *Culture, Medicine, and Psychiatry* 26:137–153.

Hinton, D. E., V. Pich, D. Chhean, and M. H. Pollack. 2004. Olfactory-Triggered Panic Attacks Among Khmer Refugees: A Contextual Approach. *Transcultural Psychiatry* 41:155–199.

Horenstein, M. 1986. Spasmophilie ou attaque de panique? *La presse médicale* 15:1230–1236.

Jones, M. 1948. Physiological and Psychological Responses to Stress in Neurotic Patients. *Journal of Mental Science* 94:392–427.

Jones, C., and R. Porter, eds. 1994. *Reassessing Foucault: Power, Medicine, and the Body.* London: Routledge.

Justin-Besançon, L., and H. P. Klotz. 1950. Étude critique de la notion de spasmophilie chez l'adulte et le grand enfant. *La semaine hopitaux de Paris* 65:3173–3190.

Katschnig, H. 1999. Anxiety Neurosis, Panic Disorder, or What? In *Panic Disorder: Clinical Diagnosis, Management, and Mechanisms.* D. Nutt, J. Ballenger, and J. Lepine, eds. Pp. 1–23. London: Martin Dunitz.

Klein, D. 1964. Delineation of Two Drug-Responsive Anxiety Syndromes. *Psychopharmacologica* 5:397–408.

Klein, D., and M. Fink. 1962. Psychiatric Reaction Patterns to Imipramine. *American Journal of Psychiatry* 119:432–438.

Klotz, H. P. 1958. *La tétanie chronique ou spasmophilie.* Paris: Expansion.

Krishaber, M. 1873. *De la névropathie cérébro-cardiaque*. Paris: Librairie de l'Academie de Médecine de Paris.

Lewis, T. 1917. Report upon Soldiers Returned as Cases of "Disordered Action of the Heart" (DAH) or "Valvular Disease of the Heart" (VDH). *Medical Research Committee*, Special Series, 8.

———. 1919. *The Soldier's Heart and the Effort Syndrome*. New York: Hoeber.

———. 1940. *The Soldier's Heart and the Effort Syndrome*. London: Shaw and Sons.

Liebowitz, M., J. Gorman, A. Fyer, D. Dillon, M. Levitt, and D. Klein. 1986. Possible Mechanisms for Lactate's Induction of Panic. *American Journal of Psychiatry* 143:495–502.

McFarland, R. A., and J. H. Huddleson. 1936. Neurocirculatory Reactions in the Psychoneuroses Studied by the Schneider Method. *American Journal of Psychiatry* 93:567–599.

McNally, R. J. 1994. *Panic Disorder: A Critical Analysis*. New York: Guilford Press.

Micale, M. S., and P. Lerner, eds. 2001. *Traumatic Pasts: History, Psychiatry, and Trauma in the Modern Age, 1870–1930*. Cambridge, UK: Cambridge University Press.

Noyes, R., and R. Hoehn-Saric. 1998. *The Anxiety Disorders*. Cambridge, UK: Cambridge University Press.

Oglesby, P. 1987. Da Costa's Syndrome or Neurocirculatory Asthenia. *British Heart Journal* 58:306–315.

Peckerman, A., K. Dahl, J. Chemitiganti, J. LaManca, J. Ottenweller, and B. Natelson. 2003. Effects of Posttraumatic Stress Disorder on Cardiovascular Stress Responses in Gulf War Veterans with Fatiguing Illness. *Autonomic Neuroscience: Basic and Clinical* 108:63–72.

Pitts, F. 1971. The Biochemistry of Anxiety. *Scientific America* 220:69–75.

Pitts, F., and J. McClure. 1967. Lactate Metabolism in Anxiety Neurosis. *New England Journal of Medicine* 277:1329–1336.

Polt, R. 1999. *Heidegger: An Introduction*. Ithaca: Cornell University Press.

Rachman, S. 1998. *Anxiety*. Hove, UK: Psychology Press.

Revel, J. 2002. *Le vocabulaire de Foucault*. Paris: Ellipses.

Rowe, P., and H. Calkins. 1998. Neurally Mediated Hypotension and Chronic Fatigue Syndrome. *American Journal of Medicine* 105:15S-21S.

Saigh, P. A., and D. J. Bremner. 1999. *Posttraumatic Stress Disorder: A Comprehensive Text*. Needham Heights, MA: Allyn and Brown.

Schondorf, R., and R. Freeman. 1999. The Importance of Orthostatic Intolerance in the Chronic Fatigue Syndrome. *American Journal of Medical Science* 317:117–123.

Schott, T. 1914. *The Balneo-Gymnastic Treatment of Chronic Diseases of the Heart*. Philadelphia: Blakiston.

Sidoun, P., R. Fontaine, and G. Falaudi. 1989. Spasmophilie, attaques de panique, et névrose hystérique. *Le Concours Médicale* 17:111–124.

Skerritt, P. W. 1983. Anxiety and the Heart: A Historical Review. *Psychological Medicine* 13:17–25.

Smith, C. 1934. *That Heart of Yours*. Philadelphia: Lippincott.

Taylor, C., and G. Brown. 1944. Some Observations on the Validity of the Schneider Test. *Journal of Aviation Medicine* 13:214–231.

Taylor, S. 2000. *Understanding and Treating Panic Disorder: Cognitive-Behavioural Approaches*. West Sussex, UK: Wiley.

Visker, R. 1995. *Michael Foucault: Genealogy as Critique*. London: Verso.

Westphal, C. 1988. *Westphal's "Die Agoraphobie" with Commentary: The Beginnings of Agoraphobia.* Lanham, MD: University Press of America.

Wheelwright, J. 2001. *The Irritable Heart: The Medical Mystery of the Gulf War.* New York: Norton.

Whishaw, R. 1939. A Review of the Physical Condition of 130 Returned Soldiers Suffering from the Effort Syndrome. *Medical Journal of Australia* 16:891–893.

Young, A. 1995. *The Harmony of Illusions: Inventing Post-Traumatic Stress Disorder.* Princeton, NJ: Princeton University Press.

Part III

Cultural Variations in Panic Disorder

6

Comparative Phenomenology of 'Ataques de Nervios,' Panic Attacks, and Panic Disorder

Roberto Lewis-Fernández, Peter J. Guarnaccia, Igda E. Martínez,
Ester Salmán, Andrew B. Schmidt, and Michael Liebowitz

THIS VOLUME PRESENTS an opportunity to use anthropological research on panic-like episodes to expand psychiatric understandings of panic disorder and to raise issues concerning the cross-cultural applicability of *Diagnostic and Statistical Manual* (*DSM*) diagnoses. The tension between psychiatric universalism and cultural specificity has been only partially examined for the anxiety disorders. Good and Kleinman's 1985 chapter "Culture and Anxiety" sets out the issues with which we grapple today: "The cross-cultural research . . . makes it abundantly clear that anxiety and disorders of anxiety are universally present in human societies. It makes equally clear that the phenomenology of such disorders, the meaningful forms through which distress is articulated and constituted as social reality, varies in quite significant ways across cultures" (Good and Kleinman 1985:298).

Since we began our research on *ataques de nervios*, the question of the relationship between *ataques* and panic have both informed and haunted our efforts. One of the issues we have explored both epidemiologically and clinically is the relationship between experiencing an *ataque de nervios* and meeting the criteria for panic disorder (along with other psychiatric diagnoses). At the same time, since the beginning of our work and continuing to the present, many investigators and clinicians have assumed that *ataques de nervios* are *just* a cultural label that Puerto Ricans and other Latinos use for panic attacks, often with the assumption that Latinos are misinformed about their own experience when they use the term *ataque de nervios*.

Our research benefits from a close working relationship with Dr. Byron Good, coeditor of this volume. The work of this chapter's two senior authors on the relationship between anxiety and *ataques de nervios* began under his mentorship. This chapter returns directly to the issues of the comparative phenomenology of *ataques* and panic that we started examining in collaboration with Dr. Good.

The study reported in this chapter began by turning some of the previous approaches to understanding the relationship between *ataques de nervios* and panic attacks and panic disorder on their heads. We started with a detailed symptomatic phenomenology of *ataques de nervios* assessed on the terms of those who experience such *ataques*. We then asked what features of *ataques de nervios* make them more equivalent to panic attacks and panic disorder, and what features distinguish *ataque* episodes that do not conform to panic criteria. This approach allows us to challenge the simplistic equation of panic with *ataques*. It provides us with the opportunity to specify the range of *ataque* experiences prior to labeling them as such, in relation to panic attacks and panic disorder, and in relation to other emotional experiences and psychiatric disorders. This chapter presents the results of our look at *ataque* from the perspective of panic phenomenology, or more formally, the similarities and differences between *ataques de nervios* and the clinical architecture of panic attacks and panic disorder.

Phenomenologies of 'Ataques De Nervios,' Panic Attacks, and Panic Disorder

To carry out a valid comparison, it is important to distinguish at the outset between panic attacks and panic disorder, because these two psychiatric entities are likely to bear different relationships to *ataque de nervios*. A separate category for panic attacks was first established in the *DSM–IV* (APA 1994) on the basis of the recognition that these episodes can occur in the context of several psychiatric diagnoses, not just panic disorder (Liebowitz 1996). For example, persons suffering from social phobia often experience panic attacks when confronted with a dreaded social situation, such as public speaking. Because these panic attacks are not unexpected in a person with this phobia, they are considered "cued" and do not merit a separate panic disorder diagnosis. Likewise, sudden episodes of acute anxiety that correspond to the clinical phenomenology of panic attacks and that occur in situations that would be frightening to anyone (such as military combat) are still labeled panic attacks, but because they are not considered unexpected, they also are not diagnosed as panic disorder. Thus, the first criterion of panic disorder as defined in the *DSM–IV* is the presence of panic attacks that arise *recurrently* and *unexpectedly*, that is, in more than one unexpected situation. The notion is of a bodily danger signal gone wrong, like a fire alarm going off when there is no fire. This definition demarcates panic disorder from other psychiatric diagnoses and highlights the presumed biological nature of the disorder.

Ataque, on the other hand, is paradigmatically a reaction to a stressful situation, such as family conflict or some other very troubling event, and is therefore typically cued and thus conceptually distinct from panic *disorder*. The similarity to panic *attacks*, however, hinges not on the issue of whether the episode is unexpected, but rather on the phenomenological relationship between the two categories. That is, from an empirical standpoint, how well do *ataques* match the other formal characteristics of panic attacks, such as rapid peaking of symptoms (*crescendo*) or displaying a minimum of four symptoms out of a predefined list of thirteen? The empirical overlap between *ataque de nervios* and panic attacks and panic disorder is what we set out to discover in the study discussed in this chapter. First, however, we turn to the results of previous studies on the panic-*ataque* relationship.

Previous Studies of the Relationship Between 'Ataques' and Panic Disorder

In previous epidemiological research on the relationship between reporting an *ataque de nervios* and meeting the panic criteria in the Puerto Rico Disaster Study, there was a strong correlation between reporting *ataques* and fulfilling diagnostic interview schedule criteria for panic disorder (see Table 6.1) (Guarnaccia et al. 1993). Those who reported an *ataque de nervios* were twenty-five times more likely to meet the criteria for panic disorder than those who had not reported an *ataque*. These subjects were very likely those who labeled any and all of their panic

Table 6.1 Relationship between reports of *ataque de nervios* and psychiatric diagnoses in the Puerto Rico Disaster Study ($N = 912$)

Psychiatric Diagnosis	No *Ataque* n = 767 (84%)	*Ataque* n = 145 (16%)	*Odds ratio*
Depression (5%)	19 (2%)	29 (20%)	9.84
Dysthymia (12%)	67 (9%)	40 (28%)	3.63
Generalized anxiety (18%)	108 (14%)	55 (38%)	3.73
Panic disorder (2%)	3 (0.4%)	13 (9%)	25.08
PTSD (6%)	29 (4%)	25 (17%)	5.30
Any affective disorder	49 (6%)	43 (30%)	6.18
Any anxiety disorder	109 (14%)	58 (40%)	4.02
Any DIS diagnosis	214 (28%)	91 (63%)	4.35

NOTES: The number in parentheses after each psychiatric variable indicates the percentage of that diagnosis in the total sample. The number in parentheses within the categories "no *ataque*" and "*ataque de nervios*" indicates the percentage of patients meeting Diagnostic Interview Schedule (DIS) criteria for that diagnosis. The odds ratios reflect how much more likely it is that someone who reported an *ataque de nervios* met the criteria for that diagnosis.
SOURCE: Adapted from Guarnaccia et al. 1993.

episodes *ataques de nervios* and did not distinguish between cued and uncued attacks (or in our terms, between *ataque de nervios* and panic attacks that qualified as panic disorder). At the same time, it is important to note that the proportion of *ataque* sufferers who met the criteria for panic disorder was only 9 percent, and that there were strong associations between *ataques de nervios* and other anxiety and depressive disorders.

In an earlier clinical study at the New York State Psychiatric Institute (NYSPI), Liebowitz and colleagues (1994) also demonstrated an overlap between *ataque de nervios* and panic disorder. Out of a total of 156 (mostly Dominican) patients coming to an anxiety disorder clinic for treatment, 109 (70 percent) had had at least one *ataque* in their lifetime. Of these 109, 45 could be diagnosed with panic disorder. Of these 45, 9 distinguished between their panic disorder episodes and their *ataques de nervios*, "or were unclear in this regard" (Liebowitz et al. 1994:873). This means that of the 109 with *ataque*, between 33 percent (n = 36) and 41 percent (n = 45) were calling *ataque de nervios* what psychiatrists would label as panic disorder, and 59 percent to 67 percent of the people with *ataques* in this specialty clinic did not have panic disorder.

Phenomenologically, there were also some phenomenological differences between *ataque* and panic disorder. Briefly, among patients with primary panic disorder (n = 58), those who reported *ataques* (n = 45) were five times more likely than those who did not report *ataques* to complain of dizziness (*mareos*) as a panic symptom. Of the fifty-eight with primary panic disorder, the thirty-six who referred to their experiences as *ataque* were sixteen times more likely than the thirteen patients who denied having *ataque* to report fear during an episode, and thirty-four times more likely to be depressed before an episode. Finally, among patients without panic disorder, those with *ataque* were more likely than those without *ataque* to endorse several symptoms from the panic list; that is, they were four times more likely to report sweating, six times more likely to report depersonalization, four times more likely to report fear of going crazy, and five times more likely to report fear of losing control. These data show that experiencing *ataque* adds phenomenological difference to panic experience. The overlap of panic symptoms experienced by patients with *ataques* and without panic disorder indicates that these symptoms are common to both syndromes rather than panic-related in any particular way. It was precisely the question of whether these common symptoms signal other phenomenological similarities that gave rise to the current study.

Even more fine-grained phenomenological distinctions emerged when the investigators compared *ataques* that arose in persons with panic disorder, depression, or other anxiety disorders (Salmán et al. 1998). *Ataques* in persons with panic disorder (n = 45) resembled panic episodes more closely than *ataques* in the other groups. These *ataques* were characterized by significantly more reports of panic symptoms (most notably asphyxia, fear of dying, and fear during the attack) than *ataques* in depressed subjects or in the other anxiety group (which reported chest pain and dizziness). Panic subjects with *ataques* were also significantly more likely than respondents with other anxiety disorders to report feeling depressed before an *ataque*. By contrast, *ataques* in persons suffering from depression ($n = 33$) were characterized by more anger and emotional lability than *ataques* in the other clinical groups, including significantly more reports of screaming, crying, anger, becoming aggressive, and breaking things. *Ataques* in the subgroup of subjects with other anxiety disorders ($n = 24$) were not characterized by outstanding symptoms. These findings suggest that the phenomenology of *ataque* is intimately connected with the specific form of psychopathology associated with the episode. One possible interpretation is that a proportion of respondents labeled panic disorder episodes as *ataques*, but other possibilities include that common vulnerabilities underlie both panic and *ataque*, or that the appearance of one disorder predisposes a person to developing the other (Salmán et al. 1998).

Finally, a study conducted among a convenience sample of female Puerto Rican psychiatric outpatients in Massachusetts found a significant association between frequency of *ataques de nervios* and lifetime rates of panic disorder and dissociative disorder (Lewis-Fernández et al. 2002). Lifetime rates of posttraumatic stress disorder (PTSD) were also two to three times higher among patients with recurrent *ataques* than among those with fewer or no *ataques*, but this difference did not reach statistical significance. Overall, 14 percent of patients who reported *ataques* also fulfilled the criteria for panic disorder on the Structured Clinical Interview for *DSM–III–R* (SCID), and the rate of panic disorder reached 38 percent among subjects who reported six or more *ataques* in their lifetime. Of note, *ataque* frequency was not associated with degree of exposure to childhood trauma (including physical or sexual abuse), which was uniformly high across all subject cohorts, but was significantly associated with clinician-rated and self-report measures of dissociative symptoms and disorder. These associations suggest that recurrent *ataques* may signal the presence of psychiatric disorders characterized by dissociative symptomatology, including panic disorder (Stein et al. 1996).

In summary, previous research on the panic-*ataque* relationship suggests strongly that a proportion of persons with *ataques* are using the cultural label to indicate experiences that psychiatrists would diagnose as panic disorder. However, the majority of subjects with *ataques* in previous studies described episodes that do not fulfill criteria for panic disorder, clearly indicating the greater inclusiveness of the *ataque* label. A third small subgroup appears to distinguish between aspects of their experience, accepting the panic label for certain episodes but describing others as *ataques de nervios*. The basis for their distinction remains unclear, although it seems to occur in persons exposed to the professional health care system who are attempting to reconcile a diagnosis of panic disorder with their *ataque* self-label. Finally, all of the research has focused on the relationship between *ataques* and panic disorder, neglecting the comparative phenomenology of *ataque* and panic attacks.

In the current study, we ask people questions about what they experience in *ataques* and then we examine whether what they experience is the same as the key phenomenological features associated with panic attacks and panic disorder. That is, we examine how much like panic *ataques* are in terms of their formal features. The key phenomenological elements of panic attacks that we examined include (1) fear experiences during an episode, (2) number and type of symptoms, and (3) crescendo (shorter than ten minutes). The panic disorder elements we examined were (4) recurrence, (5) unexpectedness, and (6) sequelae of attacks.

Methods

This study was carried out within the Hispanic Treatment Program of the Anxiety Disorders Clinic (ADC) at the NYSPI. The ADC is a clinical research unit directed by Dr. Michael Liebowitz, a prominent anxiety disorders researcher. The Hispanic Treatment Program started in 1990 to serve the large and growing Latino, particularly Dominican, community that surrounds the NYSPI in northern Manhattan.

The study was designed to provide a multidimensional perspective on the experience of *ataques de nervios* and its relationship to mood and anxiety disorders. The specific aims of the larger research project were to study the self-labeling of *ataque de nervios* by Puerto Rican and Dominican patients seen in a variety of health and mental health care settings, and to determine via structured diagnostic interview the range of psychiatric features and disorders found in people with *ataques*, with a particular focus on panic disorder.

Subjects were recruited from persons seeking treatment in the Hispanic Treatment Program for anxiety, depression, or both who were then screened for having had an *ataque de nervios*. New subjects were also recruited specifically for treatment of their *ataques de nervios*; recruitment was done through flyers and through referrals from other mental health and medical services within the large Columbia University medical system that surrounds the NYSPI.

For the purposes of this chapter, the results of three different interviews were used. The first interview used the Explanatory Model Interview Catalogue (EMIC) that the authors developed specifically for studies of *nervios* and *ataques de nervios* among Puerto Ricans and other Latinos based on a format developed by Mitchell Weiss (1997). The EMIC is a clinician-rated instrument designed to elicit key features of cultural syndromes, including precipitants, symptomatology, perceived causes, illness course, and help-seeking. The focus of the *ataque* section was on the best-remembered *ataque*. The EMIC was also designed to allow for direct assessment of the relationship between *ataque* experiences and panic attacks and panic disorder on the basis of *DSM–IV* criteria. In addition to being queried for detailed information about the best-remembered *ataque*, subjects were also asked whether all, some, or none of their *ataques* were provoked by a stressful event.

The second interview was the SCID (Spitzer et al. 1992). This interview is designed to be used by clinicians to standardize their psychiatric assessments of patients according to *DSM* criteria. Subjects are rated according to whether they met the criteria for a range of psychiatric disorders and whether their symptom levels were below or at threshold levels to meet the diagnosis.

The interviewers who did the EMIC and SCID were blind to the results of each others' assessments.

The final interview was an integrative interview that took the results of both the EMIC and the SCID and sorted out the sequencing and the interaction of the cultural experiences with the episodes of psychiatric disorder. This interview was carried out by Michael Liebowitz, director of the ADC, and Ester Salmán, a Cuban-American *ataque de nervios* researcher and ADC staff member.

There is one limitation and one methodological difficulty that should be pointed out about our approach. The limitation is that we based the EMIC design on *DSM–IV* panic criteria, but the Spanish translation of the SCID for *DSM–IV* did not become available in time, requiring use of the *DSM–III–R* version. Therefore, in this chapter we use *DSM–IV* criteria to determine how many *ataques* conform to panic phenomenology, but we then compare the *ataques* that we determined are panic-like to panic disorder diagnoses based on *DSM–III–R* criteria. Some of the differences discovered by this approach are bound to be due to differences across the two sets of *DSM* criteria rather than to true differences between *ataque* and panic phenomenology. Luckily, *DSM–III–R* and *DSM–IV* panic criteria do not differ fundamentally. The criteria for panic attacks are the same, even if these were described separately for the first time in *DSM–IV*. In *DSM–III–R* it was possible to meet the panic disorder criteria either after a single unexpected attack that was followed by at least a month of persistent fear about having another attack, or by having four attacks within a four-week period, at least one attack of which was unexpected. *DSM–IV* changed the criteria to require at least two unexpected attacks, as well as to require that at least one of the attacks have specified severity sequelae, but it eliminated the alternative criterion of attack frequency (four attacks in four weeks). In the discussion section of this chapter we comment on the degree of potential confounding introduced by these changes in panic disorder criteria.

Finally, the methodological difficulty inherent in our approach is that the EMIC and the SCID do not follow identical procedures for establishing syndrome phenomenology, and thus potentially introduce methodological variance into the findings. In the EMIC we focus on a single prototypical *ataque*, including more questions about context and causation than are contemplated in the diagnostic interview, and obtain only secondary information across all of the respondents' *ataque* episodes. The SCID, on the other hand, primarily asks the subject to respond on the basis of a mental sum of all the episodes under evaluation (for example, "Have you ever had one that just seemed to come out of the blue?"), and focuses only secondarily on a prototypical attack. Differences found between the two interviews on whether a respondent's *ataques* met panic disorder criteria may be due to these methodological differences; for example, during the EMIC a subject may have focused on an *ataque* that did not meet the crescendo criterion but may have reported in the SCID other *ataques* that met panic disorder criteria. The potential impact of these different approaches on our findings is also mentioned in the chapter's closing discussion.

The analyses presented in this chapter focus on the assessment of *ataque* experience according to panic attack and panic disorder criteria, including the frequency of panic symptoms, the key features of *ataques* that are dissimilar to panic, the association of specific phenomenological elements with these dissimilar symptoms relative to panic symptoms in *ataque* experience, and the relationship of panic disorder assessment within the *ataque* module to the SCID diagnoses of panic disorder.

Results

Ninety-two subjects were recruited into the study. Of these, sixty-six (72 percent) reported having had at least one *ataque de nervios*. Of this group, 77 percent were women and 23 percent were men (see Table 6.2), which is consistent with the over-representation of women in mental health care and among *ataque* sufferers (Guarnaccia et al. 1993). The ages of the subjects were evenly distributed, except for the relative absence of geriatric patients, who attend a different clinic at the NYSPI. Seventy-three percent of the sample were Dominican and 27 percent were Puerto Rican, reflecting the changing Latino mix of Washington Heights. All but five subjects were first-generation migrants, which is also consistent with the demographics of the surrounding community.

The first set of analyses examined key features of the *ataque* experience that would potentially distinguish between *ataques* and panic. The distinguishing features of panic attacks are (1) a discrete period of intense fear or discomfort, (2) the

Table 6.2 Demographic characteristics of subjects
with *ataques de nervios* (*N* = 66)

	N	%
Gender		
Female	51	77
Male	15	23
Age		
18–28	9	14
29–39	20	30
40–50	20	30
51–61	13	20
62–72	4	6
Ethnicity		
Dominican	48	73
Puerto Rican	18	27
Country where subject grew up*		
Dominican Republic	47	71
Puerto Rico	15	23
USA	3	5

*Data missing for one subject.

presence of four or more of the thirteen panic symptoms on the *DSM–IV* list, and (3) rapid peaking of symptoms (crescendo), defined as occurring within ten minutes. We examined subjects' reports of their best-remembered *ataque* for evidence of these characteristics. The results are presented in Table 6.3.

Sixty-four percent of respondents described becoming very afraid or frightened (*le dio mucho miedo o susto*) during their best-remembered *ataque*. This number may be interpreted as a strict evaluation of the fear criterion. However, the panic attack definition also allows for a more general description of distress ("intense discomfort") as the entry criterion of a panic attack (APA 1994:395). This criterion was approximated by the item "becoming nervous" (*se puso nervioso*), which in Caribbean Spanish indicates a state of emotional upset that can include fear, anger, or unspecified distress. Seventy-nine percent of *ataque* sufferers endorsed this item, reflecting the more nonspecific nature of the symptom. Overall, 83 percent endorsed one of these two symptoms.

A scale of thirteen *ataque* symptoms was created from the EMIC items that overlapped with the symptoms of panic attacks listed in *DSM–III–R* (and reproduced unchanged in *DSM–IV*) (see Table 6.3). The general list of symptoms from

Table 6.3   Diagnostic features of panic attacks occurring during *ataques de nervios* (*N* = 66)

	N	% positive
Fear during episode		
Very afraid or frightened	42	64
Becoming nervous	52	79
Either afraid/frightened or nervous	55	83
The thirteen panic symptoms		
Heart palpitations	50	76
Sweating	37	56
Trembling/shaking	46	70
Shortness of breath	39	59
Choking	37	56
Chest pain/discomfort	37	56
Nausea/desire to vomit	26	39
Dizziness/faintness/light-headedness	46	70
Derealization/depersonalization	17	26
Fear of losing control/going crazy	51	77
Fear of dying	37	56
Numbness/tingling (paresthesia)	22	33
Chills/hot flushes	37	56
Four or more symptoms	49	74
Crescendo		
Less than ten minutes	29	44
Duration of episode		
One hour or less	40	64
Met all three panic attack criteria*	24	36

*Presence of fear/discomfort during attack; four or more symptoms; crescendo less than ten minutes

which these thirteen symptoms were extracted was developed to include the common symptoms of *ataques* identified in previous research, as well as the symptoms of panic attacks, so that direct comparisons between these experiences could be made. Respondents with *ataques* reported a large number of panic-like symptoms during these episodes. However, as stated earlier, symptom overlap indicates that these experiences are related but does not establish that *ataques de nervios* and panic attacks are the same phenomenon. Overall, panic symptoms are quite frequent in *ataques de nervios*, and it has been this pattern of overlapping symptoms that has led to the overly simplistic equating of the two phenomena. Specifically, the criteria for panic attacks require that four or more of the thirteen panic symptoms be present during attacks. Seventy-four percent of respondents fulfilled this criterion with regard to their best-remembered *ataque*.

A key issue in terms of comparative phenomenology is the speed with which the symptoms develop. The psychiatric model of panic posits that once an attack begins, the neurochemical processes trigger a rapid crescendo of symptoms that peak in less than ten minutes. Forty-four percent of *ataques* reached their peak in that time frame; the rest developed over a longer period. A related factor, but not one of the panic criteria, is that panic attacks tend to last a short time. About two-thirds of *ataques* had a brief duration, lasting an hour or less.

To be diagnosed as panic attacks, *ataques* must fulfill the three criteria discussed earlier. Only 36 percent of subjects met all three criteria with respect to their best-remembered *ataque*. This percentage includes subjects who reported either being "very afraid" or feeling "nervous" during their *ataque*, thus approximating the more inclusive features of the panic attack fear criterion. The phenomenological element that most distinguished *ataques* from panic attacks was a crescendo lasting longer than ten minutes, which occurred in fifteen subjects who otherwise met the panic attack criteria, or 23 percent of the sample. This degree of overlap indicates that even at the level of panic attacks, many *ataques* display a phenomenology distinct from panic episodes. At the same time, a distinct subset of *ataques* appear more like panic episodes than like the prototypical *ataque de nervios* described in our previous research (Guarnaccia et al. 1996; Lewis-Fernández 1996).

Some of these prototypical *ataque* features are listed in Table 6.4. A scale of eight symptoms was extracted from the list of EMIC symptoms to describe aspects of *ataque* experience commonly reported in past *ataque* research that are less typical of panic presentations. The data show that these atypical panic symptoms are part of many *ataque* descriptions. In addition, in 82 percent of cases, people were with the person during his or her *ataque*, indicating the social nature of *ataques*. In 54 percent to 58 percent of the cases, respondents reported feeling better and relieved (*me desahogué*) after the *ataque*, which contrasts with the feeling of considerable fear of having another episode that is frequently experienced after a panic attack. These characteristics of *ataques* highlight their distinctiveness from panic attacks.

We next sought to distinguish *ataques de nervios* from panic attacks that occur in the context of panic disorder. One of the key differences between *ataques de nervios* and panic attacks within panic disorder is that *ataques* are prototypically provoked while recurrent spontaneous episodes are the hallmark feature of panic disorder. In large clinical populations, up to half of all panic disorder episodes occur

Table 6.4 Prototypical *ataque* features occurring during or after the person's *ataque de nervios* (*N* = 66)

	N	% positive
Eight *ataque* symptoms		
Loss of control	49	74
Screaming a lot	39	59
Crying attack	45	68
Rage	30	46
Aggressiveness/breaking things	26	39
Suicidal ideation/attempt	9	14
Seizure-like episodes	10	15
Amnesia after attack	11	17
People present	54	82
Felt better after	36	54
Felt relieved after	38	58

in situations in which the patient does not expect to have a panic attack (Ballenger and Fyer 1996). According to the *DSM–IV*, panic disorder episodes must fulfill the criteria for panic attacks and occur more than once when not expected, and at least one attack must be followed by one month (or more) of one (or more) of the following sequelae: persistent concern about having a future attack, worry about the implications or consequences of the attack, behavior change as a result of the attack, or some combination of these. Table 6.5 shows the proportion of best-remembered *ataques* that fulfilled each of these criteria.

In terms of recurrence, 77 percent of subjects reported more than one *ataque* over their lifetime, suggesting that persons who seek medical help for their *ataques* tend to do so after multiple episodes. The question of whether the *ataques* described were unexpected was addressed in two ways. First, respondents were asked whether the *ataque* they described was provoked by something, and if so, whether it was provoked by something bad happening, by a life change, or after the death of a loved one. Twenty-six percent reported that their best-remembered *ataque* was unprovoked. Among provoked situations, in thirty-nine cases the *ataque* was due to a major life event, and in six cases it was due to the death of a loved one. Examples of provoked *ataques* include an *ataque* experienced by a woman after being criticized by her boss for bumping into a coworker and spilling some papers, in the midst of which she quit her job, and another experienced by a person during an argument with her husband over his infidelity. An example of an unprovoked *ataque* occurred during an otherwise uneventful bus ride to another city. Second, subjects were asked if all, most, or none of their *ataques* occurred out of the blue (*sin razón, como de la nada*), that is, unprovoked by upsetting situations. Thirty-five percent of respondents reported that all or some of their *ataques* were unprovoked; in terms of this dimension, then, these *ataques* might more likely be panic episodes labeled as *ataque*. In more than half the cases of provoked *ataques*, onset occurred either immediately after or within a day of the precipitating event.

The last criterion of panic disorder we examined with respect to *ataque* phenomenology was the presence for at least one month of one of the three sequelae mentioned earlier. The proportion of *ataque* subjects reporting each sequelae is listed in Table 6.5. Overall, 80 percent of subjects experienced at least one sequelae of the necessary duration after an *ataque*.

When we examined what proportion of subjects who had *ataques* resembling panic attacks (36 percent) also met the criteria for panic disorder listed earlier, only 17 percent of all *ataque* subjects fulfilled panic disorder criteria with respect to their *ataques*. We included in this number subjects who reported that at least some of their *ataques* were unprovoked (35 percent), rather than only those whose

Table 6.5 Diagnostic features of panic disorder occurring during *ataque de nervios* (*N* = 66)

	N	% positive
Recurrence		
Two or more *ataques* per lifetime	51	77
Unexpected		
Best-remembered *ataque* unprovoked	17	26
All or some *ataques* unprovoked	23	35
Sequelae lasting one month or more		
Fear or concern about having another attack	47	71
Worried about implications or consequences of attacks	44	67
Behavior change related to attacks	44	67
At least one sequelae present	53	80
Lag between precipitant and *ataque*		
Immediate	15	23
Within a day	22	33
Met all panic disorder criteria*	11	17

*Met criteria for panic attacks, had more than one *ataque*, at least some of the *ataques* were unprovoked, and had at least one type of sequelae after the attacks, lasting a month or more.

best-remembered *ataque* was unprovoked (26 percent), in order to cast the widest possible net for an overlap with panic disorder. Thirty-five percent of respondents (n = 23) had *ataques* that would have met *DSM–IV* criteria, except they were provoked by stressful events (n = 8), lacked a rapid crescendo (n = 8), or differed from panic disorder in terms of both of these characteristics (n = 7).

We next sought to compare the relationships between the number and type of symptoms experienced during an *ataque* to some of the key defining features of panic and to some of the characteristic features of *ataque* that are less typical during panic episodes. The results are presented in Table 6.6. Our hypotheses were, first, that phenomenological characteristics typical of panic disorder (such as unprovoked attacks and rapid crescendo) would be significantly associated with higher rates of symptom endorsement on the scale of thirteen panic symptoms, and second, conversely, that characteristics more typical of *ataques* than of panic (such as provoked attacks and feeling relieved afterward) would be associated with higher endorsement on the scale of typical *ataque* symptoms that are unusual in panic.

The first hypothesis was strongly supported. Subjects who experienced fear or nervousness during their episodes, whose *ataques* were either always or sometimes unprovoked, and who experienced certain specific sequelae for at least a month and did not feel better or relieved after their episodes were significantly more likely to report more panic symptoms during their *ataques*. There was also a trend association between the presence of rapid crescendo and higher endorsement of panic symptoms. These findings show that it is possible to identify within *ataque* experience a subgroup of *ataques* in which the key features of panic disorder run together, suggesting a profound phenomenological similarity with panic disorder.

The second hypothesis was only partially supported. There was a trend (p=0.06) that, if the best-remembered *ataque* was provoked, the respondents were more likely to report more *ataque* symptoms during their episode. However, subjects who reported fear or nervousness and who experienced distressing sequelae were significantly more likely to endorse both kinds of symptoms, and more *ataque* symptoms were endorsed by subjects with recurrent *ataques* than by those with single *ataques*, suggesting that, rather than being signs of episodes distinct from panic disorder, the *ataque* symptoms listed could represent instead nonspecific indicators of *ataque* severity or general characteristics of *ataques*, independently of their relationship to panic.

Finally, we examined the relationship between experiencing *ataques* that fit all the criteria for panic disorder within the EMIC and a diagnosis of panic disorder in the same individual using the SCID (see Table 6.7). SCID interviews were performed on ten of the eleven individuals whose *ataques* fit the criteria for panic disorder on the EMIC, and six of these were positive for panic disorder. The SCID interviewers diagnosed an additional fourteen subjects as suffering from panic disorder. Eight of the fourteen individuals were identified as subthreshold on the EMIC because they met all of the panic disorder criteria except all their *ataques* were provoked or the crescendo of the best-remembered *ataque* took longer than ten minutes, or both. It would appear that these subjects' *ataques* resemble panic episodes closely, and that these subjects either focused on different episodes or re-called the same *ataques* differently in each interview (information variance). The other fourteen individuals who were subthreshold on the EMIC also did not meet full panic criteria on the SCID and probably constitute persons with *ataques* that differ more substantially from panic characteristics. The explanation for the other six cases of panic disorder based on the SCID is not clear. One possibility based on case material is that people had panic episodes that both the subject and the clinician identified as distinct from *ataques de nervios*.

We collapsed the subthreshold cases into the absent category in order to calcu-late the correlation between the EMIC and the SCID in diagnosing cases of panic disorder. This was found to be statistically significant (Pearson chi-square = 3.84, p = 0.05), indicating that both interviews were identifying essentially the same subgroup of patients as suffering from panic disorder.

Out of the sixty subjects in our sample who received SCID evaluations, twenty were diagnosed with panic disorder. Exclusively on the basis of the clinicians' as-sessment, the overlap between panic disorder and *ataque de nervios* in this data set is determined to be 33 percent.

Discussion

It should be clear at this point that the position that *ataques de nervios* are only cul-turally inflected panic attacks is not tenable. Our EMIC findings show that only about a third of *ataques* fulfill *DSM–IV* criteria for panic attacks. In terms of panic disorder, which requires the presence of additional clinical features, the overlap using this approach is even smaller. EMIC assessments show that when subjects are asked about the clinical elements of panic with respect to their *ataque* experiences, only 17 percent of *ataques* fulfill *DSM–IV* criteria for panic disorder.

The overlap between panic disorder and *ataque* increases to 33 percent when SCID evaluations are used to diagnose panic episodes on the basis of *DSM–III–R* criteria, a similar proportion to the 33 to 41 percent range of overlap found in a previ-ous study by our group (Liebowitz et al. 1994). Although not large, the discrepancy in rates of overlap obtained with our two interviews (17 percent versus 33 percent) suggests that the methodological differences between the EMIC and the SCID out-lined earlier did impact somewhat the process of diagnosing panic disorder. Whether this result is due to the two sets of *DSM* panic criteria used or to differences in the

Table 6.6 Relationship between the number and type of symptoms during an *ataque* and other phenomenological features of panic episodes and *ataque*

	N	Panic Symptoms			Ataque Symptoms		
		Mean	t value	p value	Mean	t value	p value
Fear or nervousness during *ataque*							
Present	55	8.3	-5.65	0.0001 **	3.6	-2.99	0.004 **
Absent	11	2.3			1.8		
Crescendo							
≤ 10 minutes	29	8.4	-1.63	0.11	3.6	-0.48	0.63
> 10 minutes	31	6.8			3.4		
People present during *ataque*							
Yes	54	7.7	-0.79	0.43	3.4	0.25	0.81
No	8	6.6			3.6		
Felt better after *ataque*							
Yes	36	6.7	2.76	0.008 **	3.5	-0.12	0.91
No	27	9.0			3.4		

	n		t	p		t	p
Felt relieved after *ataque*							
Yes	38	6.7	2.89	0.005 **	3.7	-0.10	0.32
No	24	9.1			3.2		
Lifetime number of *ataques*							
One	15	6.2	-1.24	0.22	2.4	-2.15	0.035 *
Two or more	51	7.6			3.6		
Precipitant							
Best-remembered *ataque* provoked	46	7.3	1.40	0.17	3.7	-1.92	0.06
Best-remembered *ataque* unprovoked	17	8.7			2.8		
All *ataques* provoked	33	6.6	-3.75	0.0001 **	3.9	1.25	0.22
All/some *ataques* unprovoked	23	9.7			3.3		
Month-long sequelae afterward							
At least one	53	8.4	-5.35	0.0001 **	3.6	-2.90	0.005 ••
None	13	2.9			2.0		

NOTE: The *t* tests were used to assess the difference in the scale means between the comparison groups. Sample size may vary due to missing data.

*p < .05, **p < .01

Table 6.7   Comparison of panic disorder assessments from EMIC and SCID interviews

		SCID			
		Absent	Subthreshold	Threshold	Total
EMIC	Absent	22	0	6	28
	Subthreshold	12	2	8	22
	Threshold	3	1	6	10
	Total	37	3	20	60

order and emphasis of the interview questions is unclear from our data. However, the EMIC-based approximations to panic disorder correlate significantly with the SCID diagnoses, indicating that these two assessment approaches identify essentially the same clinical phenomenon. Moreover, the issue of different *DSM* criteria does not affect the overlap between *ataques* and panic attacks, because the criteria remained basically unchanged across the two editions of the *DSM*.

The absence of a one-to-one correlation between panic and *ataque* is consistent with past research, which indicates that *ataque* is a more inclusive construct than panic disorder. *Ataques* occurring in the context of depression are associated not with panic features but rather with anger and emotional lability, thus resembling anger attacks more closely than panic disorder (Fava et al. 1990; Salmán et al. 1998). Significant overlap was found in a clinical sample not only between recurrent *ataques* and panic disorder, but also between recurrent *ataques* and dissociative disorders, and there was a trend association with PTSD (Lewis-Fernández et al. 2002, 2005). Finally, epidemiological research showed associations between *ataque* and major depression, dysthymia, generalized anxiety disorder, and PTSD, in addition to panic disorder (Guarnaccia et al. 1993). *Ataque* and panic are not different names for the same experience, but rather alternate constructs that indicate ranges of experience that partially overlap and whose degree of similarity can be empirically established.

Our EMIC data allow us to identify the formal features that characterize *ataques* that are distinct from panic attacks and panic disorder. The advantage of our approach is that the cultural syndrome was taken seriously on its own terms, examined in detail, and only then compared to the full phenomenological description of the psychiatric disorder. Tables 6.3 and 6.5 suggest that, out of the list of panic characteristics, two formal features—absence of a stressful precipitant and a rapid crescendo—constitute the main phenomenological differences between *ataque* episodes that fulfill panic disorder criteria and those that do not. The individual frequencies of these diagnostic elements during *ataque* episodes were 35 percent and 44 percent respectively, which is much lower than the frequencies of the other formal criteria studied—fear or intense discomfort during the attack, the presence of four or more symptoms from the panic list, recurrence, and at least one sequelae of one month duration—which ranged from 74 percent to 83 percent. From the perspective of panic phenomenology, 23 percent of the sample experienced *ataques* that met all the panic attack criteria except for the presence of rapid crescendo. In terms of panic disorder, 35 percent of respondents had *ataques* that would have met *DSM–IV* criteria, except they were provoked, had a slow crescendo, or were distinct from panic episodes in terms of both characteristics. These findings suggest that *ataques* often share individual phenomenological features with panic episodes, but these features do not necessarily run together during the *ataque* experience.

When we examined the EMIC data from the perspective of past research on prototypical *ataque* features rather than on panic characteristics, we also found that certain features distinguished those *ataques* that did not resemble panic episodes from those that did. Patients who reported feeling better or relieved after their episodes endorsed significantly fewer panic symptoms than subjects who did not report this, suggesting that feeling relief after an episode is a sign of an *ataque* that does not fulfill panic criteria. In addition, there was a statistical trend for provoked episodes to be associated with a larger number of prototypical *ataque* symptoms, suggesting that the presence of a precipitant is associated with *ataque* phenomenologies distinct from panic disorder. However, the presence of certain formal features during episodes—such as the experience of fear, month-long sequelae, and recurrence—was significantly associated with a larger mean number of both prototypical *ataque* and panic symptoms. This result could indicate that what we have considered prototypical *ataque* symptoms should be seen instead as nonspecific markers of episode severity. Alternatively, it could mean that these formal features are not exclusive to *ataques* that fulfill panic disorder criteria, but rather are characteristic of most *ataques*, independently of their relationship to panic.

These analyses provide important indicators for distinguishing the features that are shared between *ataques* and panic disorder from those that are not. *Ataques* that are distinct from panic disorder episodes appear to be provoked by some important life event, to peak in longer than ten minutes, and to be followed by a sense of relief rather than by intense fear or dread. On the other hand, features that seem common to both *ataque* and panic disorder include recurrence of attacks, the experience of fear or nervousness during an episode, and anticipatory or behavioral sequelae afterward. These indicators confirm some of the distinctions included in the Glossary of Culture-Bound Syndromes that appeared in Appendix I of *DSM–IV* (APA 1994:845) and provide some guidance to clinicians on how to diagnose patients presenting with *ataques de nervios*.

One key difference between *ataque* and panic that needs to be taken into account by clinicians intent on treating someone suffering from *ataques* is the very different emphases given by the popular and the professional perspectives to the issue of provoked episodes. What is evident about the current definition of panic disorder is that for contemporary mental health professionals the most interesting kind of anxiety attack is the one that is unprovoked. From the professional perspective, this emphasis is seen to facilitate clarification of the neurophysiological and cognitive mechanisms that underlie fear and anxiety, with potentially dramatic research and treatment implications.

For the popular nosology, however, the point of the *ataque* label is to make a comment on the stressors that produced the reaction. There the point is lost if we focus on the biological aspects or the psychological mechanisms giving rise to unprovoked experience. From the local perspective, provoked attacks are more the stuff of life, of reaction to difficulty, and as such, a matter for popular discussion. Unprovoked attacks are less central, because they are much less common than provoked distress, given the wealth of adversity that surrounds the lives of most low-income Latinos. For example, Table 6.5 shows that provoked *ataques* are three to four times more common than unprovoked ones.

These different perspectives have real consequences when it comes to what treatment is expected and recommended, and to how the congruence or incongruence of treatment and expectation affects the clinician-patient relationship. If the body gone haywire is the focus, then medication has a more obvious appeal. But if the stressor is the point, then a treatment that copes with the environment is more congruent with the patient's expectations. Clinicians treating persons with *ataques* should determine the explanatory model of the patient and his or her social network in order to ensure the patient's participation in treatment. The fact that only 35 percent of the subjects in our study reported a history of unprovoked *ataques* suggests that perhaps most persons with *ataques* may expect to receive a psychosocial intervention as part of their treatment regimen (Lewis-Fernández et al. 2005).

Two clinical accounts taken from integrative interviews carried out at the ADC that consolidated the ethnographic and diagnostic material may serve to illustrate the life contexts of persons suffering from *ataques*, which in turn would help predict their treatment expectations. The first account involves a fifty-three-year-old Puerto Rican woman with a history of both *ataques* and panic attacks. Her *ataques* began before her panic episodes as a result of conflicts with her daughter, who was involved with drugs. Her *ataques* were always provoked and caused considerable distress. She also suffered intermittent, spontaneous panic attacks, but these were relatively mild and didn't occur often enough to meet the criteria for panic disorder. Her principal diagnoses on the SCID were major depressive disorder and PTSD.

The second case involves a forty-year-old woman from the Dominican Republic. Her first *ataque* occurred after the death of her daughter, who was hit by a car and killed. The subsequent nine *ataques* occurred following arguments with other people close to her. All of these episodes were provoked by some crisis in the family. Although she suffered considerable anxiety, it was not in the form of panic attacks. Her profound loss shaped her emotional life. Despite her traumatic experience, she did not meet the SCID criteria for PTSD, but instead received diagnoses of major depressive disorder and generalized anxiety disorder.

These cases indicate that social context is central not only to understanding how the person's diverse diagnoses come together as lived experience, including the person's relationship to popular syndromes such as *ataque*, but also to helping direct the clinician to the areas of the person's life and relationships that are in need of therapeutic psychosocial intervention. Ultimately, *ataque* and panic disorder are labels for overlapping categories of experience rather than mutually exclusive sets. The forms of suffering they codify are mediated similarly by social adversity, individual vulnerabilities, and cultural forces, which also give shape to the other psychiatric disorders that accompany them. An anthropologically informed psychiatric practice should neglect neither the biologically based study and treatment of anxiety states and disorders nor the social and cultural factors that influence their onset and phenomenology as well as the therapeutic expectations of sufferers.

Acknowledgments

The research for this paper was supported by a Program Project Grant of the National Institute of Mental Health. The principal investigator was Donald Klein (5 PO1 MH037592). Roberto Lewis-Fernández was supported by grants from the MacArthur Foundation's Mind-Body Network and the Nathan Cummings Foundation. Igda Martínez was supported by Project L/EARN at the Institute for Health, Health Care Policy and Aging Research. The authors would like to thank Kim Diamond, João Silvestre, Ivan Balán, Sharon Davies, Deborah Goetz, and Shu-Hsing Lin for their help obtaining and managing the data for this chapter.

References

American Psychiatric Association (APA). 1994. *Diagnostic and Statistical Manual of Mental Disorders*. 4th ed. [*DSM–IV.*] Washington, DC: American Psychiatric Association.
Ballenger, J. C., and A. J. Fyer. 1996. Panic Disorder and Agoraphobia. In *DSM-IV Sourcebook*. T. A. Widiger, A. J. Frances, H. A. Pincus, R. Ross, M. B. First, and W. W. Davis, eds. Pp. 411–471. Washington, DC: American Psychiatric Association.
Fava, M., K. Anderson, and J. F. Rosenbaum. 1990. "Anger Attacks": Possible Variants of Panic and Major Depressive Disorders. *American Journal of Psychiatry* 147:867–870.
Good, B. J., and A. Kleinman. 1985. Culture and Anxiety: Cross-Cultural Evidence for the Patterning of Anxiety Disorders. In *Anxiety and the Anxiety Disorders*. A. H. Tuma and J. D. Maser, eds. Pp. 297–323. Hillsdale, NJ: Erlbaum.

Guarnaccia, P. J., G. Canino, M. Rubio-Stipec, and M. Bravo. 1993. The Prevalence of *Ataques de Nervios* in the Puerto Rico Disaster Study. *Journal of Nervous and Mental Disease* 181:157–165.

Guarnaccia, P. J., M. Rivera, F. Franco, and C. Neighbors. 1996. The Experiences of *Ataques de Nervios:* Towards an Anthropology of Emotions in Puerto Rico. *Culture, Medicine, and Psychiatry* 20:343–367.

Lewis-Fernández, R. 1996. Diagnosis and Treatment of *Nervios* and *Ataques* in a Female Puerto Rican Migrant. *Culture, Medicine, and Psychiatry* 20(2):155–163.

Lewis-Fernández, R., P. Garrido-Castillo, M. Bennasar, E. Parrilla, A. Laria, G. Ma, and E. Petkova. 2002. Dissociation, Childhood Trauma, and *Ataque de Nervios* Among Puerto Rican Psychiatric Outpatients. *American Journal of Psychiatry* 159:1603–1605.

Lewis-Fernández, R., P. J. Guarnaccia, S. Patel, D. Lizardi, and N. Díaz. 2005. *Ataque de Nervios:* Anthropological, Epidemiological, and Clinical Dimensions of a Cultural Syndrome. In *Perspectives in Cross-Cultural Psychiatry.* A. M. Georgiopoulos and J. F. Rosenbaum, eds. Pp. 63–85. Philadelphia: Lippincott Williams and Wilkins.

Liebowitz, M. R. 1996. Anxiety Disorders. In *DSM–IV Sourcebook.* T. A. Widiger, A. J. Frances, H. A. Pincus, R. Ross, M. B. First, and W. W. Davis, eds. Pp. 397–410. Washington, DC: American Psychiatric Association.

Liebowitz, M. R., E. Salmán, C. M. Jusino, R. Garfinkel, L. Street, D. L. Cárdenas, J. Silvestre, A. J. Fyer, J. L. Carrasco, S. Davies, P. Guarnaccia, and D. F. Klein. 1994. *Ataque de Nervios* and Panic Disorder. *American Journal of Psychiatry* 151(6):871–875.

Salmán, E., M. R. Liebowitz, P. J. Guarnaccia, C. M. Jusino, R. Garfinkel, L. Street, D. L. Cárdenas, J. Silvestre, A. J. Fyer, J. L. Carrasco, S. O. Davies, and D. F. Klein. 1998. Subtypes of *Ataques de Nervios:* The Influence of Coexisting Psychiatric Diagnoses. *Culture, Medicine, and Psychiatry* 22:231–244.

Spitzer, R. L., J.B.W. Williams, M. Gibbon, and M. B. First. 1992. The Structured Clinical Interview for DSM-III-R (SCID): History, Rationale, and Description. *Archives of General Psychiatry* 49:624–629.

Stein, M. B., J. R. Walker, G. Anderson, A. L. Hazen, C. A. Ross, G. Eldridge, and D. R. Forde. 1996. Childhood Physical and Sexual Abuse in Patients with Anxiety Disorders and in a Community Sample. *American Journal of Psychiatry* 153(2):275–277.

Weiss, M. 1997. Explanatory Model Interview Catalogue (EMIC): Framework for Comparative Study of Illness. *Transcultural Psychiatry* 34(2):235–263.

7

Dizziness and Panic in China

Organ and Ontological Disequilibrium

Lawrence Park and Devon E. Hinton

IN MANDARIN CHINESE, the term for *dizziness* is *tou yun*, literally, "circular motions in the head" (*tou*, "head"; *yun*, "circular motion"). *Tou yun* indicates a variety of physical sensations, including lightheadedness, general instability, head discomfort, syncope, and true vertigo, that is, the sensation of oneself or of the surrounding world spinning. Upon describing themselves as *tou you*, patients often make circular hand motions near the head.

Dizziness is a common presenting symptom for Chinese patients. Panic is not. Chinese do not typically recount to others, "I am having panic attacks," but acute episodes of distress resembling Western panic are discernable. In one study of patients with neurasthenia—a common professional and popular illness category in China—35 percent were found to have panic disorder (Kleinman 1982). Panic is experienced in China, but it manifests in locally specific forms.

Distress ontology is influenced by the theoretical models available to individuals to understand their suffering. Kleinman employs the concept of *explanatory model* to refer to "the notions about an episode of sickness and its treatment that are employed by all those engaged in the clinical process" (1980:105). Such explanatory models often emerge from fundamental principles of a culture (Good 1994); epistemic systems provide the theoretical framework for shaping how individuals explicate, experience, and create meaning from suffering. Two unique systems of medical understanding coexist in contemporary China: biology-based Western medicine and traditional Chinese medicine (TCM). TCM is an indigenous system of medicine, developed empirically over the past four thousand years of Chinese history and intimately related to traditional Chinese thought. Western biomedicine, by contrast, is a relative newcomer, having been introduced in China within the past two to three hundred years.

Preliminary ethnography in a Chinese psychiatric clinic by this chapter's first author revealed that panic patients often had dizziness as a presenting complaint, and that the experience of dizziness and panic was shaped by TCM, an indigenous theory focusing on the functioning and interaction of the *zang fu*, that is, the organs—such as the heart (*xin*), liver (*gan*), spleen (*pi*), kidney (*shen*), lung (*fei*), and gallbladder (*gan dan*)—as conceptualized within TCM. The first author found that depending on the disequilibrium of the implicated organ, dizziness-focused panic varied greatly in terms of associated mental and physical symptoms, interpersonal meanings, and treatment, and that the degree of dizziness and panic corresponded to the state of disequilibrium of the organ system as well as to the instability of the social, interpersonal, and environmental context of the patient.

In this chapter, we first present the results of a clinical survey of psychiatric disorders that demonstrates dizziness to be characteristic of Chinese anxiety states, most particularly panic. We then present three representative cases of dizziness-focused panic that involve the traditional Chinese organ systems of *liver*, *kidney*, and *heart*, respectively. In these cases, dizziness and associated symptoms intensify to the point of panic, with dizziness and panic serving as experiential analogs of general disharmony and disequilibrium. In the discussion section of the chapter, we illustrate how in the Chinese context dizziness serves as a key symptom, and that it may precipitate panic by its semantic networks (such as dizziness-related metaphors and ethnophysiology), by its links within the sociosomatic reticulum (that is, dizziness as an embodiment of social, economic, political, and existential distress, an embodiment guided by metaphor and other processes), and by its importance in local biology (that is, a strong predisposition to actually experiencing dizziness through biological mechanisms).

Methods

Tianjin Mental Health Hospital is a three-hundred-bed psychiatric hospital in Tianjin, an industrial city of approximately ten million inhabitants in northeastern China. The hospital is a secondary-care facility within the biomedical system of health care delivery. Its staff of ten physicians were all trained in the Western biomedical model, including specialized training in psychiatry. Diagnosis is made by physicians using the *Chinese Classification of Mental Disorders* (*CCMD-II*), which is based on the *International Statistical Classification of Diseases* (*ICD-9*; Lee 1996; Zheng et al. 1994). Typical treatments include psychopharmacology (tricyclic antidepressants, benzodiazepines, antipsychotics), psychotherapy (cognitive-behavioral, psychodynamic, supportive), insulin-shock therapy, and an assortment of milieu-based techniques (music therapy, art therapy, electrical therapy).

The study investigated the diagnosis and illness experience of patients who consecutively presented to Tianjin Mental Health Hospital over a three-month period. The first author, a Western-trained psychiatrist, used the *DSM–IV* to assess diagnosis, and a semistructured-interview format to investigate presenting symptoms, associated symptoms, course of illness, treatment response, and patient beliefs about diagnosis, illness etiology, and prognosis. Interviews were audio-recorded and transcribed. Of eighty-two possible study participants, eighty agreed to participate. Consent was obtained prior to study participation.

Results

The *DSM–IV* diagnosis of the eighty participants is presented in Table 7.1. Fifty-one percent of the patients had an anxiety-disorder diagnosis, with 13 percent of all patients meeting *DSM–IV* criteria for panic disorder. Dizziness was a prominent presenting complaint for 33 percent (26/80) of the entire sample, and it was particularly associated with anxiety states: among patients with generalized anxiety disorder, 50 percent (10/20) had prominent dizziness as a presenting complaint; among panic disorder patients it was 80 percent (8/10).

Table 7.1 Distribution of psychiatric disorders in Tianjin, People's Republic of China

Diagnosis	Number of patients	Percentage of total patients (N = 80)
Major depressive disorder	22	28
GAD	20	25
Schizophrenia	11	14
Panic disorder	10	13
OCD	9	11
Adjustment disorder	8	10
Phobias	5	6
Personality disorder	4	5
Somatoform disorder	1	1
Epilepsy	1	1
Mental retardation	1	1
Dementia	1	1

NOTE: Total percentage of diagnosed disorders is greater than 100 percent because some patients had multiple diagnoses. GAD means generalized anxiety disorder, OCD means obsessive-compulsive disorder.

Cases

Analysis revealed that most of the ten patients with panic disorder had periodic dizziness that ultimately—after months or years—resulted in episodes in which the dizziness escalated to panic. In several other cases, the first experience of dizziness escalated to panic. The patients with panic disorder thought the cause to be various organ disturbances. The following three cases are representative of the experience of dizziness and panic in China, with each patient attributing the disorder to a TCM-defined pathophysiological process involving a particular organ. As shown later, despite similarities at a general level (that is, in the fact of having panic), each patient's dizziness and panic experience was quite different from the others, depending on the implicated organ.

Case 1: Flaring of Liver-Fire ('Gan Huo Shang Yan')

Ms. X was forty-six years old at the time of her presentation to the clinic. She lived in Beijing with her husband, daughter, and son, working in a government construction work unit as an architect.

She had been treated at a psychiatric clinic several years prior to the current presentation and had been diagnosed with neurasthenia (literally, "nerve weakness," or *shen jing shuai ruo*). At that time she felt increasingly distressed after her work group refused her request to pursue a master's degree at the planning institute. Underlying her desire to pursue further education was the feeling of falling behind her peer group—a feeling that, compared to her index peer group, her standing in society was falling. This conflict with her work-unit leaders and the turmoil in the workplace resulted in insomnia and dizziness. As conflicts at work increased, so too did her distress and frustration. The work unit finally allowed her to transfer to another work unit that would give her permission to return to school.

Upon returning to the planning institute, she was unpleasantly surprised by the increased level of stress and competition. Compared to what she described as the "harmony and equality" of the Cultural Revolution and her undergraduate college days, she experienced competition between herself and her current peers, and felt like she was "falling behind" again. "Before, we all worked together. We all felt happy together or unhappy together. But now things are different." The competitive atmosphere led to insomnia and dizziness. Ms. X sought treatment from both TCM and Western medical practitioners. Her symptoms remitted only after psychiatric hospitalization and transfer to yet another work unit. Since that time she has suffered intermittently from insomnia and dizziness, but until the current presentation she had not been hospitalized.

The recent worsening occurred when Ms. X's work unit, because of her slow progress in her studies, denied her request to continue her studies. She once more requested transfer to a different work unit. The escalation of personal conflicts and arguments at her work unit was accompanied by an intensification of anger, anxiety, and irritability. These symptoms were superimposed on her chronic symptoms of insomnia and dizziness. Her symptoms worsened upon going to an architectural exhibition in Beijing; while there she felt extremely angry, and upon returning home her anger and irritability did not subside but rather intensified. She began to experience headaches and neck pains. Anything that reminded her of work or career exacerbated her distress. One day, while drafting at home, Ms. X felt very nervous, and this anxiety increased, leading to an attack of dizziness, headache, body aches, tremulousness, and sweating.

The attacks became more frequent and severe. During these acute attacks, her chronic dizziness became far more severe, reaching the point of panic. The attacks occurred frequently at work. Just thinking about the conflicts at work, whether she was actually at work or just drafting at home, caused an attack. She became increasingly nervous, her insomnia worsened, and she developed agoraphobia-like symptoms. Being on the street often made her so nervous that she had to return home; she found it almost impossible to leave the house, even to buy food at the market.

To treat her symptoms, Ms. X first went to a TCM practitioner; he diagnosed "flaring of liver-fire" (*gan huo shang yan*). Supporting this diagnosis, palpation of the wrist revealed a pulse that was full, wiry, and rapid, and examination of the mouth revealed a tongue with a yellow coating. Other typical diagnostic signs included outbursts of anger, headaches, dizziness, disturbed sleep, and rubor (redness) of the eyes, face, and tongue. Herbal medications (such as *long dan xie gan*) were prescribed to treat the liver-fire and insomnia, but without significant benefit.

Already familiar with the Western psychiatric system from her previous admission for neurasthenia, Ms. X sought treatment at Anding Hospital; from there she was referred to Tianjin Mental Health Hospital for hospitalization. Ms. X was diagnosed with anxiety and panic attacks, and prescribed amitriptyline and benzodiazepines to be taken on an as-needed basis. In addition to pharmacotherapy, she received cognitive therapy and biofeedback. At the time of the interview, no significant symptom improvement had occurred, and she was losing hope of recovery.

From Ms. X's perspective, her illness was caused by the work unit's not allowing her to continue her education. She felt it was unfair to hinder her career advancement, and that this hindrance led to chronic discord with the work-unit leaders. Arguments with others in her work unit, general societal pressures, and fears of sinking social standing all combined to cause her feelings of instability and inequity, which translated to a physical sensation of dizziness. External turmoil was experienced as internal disequilibrium.

Ms. X made sense of her suffering primarily through traditional beliefs, stating that it was the conflicts that led to her illness. According to TCM, as the conflicts increased, Ms. X experienced increasing anger, that is, "rising *qi*" (*sheng qi*), which corresponded to the liver-fire pathology, a common manifestation of excess rising *qi*. With increasing anger, the liver-fire rose to the head and exacerbated the sensation of dizziness. Fueled by the chaos and turmoil of the external situation, anger and dizziness intensified and ultimately led to the onset of panic symptoms.

Panic, for Ms. X, was a state of excessive mental agitation resulting in extreme disequilibrium—a feeling of being completely overwhelmed on every sensory level. Associated with the panic were agoraphobia symptoms, which served to isolate Ms. X in her home, which effectively decreased her interpersonal contact and the possibility of turmoil but did not lead to reduction of dizziness and panic. Although she attempted to obtain relief from both TCM and Western practitioners, her understanding of her suffering was firmly rooted in the traditional belief system.

Case 2: Deficiency of Kidney-Yin ('Shen Yin Xu')

Ms. Y, a thirty-two-year-old married woman with no previous psychiatric history, lived with her husband and twelve-month-old daughter in Tianjin, where she worked as an accountant for a private business. Her symptoms began six months prior to presentation. She began feeling fatigue and lower back pains, and she ascribed these symptoms to "kidney weakness" (*shen xu*). Six months prior to the onset of the symptoms, Ms. Y gave birth to a baby daughter. She felt herself predisposed to kidney weakness because of giving birth at the advanced age of thirty-one years. After the infant's birth, Ms. Y had to care for her and continue her work as an accountant. She also referred to her illness as "obstruction in the heart" (*xin li zhang ai*), a popular lay term used to describe general psychological distress. Her own feelings of being more pressured emerged, she asserted, in parallel with changes in Chinese society, such as technological advances, and increasing financial competition, which increased her fear and uncertainty.

After six months of maternity leave, Ms. Y was required to return to her job. She felt great fear and uncertainty about the return to work because of the rapidity of change in the workplace, and in Chinese society more generally. She found that the work unit had been restructured and she no longer felt able to do her assigned tasks. Ms. Y heard her work-unit leaders making comments about younger workers being better than older ones. Fearing the loss of her position, she requested transfer to a different job but was denied; moreover, Ms. Y began feeling increasingly fatigued from caring for her child while simultaneously working. The more she thought about her work predicament, the more fearful she became about her career future and her ability to care for her child.

Ms. Y began to experience frequent headaches, another sign of kidney disorder. Then one day at work she experienced intense body aches and severe dizziness that worsened to a state of terror, severe agitation, and confusion. After that initial episode, Ms. Y did not go to work for a period, but the episodes began to occur at home as well. She became quite hopeless, losing her appetite and having frequent crying spells throughout the day. Her hopeless feelings developed into depression, and at one point she even contemplated suicide.

Initially Ms. Y sought treatment from a TCM practitioner. It was suspected that her symptoms were related to her postpartum state, and she was diagnosed as having a deficiency of *yin* in her kidney (*shen yin xu*), or in both her kidney and her spleen (*shen pi yin xu*). Kidney involvement was indicated by the fact that the illness was precipitated by parturition and work stress. The TCM physical examination was consistent with kidney-*yin* deficiency: a red tongue with no coating, and a floating and rapid pulse. Spleen involvement was implicated by depressed mood and poor appetite. Herbal treatment (*shan yao* and *tu si zi*) was prescribed to increase *yin* in the kidney and spleen. With herbal treatment, her symptoms initially remitted.

After these therapeutic interventions, Ms. Y returned to work, but under the stress of work combined with caring for a newborn child, she quickly suffered a recurrence of symptoms, particularly fear, dizziness, and headache. She returned to the TCM practitioner at her work unit; he again diagnosed deficiency of kidney-*yin* and suggested acupuncture to increase it. The four acupuncture points to be targeted (*guan yuan, tai xi, zhao hai,* and *yin gu*) were located on meridians related to particular organ systems.

Ms. Y's symptoms remitted after several acupuncture treatments, but again quickly returned after stopping treatment. This time she did not want to go back to the TCM practitioner. After her sister advised seeking treatment at a Western psychiatric facility, she went to the outpatient psychiatric clinic and was admitted to Tianjin Mental Health Hospital. She was diagnosed with panic-type anxiety and with depression, and was started on amitriptyline and given cognitive therapy. Significant improvement was noted from these treatments.

As in the first case presented, Ms. Y viewed her illness through the TCM explanatory model; however, unlike Ms. X, she considered her dizziness to represent a state of weakness or deficit. The patient reported her difficulties as resulting from multiple stressors in her life; the most significant initial stressor, from her perspective, was the late age of childbirth. In addition, she identified mental and physical overwork, as well as fear, as contributing to her illness. Back soreness, given the physical proximity to the kidneys, is commonly viewed as a symptom of kidney weakness. The stress of simultaneously working and caring for her child continued to weaken kidney-*qi* (and kidney-*yin*). She began to experience more general body aches and dizziness. Also, according to TCM physiology, the internal physiological stress of childbirth and the external stressors of childrearing and work led to kidney weakness. Parturition depleted *jing* (sexual essence), a substance stored in the kidney. Chronic overwork, particularly mental overwork, diminished the kidney-*yin*. Deficiency of kidney-*yin* resulted in fearfulness, mouth dryness at night, soreness of the back and waist, body aches, and dizziness. According to TCM, "kidney-*yin* deficiency (and *yin* deficiency in general) leads to a state where the marrow is not sufficiently nourished. When the marrow is weak, it is unable to rise to nourish the brain. This can result in dizziness" (Veith 1949).

Case 3: Heart Weakness ('Xin Xu')

The forty-two-year-old Mr. Z lived with his wife and one child in Tianjin, where he operated a silverware kiln at a tableware factory. His symptoms began suddenly one month prior to presentation. While at home he experienced the acute onset of a sensation that his heart was "twitching." He did not note any acute precipitant for the episode. Although for several years prior to this experience Mr. Z had experienced several symptoms—intermittent dizziness, mild palpitations, pressure on the chest, difficulty breathing—he had not sought out any treatment. Several days after his first panic attack, he had another episode of the sudden onset of "heart twitching," dizziness, shortness of breath, and anxiety. The symptoms intensified until he had difficulty breathing and felt paralyzed, as if about to die. Most of the symptoms resolved after several minutes, but numbness and the inability to speak continued for approximately one hour. Mr. Z thought his distress might be a result of heart weakness (*xin xu*). He went to a Western hospital for a medical checkup. An electrocardiogram was done and demonstrated no abnormality, so he was discharged to home without any treatment.

Mr. Z continued to have episodes of dizziness, palpitations, and a sensation of "stuffiness in the chest." He also developed chronic tremulousness and became too anxious to sleep soundly. He began to drink large amounts of alcohol at night to fall asleep, which was marginally successful. He became more irritable and developed a fear of noisy and crowded places. Mr. Z was unable to leave his apartment because he found the street too crowded and "disgusting." His agitation increased to the point that he was bothered by his wife and child watching television, because it was "too noisy and disorderly."

Because acute panic episodes continued to occur once or twice a week, Mr. Z sought treatment at Western medical clinics, but no medical cause was identified, and all other treatments he received, including nitroglycerin and atropine (medications usually given for a serious heart condition), were ineffective. He then went to see a TCM practitioner, who diagnosed his condition as "unpeaceful heart" (*xin zhang bu an*), a condition resulting from a weakness of *yin* and *yang* in the heart (*xin yin yang xu*). Typical of unpeaceful heart, and of heart weakness, were palpitations, chest pressure, dizziness, and shortness of breath. Mr. Z was prescribed acupuncture and herbal medicines, which resulted in minimal improvement. One of the TCM practitioners recommended that he go to see a mental health care practitioner. Upon presenting to Tianjin Mental Health Hospital, Mr. Z had suffered five more panic attacks in the previous month. He was admitted to the hospital and treated with amitriptyline and benzodiazepines, resulting in improvement.

Mr. Z believed that his illness was a result of multiple hardships in his life. He was born in Beijing and at fifteen years of age his family moved to Gansu province in Western China, during the Cultural Revolution. Life was very difficult. Often he did not have enough to eat, and his father was not allowed to live with the family but instead was subjected to the indignity of having to live in a cowshed. After residing in Gansu for two years, Mr. Z lived in various other places in China, including Tang Shan. While he was living in Tang Shan, a major earthquake struck the area, resulting in great destruction and many deaths. Although Mr. Z and his family were not injured, he looked back on this event as extremely upsetting, as an indicator of the overall turmoil of his life. He considered that his "fate [was] bad," that bad luck predisposed him to encountering situations of chaos, adversity, and disharmony.

Mr. Z thought that the arduous nature of his work was the proximal reason for developing heart weakness. Work pressure led to significant mental and physical strain. Because the tableware factory was exporting products to the United States, the demand for quality was very high. His work was strenuous and involved laboring in very hot conditions, which he thought predisposed him to heart instability and weakness. Several days prior to his initial panic episode, his work-unit leader said something that deeply upset him—that he needed "first-rate workers" to meet quality and production goals, and that younger workers were better because they were stronger.

According to Mr. Z, the combination of these physical and mental pressures overloaded and ultimately weakened his heart. The remarks of his work-unit leader served as the acute precipitant of the panic attacks. From Mr. Z's perspective, he was having a problem with his heart. He went to both Western and TCM practitioners, who treated him for heart problems but to no avail. Mr. Z also identified a number of areas of instability in his past life that contributed to his present illness. Reminiscing about his past, he described instability in family life and social upheaval. He also described the destruction and instability of environmental events, that is, the Tang Shan earthquake, as indicative of disharmony throughout his life.

From Mr. Z's perspective, which was derived from TCM, his distress resulted from heart deficiency. His heart efficiency was impaired so that blood was unable to nourish the brain adequately, resulting in dizziness; as the deficiency state worsened, anxiety and agitation occurred, and increased to the point of extreme agitation, panic, and confusion. Dizziness indicated that the heart was deficient and unable to support other organs. Owing to the heart's relationship to activation states, Mr. Z's dizziness was accompanied by anxiety and agitation. As the heart became too weak to support the brain, panic attacks mixed with symptoms of confusion and paralysis ensued.

Discussion

Dizziness was a common aspect of dysphoria among patients treated at the Tianjin Mental Health Hospital in China and was strongly associated with anxiety states, especially panic disorder. Among all patients, 33 percent presented with prominent dizziness; among patients with panic disorder it was 80 percent. The three cases just presented illustrate how dizziness may result from the experiencing of disharmony and disequilibrium, how it may escalate to panic, and how its attribution to a specific organ system implicates certain pathophysiological processes and has specific interpersonal meanings. Excessive conflict, progressive depletion, and chronic overload led to disequilibrium in any of various organ systems, and to organ-caused dizziness, and as disharmony and disequilibrium increased, symptoms became greater in number and intensity, to the point of panic. The initial symptom constellation included dizziness, a sensation resulting from the experience of disequilibrium; and as disequilibrium intensified, the symptoms became more severe, and different types of symptoms resulted until distress culminated in panic.

Dizziness as Paradigmatic Symptom in China

Kleinman and Kleinman (1994) have described dizziness as one of three paradigmatic symptoms in China (along with exhaustion and pain). They claim that "dizziness, a common though usually unmarked symptom of neurasthenia and other chronic fatigue syndromes in the West, carries particular salience in Chinese society, where the Chinese medical tradition emphasizes balance and harmony as constitutive and expressive of health" (1994:715). In China, they further explain, dizziness is an embodiment of social suffering and trauma:

> To be dizzy (or vertiginous; Chinese patients do not make a distinction between the two) is to be unbalanced, to experience malaise, to be dis-eased. Dizziness was understood by our informants to be the embodiment of alienation, the felt meaning of delegitimation in their local words. The broken moral order of local worlds was quite literally dizzying. To experience dizziness was to live and relive the memory of trauma. [Kleinman and Kleinman 1994:715]

Dizziness and Panic in China: The Symbolic and Biological Bridges of the Sociosomatic Reticulum

Why is dizziness a key aspect of the Chinese distress ontology, particularly its anxiety ontology? In this section we try to answer this question, examining dizziness in the Chinese context from the perspective of biology, ethnophysiology, metaphor, natural and built environment (that is, the environmental surround), and socioeconopolitical context. Put another way, if dizziness constitutes a key part of the sociosomatic reticulum in China, what are the specific "symbolic bridges" (Kleinman and Kleinman 1985)—and local biological mechanisms—by which dizziness links social processes and trauma to bodily and personal experience? To answer these questions requires an examination of dizziness's "semantic networks" (Good 1977), its link to biology, environmental surround, and social context.

Biology and Dizziness   Scientific studies show Chinese populations to be much more predisposed than Western populations to experiencing dizziness, as evidenced by a greater sensitivity to the spinning motions of a surrounding drum (see Chapter 3). The reasons may be biological, cultural, or a combination of both. This local biology would be expected to result in increased sensitivity to dizziness triggers (such as seeing a spinning object, being in a complex visual situation, or the back-and-forth turning of the head), a tendency to experience dizziness when distressed, and increased conditioning of dizziness to traumatic events, all of which would have profound effects on the ontology of anxiety and panic (Hinton and Hinton 2002).

The Ethnophysiology of Dizziness and Panic: The Zang Fu System   TCM is a complete system of medicine, comprising a physiology based on fundamental substances and *zang fu*, a theory of pathogenesis, and a method of diagnosis and treatment. The fundamental concepts of TCM, such as its theories about *zang fu* functioning, are common knowledge to both TCM practitioners and laypersons. Although Western biomedicine has made significant inroads into Chinese culture, traditional Chinese beliefs still play the primary role in shaping the meaning and experience of suffering. Most distressed Chinese will not hesitate to seek treatment from either institution, but when asked about their understanding and experience of suffering, explanations invariably remain rooted in traditional models. Five organs—each corresponding to one of the five elements, to a "role," and to certain functions (see Table 7.2)—play a key role in the TCM physiology. We now describe in more depth the functions and correspondences of the three organs (liver, heart, and kidney) that played a major role in the three cases.

The liver (*gan*) corresponds to the wood element. Wood is associated with storage and growth (Porkert and Ullmann 1982:97); analogously, the liver is said to store and regulate blood, and to maintain the smooth flow of *qi* and blood throughout

Table 7.2 Organ functions and correspondences

Organ	Element	Activity	Role
Kidney	Water	Stores *jing* (life essence) Controls reproduction and development Regulates water metabolism Controls and promotes inspiration	Mighty official
Liver	Wood	Regulates the flow of *qi* and blood Stores blood Ensures a free-and-easy internal environment	Commander
Heart	Fire	Controls circulation Controls mental activities Produces and houses *shen* (mind)	Prince
Spleen	Earth	Dredges and regulates water passages Coordinates all visceral activities Controls respiration and *qi* (vital energy)	Censor
Lung	Metal	Transforms food into pure essence Sends pure essence upward Maintains blood in the vessels	Minister

the body (Kaptchuk 1983). Because of the liver's regulation of key substances in the body, early TCM texts refer to the liver as the "commander." The liver's role in anger is known by both TCM practitioners and the general population. If the liver is out of harmony, then *qi*—or fire as the manifestation of excess *qi*—may rise into the chest and head. As a result, emotions become out of balance, and this leads to irritation and anger. As irritation and anger intensify, the liver's *qi* and fire may ascend along the meridian to damage the head and eyes, causing "dizziness, distending pain in the head, flushed face and congestion of the eyes" (Liu and Hyodo 1994:274). Liver-fire may worsen and result in anxiety, irritability, stroke, and death (Beijing College of Traditional Medicine 1980:332). Other factors that may adversely affect the liver are wind, dampness, and spicy or greasy food; also, a wind may hit the body and harm the liver, causing the acute onset of anger attacks, neck stiffness, headache, and dizziness (Liu and Hyodo 1994:277).

The heart (*xin*) corresponds to the fire element. Because it controls the circulation, the heart is considered the "prince" of the organs (Porkert and Ullmann 1982:99). The heart has a key role in respect to the emotion of joy, and a special relationship with overall mental functioning. It produces and houses *shen*, meaning "spirit" or "mind"—that is, personality, consciousness, thought, and behavior (Liu and Hyodo 1994:45). A disharmonious heart is accompanied by general mental distress, often experienced as anxiety and agitation. If the heart becomes overloaded, it will fail to nourish itself, leading to palpitations, agitation, and insomnia; if undernourished and weakened, it is unable to nourish other organs adequately,

including the brain, and this may lead to pain, insomnia, and dizziness, even delirium, coma, and death (Liu and Hyodo 1994).

The kidney (*shen*; not related to *shen* as spirit or mind) corresponds to the water
element, and because the kidney regulates water metabolism and controls reproduction and life development, it is known as the "mighty official" (Porkert and Ullmann 1982). The kidney produces and stores *jing* (life essence), which is converted
into semen. *Jing* represents the combined store of inherited and acquired energy
and is the source of an individual's constitution and endurance. The "*jing* (kidney
essence) produces marrow which generates the spinal cord and 'fills up' the brain"
(Maciocia 1989:96). Together, the spinal cord and brain are known as the "sea of
marrow" (*sui hai* [Liu and Hyodo 1994:58]). If "the kidney fails in its function of
producing marrow and filling out the brain, the result is dizziness, blurry vision,
poor memory, and tinnitus" (Beijing College of Traditional Medicine 1980); that
is, a weakened kidney cannot produce sufficient marrow to fill the spinal cord,
so the brain will not receive adequate nourishment (see Figure 7.1). According to

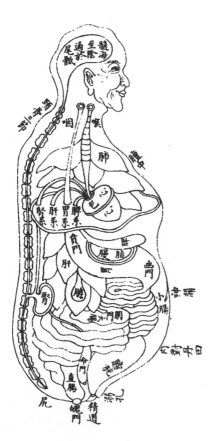

Figure 7.1 The "Sea of Marrow"
NOTES: Diagram taken from *Nei Jing* (published in
1624), the classic text on internal medicine in TCM.
On the left of the diagram, the kidney is shown
directly connected to the spinal cord, with the spinal
cord ascending to connect to the brain. The kidney
is the source of "marrow" that fills and nourishes the
spinal cord and brain. For further discussion of this
image, see Gwei-Djen and Needham 1980.

TCM, the kidney can never have too much *jing*; there are no excess states of the kidney. Many processes, such as overwork, stress, fear, anxiety, and startle, as well as pregnancy, childbirth, and excessive sexual activity, may weaken the kidney and directly deplete *jing*. A weakened kidney and depleted *jing* predispose a person to being timid and fearful; to having symptoms such as dizziness, tinnitus, and deafness; and to panicking (Liu and Hyodo 1994).

Within the overall organ physiology, each organ either promotes or inhibits another organ because of its relationship with an element. This is usually depicted as two cycles (see Figure 7.2). In promotion, one element increases the activity of another: wood promotes fire, fire promotes earth, earth promotes metal, metal promotes water, and water promotes wood. In the control relationship, the effect is one of restriction: wood controls earth, earth controls water, water controls fire, fire controls metal, and metal controls wood. In a manner analogous to the relationships among the five elements, the five organs also demonstrate the interactive cycles of promotion and control in that the activity of each organ is promoted by another organ and controlled by a second (see Figure 7.3).

As described earlier, the master image of health in TCM is that of the harmonious and balanced operation of multiple interlocking cycles of the *zang fu*, a system that also includes the *zang fu*'s associated meridians, with interconnected channels that carry *qi* and blood, linking together the *zang fu*. *Qi* flows within and between organ pairs and their meridians, transferring and transmuting energy as it circulates. For the proper functioning of *qi* and the organ system, there must be harmony and balance not only within the body, but also on multiple nonsomatic levels. The Chinese *zang fu* physiology is not confined to the physical space within

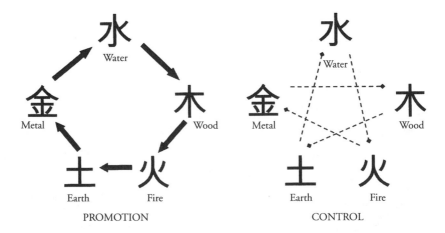

Figure 7.2 The relationship of the five elements

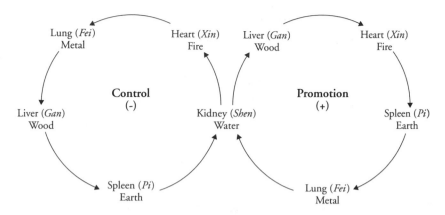

Figure 7.3 The relationships among the five elements and the five organs

the human body or to its mechanical functioning; it has physical, mental, interpersonal, and environmental correlates, all of which may disturb it. When any part of the system—from the body to the emotions to interpersonal relationships to the natural environment—becomes disturbed, so too does the organ system. The physical sensation of dizziness corresponds to initial *zang fu* disequilibrium, and as disequilibrium and disharmony intensify, the physical sensation of dizziness may develop into the more distressing and intense sensation of panic.

Mental states, interpersonal interactions, sociocultural context, political conditions, and environmental variables are all linked within the five-elements theory and that of *zang fu*. Within this system, mental states, that is, emotions and cognitions, may take on various roles; they may be indicators of balanced healthy functioning, symptoms of unbalanced pathological functioning, etiological agents that disrupt balance, or therapeutic agents that restore balance. Anxiety and panic states are indicators that something is amiss. Insofar as they represent a generic state of heightened arousal, anxiety and panic may be related to disharmony of any of the *zang fu*. For the individual, however, the experience of anxiety- and panic-related distress depends on which organ system is out of balance. The sensation of anxiety and panic is shaped by the emotional state and by the pathophysiology that is affiliated with the implicated organ.

Within TCM, primary emotional states correspond to particular organs (see Table 7.3). In contrast to the Cartesian split of mind and body, in TCM the major emotions are closely related to the *zang fu* (see, for example, Zhang 2007). The kidney is related to fear; the heart, to joy; the liver, to anger; the lungs, to grief; and the spleen, to rumination. The gallbladder, in close relationship with the liver, also plays a special role in respect to courage. Specific organ imbalances are associated

Table 7.3 Organs and mental state

Organ	Element	Mental State
Kidney	Water	Fear
Heart	Fire	Joy
Liver	Wood	Anger
Lung	Metal	Grief
Spleen	Earth	Rumination
Gallbladder	Wood	Courage

with specific emotions. Kidney deficiency states are often marked by anxiety, accompanied by feelings of fear and even terror. Dysregulated states of the liver are often associated with feelings of anxiety, irritation, and anger. In lung deficiency states, the individual may experience intense sadness and grief intermingled with anxiety. When the spleen is deficient, rumination, depressed mood, and anxiety may present together.

However, not only does an organ dysfunction cause the correlated emotion, but also the experiencing of an emotion can disrupt the correlated organ. In a general sense, emotions, even those of extreme joy, are considered pathogens. Experiencing emotions too intensely, too frequently, or in an otherwise inappropriate way may lead to imbalance and disharmony. Joy may lead to disturbance of *qi* in the heart, resulting in dizziness as well as disturbance of concentration and memory; excessive joy may lead to increased agitation, delirium, stroke, and possibly death. Anger is said to cause an upward flow of liver-*qi*, which can cause blood to rise to the head, resulting in closure of the orifices of the head, which may lead to syncope and panic. Sadness and grief are said to consume lung-*qi*, which leads to demoralization. Fear causes the kidney's *qi* to become unconsolidated and to sink; this may result in urinary and fecal incontinence. Terror completely interrupts *qi*'s flow and may cause severe confusion and panic. Rumination causes stagnation of *qi*, impairing its function, and preferentially affects the heart and spleen. Disturbance of the spleen's *qi* results in gastrointestinal symptoms, including poor appetite and even anorexia.

Within the TCM theoretical model, dizziness is the experiential manifestation of the imbalance and disequilibrium of the entire system. When the interlocking cycles of *yin* and *yang* and those of the *zang fu* are thrown out of balance, the whole system begins to spin out of control. Dizziness is the initial indicator of this state. Panic may result. Various states of organ pathology, that is, various pathophysiologies, may cause dizziness; in each instance, the associated affect, symptoms, and meaning vary. In "flaring of liver-fire," the liver-fire (or *qi*) ascends to the head and results in dizziness and panic; other common symptoms include anger, insomnia, and headache. If there is a deficiency of the kidney's *yin*, dizziness will result due to decreased *yin* ascending from the kidney to the brain and to decreased marrow ascending from the kidney along the spinal cord to nourish the brain. In kidney deficiency states, common symptoms include dizziness, weakness, tinnitus, cognitive dullness, and great fear. Depletion of the heart's *yin* (or *qi*) can result in poor blood circulation and inadequate nourishment of the brain, leading to dizziness accompanied by agitation and confusion, and a weakened *shen* ("spirit" or "mind"), which will in turn cause impaired mental processing, anxiety, and agitation.

In each of the three cases described in this chapter, a different organ disharmony was implicated. Depending on the implicated organ, each patient had a very different panic ontology, including varying symptoms. Ms. X (Case 1) suffered "flaring-up liver-fire," resulting in dizziness, anger, irritability, and insomnia. Ms. Y (Case 2) suffered kidney-*yin* deficiency, resulting in dizziness, fear, fatigue, and back weakness. Mr. Z (Case 3) had heart deficiency, resulting in dizziness, agitation, confusion, palpitations, and shortness of breath. Depending on the implicated organ, dizziness evokes different dynamic interpretants, pathomechanics, interpersonal meanings, ideas of causation, and ways of redress. (Although not present in any of the three cases, if panic is precipitated by a "wind," then a very different panic ontology is embodied that is also centered on dizziness. See the later discussion of landscape.)

The Metaphoric Resonances of Dizziness

In the Chinese context, just as the social context and workplace are analyzed and experienced in terms of balance or imbalance, harmony or conflict, so too are the *zang fu*. The *zang fu* system serves as a metaphor of Chinese society, and as Chinese society has changed, so too have the ways of talking about the organ system (Taylor 2001). In TCM the terms *organ* (*zang*) and *bowels* (*fu*)

> no longer have the connotations of the pre-Han bureaucratic roles of "depots and granaries" or "palaces." Doctors in contemporary China tend to compare them with the organs (*zangpi*) described in Western biomedicine. Elisabeth Hsu points out that such direct translations, however, fail to represent their functional and spatial interrelatedness, which she compares with that of the interrelatedness of "compartments" within an administrative unit, such as the Socialist work unit (*danwei*). Such a conceptualization of the Chinese medical terms of *zang* and *fu* stresses their existence in relation to one another, a connection which cannot be derived from the Western biomedical model. [Taylor 2001:53]

The *zang fu* system is a metaphor, an icon, of the complex interrelationships of persons within the work unit and within social networks (Taylor 2001). It is a tool that primes people to enact and engage in these complex relationships, to think in terms of such complex interrelatedness, to make these social relations and political systems seem natural; at the same time, the *zang fu* system provides a somatic language for expressing a sense of disharmony and disequilibrium in respect to these relationships and politico-economic structures. TCM healing uses an organ-language that is also a relationship-language, a language that speaks of restoring healthy interrelatedness, of multiple interrelated networks and forces. The *zang fu* system provides a set of metaphors that apply both to the body and to the social and work world.

In all three cases, decreasing social, economic, and political status in the context of a rapidly modernizing society results in a global loss of stability for each patient. The fear of falling in social status seems to be embodied as vertigo in the three cases. As other scholars have noted, as Chinese society engages in explosive development and change, those who do not keep pace experience this lagging behind as a fall, as the contemplation of an abyss, leading to the somatization of distress as dizziness (Kleinman and Kleinman 1994). More generally, families who were successful before the Chinese revolution but lost property and status afterward experienced this loss as a dizzying fall. These themes were apparent in the three cases presented.

Chinese often employ somatic metaphors that lead to metaphor-guided somatization; in turn, experiencing the symptom may evoke current existential issues through metaphoric resonances. In everyday Chinese it is not uncommon to hear someone saying "unbalanced heart" (*xinlibupingheng*) or "obstruction of the heart" (*xinlizhangai*) when referring to general states of psychological distress. For a particular individual, these expressions may indicate emotion-related physiology rather than just tropes. As a system of organ functioning and corresponding physical and mental states, TCM provides an abundance of associations between mental states and other processes. Specific emotions correspond to particular organs, and often the organ or physiological entity will stand in place of the emotion. For example, in everyday communication, anger is described as "rising *qi*" (*shengqi*) or "liver-fire" (*ganhuo*), and one can be "so angry the head spins" (*aidehunletou*) (King 1989) and to the point that one can "die of *qi*" (*qisiwole*). Cowardice is referred to as having a "small gallbladder" (*danxiao*). To be put in a bad mood is referred to as "to make spleen-*qi*" (*fapiqi*). One must carefully question a patient to know whether for that person these expressions indicate a specific physiology of emotion or are only tropes. Even if the patient utilizes these expressions as tropes, the tropes may guide somatization; that is, speaking metaphorically about one's existential state as "obstruction of the heart" may result in chest pain or pressure, in "unbalanced heart," palpitations, and dizziness, and unsteadiness of gait.

Dizziness and the Environmental Surround   The creation of parallels between dizziness and spinning objects in the surrounding landscape is promoted by graphic symbolism in the Chinese language. As indicated in the beginning of this chapter, the character for dizziness contains a wheel. This symbol is an implicit metaphor: to be dizzy is to spin like a wheel. Dizziness is thus linked to an environmental image, configured as "spinning," whereas the English term *dizzy* is not so narrowly linked to vertigo, a rotational motion, the feeling that the body is spinning in space or that the things around one are spinning.

In the Chinese context, the concept of circulation has multiple environmental referents. If a person feels dizzy and attributes this feeling to a disturbance of the organ system, then environmental analogs or circulations may be evoked—from images of nature to those of the city to those of a factory, as in its geared machines. Also, environment-scapes may produce distress by acting as metaphors of other complex systems, such as social relationships, the workplace, the Communist state, or the *zang fu.*

Chinese civilization has been described as "the most circulation-minded by far" of all ancient cultures (Gwei-Djen and Needham 1980:152). As early as the second century A.D., Chinese medical scholars hypothesized that blood and *qi* circulated in the body; by way of contrast, their Western counterparts asserted that blood ebbed and flowed like the tides, a view that would persist until William Harvey's discovery of blood circulation in the seventeenth century (Gwei-Djen and Needham 1980:29, 35). From a very early time, the Chinese also utilized complex gear mechanisms, harnessing the power of moving water to actuate a waterwheel and so accomplish multiple tasks, such as milling, irrigation, metal making, driving bellows, and other vital tasks (see Needham 1956; Needham et al. 1970). The Chinese harnessed water power to construct elaborate clocks that showed the movement of the stars and the time of day, a feat accomplished in the West only at a much later date (Needham 1956; Needham et al. 1960).

The circulation of the *qi* in the body was conceptualized in hydraulic engineering terms, with acupuncture promoting flow by undoing blockages, analogous to the clearing of a water gutter (Gwei-Djen and Needham 1980:24). The body was often described in terms of nature imagery, comparing the circulations in nature to the functioning of the body, suggesting a deep relationship of interdependence of the two realms, of the *yin* and *yang* in the body and in nature, of the flows in nature and the body, of the elements in the body and in nature (Veith 1949:123). In TCM, the functioning of the body—of its elements and organs—was considered to be closely linked to various cyclical elements in nature, such as season, lunar position, and time of day (Gwei-Djen and Needham 1980:137).

Nature and its events can influence the conceptualization of the organ system, and can lead to anxiety that nature's events may dysregulate the organ system. The environment may also cause what the *DSM–IV* refers to as *agoraphobia*, a fear of going out into the world, particularly into urban spaces, a condition that results from having previously experienced panic upon going out into those spaces. Panic in urban spaces is promoted by multiple factors (Hinton 2002): the predisposition to experience dizziness, sensitivity to dizziness (that is, the degree of reactivity to dizziness once it occurs), spatial symbolism (such as long perspectival corridors evoking a feeling of void), acoustic and visual complexity, and acoustic and visual shrillness.

As described earlier in the section on biology and dizziness, Chinese seem to be particularly prone to motion sickness, and in the Chinese cultural context, dizziness has deep affective resonances, for example, due to multiple metaphors such as those about lack of balance in relationships or those concerning fear of "falling" in status. Dizziness also gives rise to catastrophic cognitions, for example, interpreting dizziness as indicating weakness and various organ dysfunctions. If dizziness is induced in an urban locality, either by the fear of having dizziness in an external locality or by other processes such as the complexity of the sensory-scape, then anxiety and panic may arise as the result of dizziness-type affective resonances and catastrophic cognitions. In China, a country undergoing intense industrialization, urban space symbolizes change and the death of the old order, and evokes the specter of rabid competitiveness and new soteriologies. Many urban spaces have just been built, adding to a sense of disorientation; and the urban space is characterized by acoustic and visual complexity and shrillness. In fact, agoraphobia first arose in Europe in the 1870s in rapidly modernizing urban landscape contexts that were considered to be new and disorienting (Hinton 2002), such as the post-Haussmann landscape of Paris.

In the case of both Ms. X (Case 1) and Ms. Y. (Case 2), vertigo and panic were often experienced upon going out into public spaces, into the modernizing cityscape, which was characterized by changing vistas and buildings, by the chaos of frenetic motions, by a multiplicity of sounds—the whir of bicycle wheels, the chatter of approaching and receding people, the chug of car engines, the zip of motorcycles, the repeated poundings of construction machinery. It is in those public spaces that dis-ease seized Ms. X (Case 1) and Ms. Y (Case 2).

Although it is not a prominent aspect of any of the three cases presented here, the fear of "winds" in the external environment plays an important role in TCM pathogenesis (as in the "wind"-caused syndrome called *bizheng*). "Wind is the cause of a hundred diseases" (Veith 1949:107), according to the *Nei Jing*, one of the classic texts of TCM (see also Kuriyama 1999; Veith 1949:110). Winds may disturb the bodily physiology, a key symptom of such disturbance being dizziness (Hinton et al. 2003). If one goes outside after bathing or while sweating, or simply if one is "weak," wind can enter the body through the pores of the skin and cause illness. Gusts of wind, an outer image of chaos, insinuate themselves through the pores of the body, wreaking inner havoc and causing disordered flow in the body. Swirling winds, attacking various parts of the body, will disrupt the internal equilibrium and may result in dizziness, pain, stroke, or even death. The experience of wind-caused dizziness and panic in China also symbolizes the social and economic vulnerability of the individual; a wind such as misfortune and capricious outer forces may suddenly strike one (Kuriyama 1999).

Dizziness as Evoker of Memory   As described in the earlier section on biology and dizziness, the increased predisposition to motion sickness found among the Chinese population would be expected to have important consequences in respect to the encoding and cued recall of traumatic events. It would be expected to result in traumatic events tending to induce strong dizziness, and in the trauma memory having dizziness as a salient aspect. It would also be expected to result in the experience of dizziness at a later time having the power to bring to mind that trauma, and conversely, in the recall of the trauma—such as upon seeing the perpetrator of the trauma—having the power to induce dizziness due to somatic flashback and other processes. The experiencing of any dysphoric event—even if not *traumatic* in the strict sense of the term—would be expected to activate these same processes, producing an extensive linking of dizziness to dysphoric memories.

Dizziness may evoke past memories: a trauma, such as a blow to the head, or a personal or familial experience of disgrace, as in "falling (or fear of falling) from a higher to lower social position" (Kleinman and Kleinman 1994:715). Many patients had also experienced or heard about the Cultural Revolution, a time when starvation to the point of dizziness and death was common.

None of the three patients discussed here were specifically asked whether dizziness evoked memories. Patients may be reluctant to talk about these issues and memories for fear of reprisal. But Mr. Z (Case 3) reported that his family experienced extreme hardship during the Cultural Revolution. In Gansu province, his family was persecuted and nearly died from starvation on numerous occasions. Mr. Z also associated his current distress with the trauma of the Tang Shan earthquake. The memory of everything becoming wobbly and unsteady, and of actual collapse, was an important dynamic interpretant of dizziness for Mr. Z. In his case, there are various levels of homology: emotional state (feeling off balance), metaphor (unbalanced heart), an organ event (in palpitations, the shaking of the chest, and the motions of the agitated, unstable heart), and a certain memory (standing on the unstable earth during the earthquake, observing the oscillations of surrounding objects).

The Interpersonal, Economic, and Political Effects of Having Dizziness   Dizziness may serve as a "form of resistance against local sources of oppressive control" (Kleinman and Kleinman 1994:715). More generally, one must inquire about what the interpersonal and economic effects are of having dizziness and of its associated pathologies, of embodying their "symbolism." In the three cases, dizziness (and the other presenting symptoms) served as an acceptable response to an oppressive work and home environment, and was effective in addressing conflicts and providing remedy. Dizziness and its associated illness categories served as an effective "weapon of the weak," creating a better life-world space to occupy, a new and better ontological niche. Ms. X's illness eventually led to her transfer to another work unit and to the opportunity to continue her education (this happened twice). Ms. Y's and Mr. Z's illnesses resulted in rest when it was sorely needed. On a political level, these three individuals' dizziness would seem to have served as an embodied protest against the structure of society, an indictment that the work of culture was not being done, a protection against disharmony, which is a key cultural value; their dizziness was an assertion of the existence of a pathology of culture, of modernity as pathophysiological. History's victims announced their dis-order in the available idiom, and did not always go silently.

The Causation of Dizziness-Centered Panic: Transducers, Ontological Resonances, and Local Biology

In the Chinese cultural context there are multiple dizziness inducers and dizziness amplifiers, such as metaphors, resulting in frequent dizziness. In the Chinese cultural context, metaphors act as *anxiety transducers* (Hinton et al. in press): they cause anxious dysphoria to be experienced as dizziness, such as when an anxious person describes his or her emotional state in tropes that configure it as spinning. Also, in the Chinese cultural context, the ethnophysiological understanding of how anxiety is produced also transduces anxiety into dizziness by ascribing anxiety to specific pathophysiological mechanisms that would be expected to produce dizziness, thus leading to a hypervigilant surveying of the body for signs of dizziness. Even mild anxiety tends to be transduced into panic due to the catastrophic cognitions produced by the ethnophysiology of anxiety and of dizziness. Similarly, in the Chinese context, metaphors and ethnophysiology act as *anger transducers*, causing anger to result in dizziness and panic (such as in describing anger as a flame that leaps up to attack the brain); and specific metaphors and ethnophysiology act as *fatigue transducers*, causing fatigue to result in dizziness and panic (as in ascribing weakness to a depletion of a kidney-produced substance that nurtures the brain). Also, in the Chinese context, *social-conflict transducers* (such as metaphors of and ethnophysiological ideas about the effects of social conflict) configure workplace and interpersonal disputes as disequilibrium and as draining one's vitality and disturbing the organs; these social-conflict transducers result in social conflict tending to produce dizziness, catastrophic

cognitions, and panic. (Transducers might also be called interpretants or forma-
tives: anxiety interpretants are the metaphors, imagery, symptoms, and various
other representations that shape the experience of anxiety, analogous to Peirce's
contention that a word's dynamic interpretants, the images it evokes, determine
its meaning; see Chapter 3.)

How ethnophysiology and metaphor transduce emotional states, fatigue, environmental events, and social conflicts into dizziness and panic was illustrated in
the cases. For example, in Case 1, dizziness was associated with a sense that the
patient was in competition and conflict with her peers and was "falling behind" (a
metaphor transducer). In Case 2, dizziness was associated with a sense of depletion
because the patient did not have enough "energy" to keep up with the rapid changes
of society and the increased demands that modern society makes on women (an
ethnophysiology transducer).

Various transducers (of social conflict, of emotional state, of environmental
contexts) along with multiple other processes outlined in the preceding sections
result in dizziness being a prominent part of the Chinese distress ontology. Predisposition to motion sickness, a modernizing environment, familial and personal
histories of trauma, overwork, stresses of competition, and emotion and social-event
transducers, these all result in the induction of dizziness and the activation of ontological resonances and pathological processes wired into the local biology, in the
production of psychological and biological disequilibrium—from the level of social
networks to organ systems to mental imagery to the brain-equilibrium system that
integrates inner ear, sight, and proprioceptive information (McCredie 2007).

Conclusion

In China, suffering is seen as part of an overall pattern of distress; the dysphoric
state manifests as a blend of physical and mental symptoms within a context of discordant interpersonal, work, or societal conditions. An initial symptom of dizziness
will intensify, and overall distress may then progress across experiential modalities.
When disequilibrium reaches its multimodal peak, the associated sensation is one
of panic. In China, distress is commonly experienced as dizziness that can develop
into acute episodes resembling Western panic attacks. These distressing sensations
occur in a unique cultural context with a distinctive set of associated symptoms,
beliefs, and purported etiologies.

Dizziness is commonly experienced in China during states of dysphoria, especially anxious dysphoria. Understood within a framework of contemporary
TCM, which configures health in terms of an aesthetic of balance and harmony,
dizziness serves as an indicator of general disequilibrium. Emotions are associated
with specific organs in the TCM organ diagnostic system, but dizziness and panic

represent general distress. Dizziness and panic may result from disturbance in any of several organs; depending on which organ is involved, a unique constellation of physical and mental symptoms results. Dizziness embodies the disharmony experienced on multiple levels: disordered physiology, discordant interpersonal relationships, tumbling social status, swirling and pernicious winds, and otherwise chaotic and unpredictable external conditions. If disharmony and disequilibrium reach an extreme level, dizziness, accompanied by other symptoms, may intensify to panic.

As illustrated throughout the chapter, dizziness has multiple dynamic interpretants. It evokes an extensive spectrum of meaning, from the level of *zang fu* disequilibrium to metaphor to environment-caused pathology. Vertigo and the feeling of imbalance have wide resonances, linking the body to the social and physical world; these symptoms play a key part in the sociosomatic reticulum, a key aspect of the distress ontology. The chapter has outlined some of the symbolic bridges (that is, semantic networks) and biological and psychological mechanisms that link personal experience to somatic symptom—in this case, to dizziness, and panic.

As illustrated throughout the chapter, dizziness serves as a key indicator of the *degree of distress*, and at the extreme, dizziness involves panic. In each of the three cases presented, the experience of dizziness serves as a somatic indicator of distress, as a key aspect of the embodiment of general anxiety, and a chronic state of dizziness is the baseline state of these three patients. When disharmony increased, both anxiety and dizziness intensified to the point of panic. To understand the role of dizziness as a *key distress-indicator*, one must determine its severity and its course over time, that is, whether it is a chronic somatic symptom or whether it sometimes intensifies to the point of panic. In the Chinese context, dizziness serves as a *key idiom of distress* (Nichter 1981), but careful phenomenology is needed to know what it is trying to say.

Dizziness is a key symptom in the Chinese context; it has a rich set of ontological resonances, from common symptom to metaphor to key physiological sign to landscape icon. Owing to these rich ontological resonances, dizziness often occurs in panic, and may cause panic. To understand panic in the Chinese context, one must do a careful analysis of dizziness, exploring its ontological resonances and phenomenology, and examining its relationship to panic.

References

Beijing College of Traditional Medicine, Shanghai College of Traditional Medicine. 1980. *Essentials of Chinese Acupuncture.* Beijing: Foreign Language Press.

Good, B. J. 1977. The Heart of What's the Matter: The Semantics of Illness in Iran. *Culture, Medicine, and Psychiatry* 1:25–58.

————. 1994. *Medicine, Rationality, and Experience: An Anthropological Perspective.* Cambridge, UK: Cambridge University Press.

Gwei-Djen, L., and J. Needham. 1980. *Celestial Lancets: A History and Rationale of Acupuncture and Moxa.* Cambridge, UK: Cambridge University Press.

Hinton, D. E. 2002. Munch, Agoraphobia, and the Terrors of the Modernizing Landscape. In *Panic: Origins, Insight, and Treatment.* L. Schmidt and B. Warner, eds. Pp. 229–252. Berkeley, CA: North Atlantic Books.

Hinton, D. E., and S. D. Hinton. 2002. Panic Disorder, Somatization, and the New Cross-Cultural Psychiatry: The Seven Bodies of a Medical Anthropology of Panic. *Culture, Medicine, and Psychiatry* 26:155–178.

Hinton D. E., T. Pham, H. Chau, M. Tran, and S. D. Hinton. 2003. "Hit by the Wind" and Temperature-Shift Panic Among Vietnamese Refugees. *Transcultural Psychiatry* 40:342–376.

Hinton, D. E., S. D. Hinton, J. R. Loeum, V. Pich, and M. H. Pollack. In press. The "Multiplex Model" of How Somatic Symptoms Generate Distress: Application to Tinnitus Among Traumatized Cambodian Refugees. *Transcultural Psychiatry.*

Kaptchuk, T. 1983. *The Web That Has No Weaver: Understanding Chinese Medicine.* New York: Congdon and Weed.

King, B. 1989. Conceptual Structure of Emotional Experience in Chinese. Ph.D. dissertation, Department of Anthropology, Ohio State University.

Kleinman, A. 1980. *Patients and Healers in the Context of Culture: An Exploration of the Borderland Between Anthropology, Medicine, and Psychiatry.* Berkeley: University of California Press.

————. 1982. *Social Origins of Distress and Disease.* New Haven, CT: Yale University Press.

Kleinman A., and J. Kleinman. 1985. Somatization: The Interconnections in Chinese Society Among Culture, Depressive Experiences, and the Meanings of Pain. In *Culture and Depression: Studies in the Anthropology and Cross-Cultural Psychiatry of Affect and Disorder.* A. Kleinman and B. J. Good, eds. Pp. 429–490. Berkeley: University of California Press.

————. 1994. How Bodies Remember: Social Memory and Bodily Experience of Criticism, Resistance, and Delegitimation Following China's Cultural Revolution. *New Literary History* 25:707–723.

Kuriyama, S. 1999. *The Expressiveness of the Body and the Divergence of Greek and Chinese Medicine.* New York: Zone Books.

Lee, S. 1996. Cultures in Psychiatric Nosology: The CCMD-2R and International Classification of Mental Disorders. *Culture, Medicine, and Psychiatry* 20:421–472.

Liu, G., and A. Hyodo, eds. 1994. *Fundamentals of Acupuncture and Moxibustion.* Tianjin, CN: Tianjin Science and Technology Translation and Publishing.

Maciocia, G. 1989. *The Foundations of Chinese Medicine.* London: Churchill Livingstone.

McCredie, S. 2007. *Balance: In Search of the Lost Sense.* New York: Little, Brown.

Needham, J. 1956. *Science and Civilization in China.* Volume 2: *History of Scientific Thought.* Cambridge UK: Cambridge University Press.

Needham, J., L. Wang, and J. Derek. 1960. *Heavenly Clockwork: The Great Astronomical Clocks of Medieval China.* Cambridge, UK: Antiquarian Horological Society.

Needham, J., W. Ling, L. Gwei-Djen, and H. Ping-Yu. 1970. *Clerks and Craftsmen in China and the West.* Cambridge, UK: Cambridge University Press.

Nichter, M. 1981. Idioms of Distress: Alternatives in the Expression of Psychological Distress: A Case Study from Southern India. *Culture, Medicine, and Psychiatry* 5:379–408.

Porkert, M., and C. Ullmann. 1982. *Chinese Medicine.* New York: Henry Holt.

Taylor, K. 2001. A New, Scientific, and Unified Medicine. In *Innovations in Chinese Medicine.* E. Hsu, ed. Pp. 343–369. Cambridge, UK: Cambridge University Press.

Veith, I. 1949. *The Yellow Emperor's Classic of Internal Medicine.* Berkeley: University of California Press.

Zhang, Y. 2007. *Transforming Emotions with Chinese Medicine: An Ethnographic Account from Contemporary China.* Albany: State University of New York.

Zheng, Y., K. Lin, J. Zhao, M. Zhang, and D. Yong. 1994. Comparative Study of Diagnostic Systems: Chinese Classification of Mental Disorders—Second Edition Versus DSM–III–R. *Comprehensive Psychiatry* 35(6):441–449.

8

Gendered Panic in Southern Thailand

'Lom' ("Wind") Illness and 'Wuup' ("Upsurge") Illness

Pichet Udomratn and Devon E. Hinton

---•

PANIC VARIES RADICALLY depending on how it and its somatic symptoms are labeled, and on the illnesses it is thought to indicate. In this chapter we examine the relationship between panic disorder (PD) and certain illness categories in Southern Thailand. As the chapter illustrates, cultural beliefs and practices profoundly shape the panic experience. Assessing for the presence of *Diagnostic and Statistical Manual* (*DSM*) criteria is just the beginning of the exploration of panic phenomenology in a particular culture; it is a view from the outside, not a description of panic's inner workings, which are culturally (and individually) variable.

The material in the current chapter is drawn from cases treated by the first author, Dr. Pichet Udomratn. Dr. Udomratn works as a psychiatrist in a university hospital clinic in Southern Thailand. Many of his patients come from rural areas. For the present chapter, he chose cases he believed to be typical of how PD manifests in Southern Thailand. The second author, Dr. Devon E. Hinton, an anthropologist and psychiatrist, has performed extensive fieldwork in Thailand, mainly in Northeastern Thailand (Hinton 1999).

Thailand consists of four main cultural areas designated on the basis of language: Northern Thailand, Northeastern Thailand, Central Thailand (that is, Bangkok and its surrounding area), and Southern Thailand. In each area, the dialects are quite different, although mutually understandable to a large degree. Southern Thailand has certain unique features, including a large Islamic minority and an extensive rubber industry.

This chapter investigates certain questions in respect to panic experience in Southern Thailand. Which illness syndromes overlap with PD? Are the somatic symptoms that occur in panic attributed to the pathomechanics of a specific ethnophysiology? Do men and women have different forms of panic? Are the panic attacks of men and women attributed to different etiologies and physiologies? And if panic does vary by gender, how does it perpetuate, and construct, gender stereotypes?

Background

Before we turn to an examination of the cultural construction of panic in Thailand, we first discuss how the *DSM* was introduced into Thailand and review studies conducted in Thailand on rates of panic, including those that examine gender differences.

The Introduction of Panic Disorder into Thai Psychiatry

The term *panic disorder* is a relatively new import to Thailand. When the American Psychiatric Association introduced the category of PD in *DSM–III* (APA 1980), recognizing it for the first time as a discrete psychiatric entity, most Thai psychiatrists were reluctant to identify it in their patients. Many of the Thai psychiatrists who had trained abroad had gone to the Maudsley Hospital in London, a bastion of the *International Statistical Classification of Diseases* (*ICD*). In the *DSM–III* (1980), the *DSM–II* category *anxiety neurosis* was divided into PD and *generalized anxiety disorder* (McNally 1994:4); in the *ICD-9* (WHO 1978), these two disorders were lumped together under the diagnosis *anxiety states* (a category similar to *anxiety neurosis* in the *DSM–II*).

When the *DSM–III* was initially published, the first author of this chapter was a psychiatry resident in Bangkok. One of his patients could have been diagnosed with PD according to the *DSM–III* criteria, but his advisor—a senior psychiatrist who had been trained in England—asserted the correct diagnosis to be *anxiety states*. Only after finishing his psychiatric training and passing the National Board Examination in Psychiatry did the first author finally become confident in diagnosing PD. In addition, upon joining the staff at Prince of Songkla University (PSU), the first author learned a great deal from Dr. Boonnum Wongchaowart—a Thai psychiatrist with a diploma from the American Board of Psychiatry and Neurology—who introduced many new American concepts to Thai psychiatrists at PSU, including the American view (*DSM–III* and *DSM–III–R*) of PD. Many conversations on PD with Dr. Wongchaowart clarified the first author's thinking about the relevance of the diagnosis in the Thai context.

Rates of Panic Disorder in Thailand:
Community Versus Psychiatric Clinic Samples

In a national cross-sectional community survey using the Mini-International Neuropsychiatric Interview, 11,700 adult participants were selected by a stratified two-stage cluster sampling (Udomratn 2006). The one-month prevalence rate of PD was 0.4 percent. Another national survey using the Composite International Diagnostic Interview, with a sample size of 7,149, found the lifetime prevalence of PD to be 1 percent. In that study, when analyzed by region, Northeastern Thailand had the highest rate (1.7 percent), followed by the Northern (1.1 percent), Central (0.5 percent), and Southern (0.4 percent) regions (Bunditchate et al. 2001; Udomratn 2004).

Several surveys of PD rates in Thailand have been conducted in psychiatric clinics (see Table 8.1). A yearlong study of patients who presented at the psychiatric outpatient clinic of Ramathibodi Hospital in Bangkok found 4.1 percent (26/665) to be diagnosable with PD (Nilchaikovit 1988); a retrospective study of newly presenting psychiatric patients at a Bangkok clinic during a five-year period found that only 2.1 percent (120/5,608) were diagnosed with PD (Silpakit and Sukanich 1992). In contrast, at a psychiatric clinic at Songklanagarind Hospital in Southern Thailand, 12.4 percent (80/644) of the patients first presenting for treatment were diagnosed as having PD during a one-year period (Udomratn 2000).

These studies show that *DSM*-defined PD can be identified in community and clinic populations in Thailand. They also show differences in rates across regions. Future studies will need to be done to determine if rates differ after controlling for variables that influence PD rates, such as age, gender, comorbid medical conditions, and economic status (leading to more stress and hence panic). These regions are quite different culturally, so panic rates may vary as a result of differences in the interpretation of PD symptoms, with the local ethnophysiology and cultural syndromes in one region leading to more catastrophic cognitions; or PD-type illness and its associated syndromes may be more accepted and effective as an "idiom of

Table 8.1 Summary of Thai epidemiological data from psychiatric clinics in respect to the rate of panic disorder

Author	Year of Study	%	Rate	Criteria Used
Nilchaikovit	1988	4.1	(26/665)	*DSM–III*
Silpakit and Sukanich	1986–1990	2.1	(120/5608)	*DSM–III*
Udomratn	1991	12.4	(80/644)	*DSM–III–R*

186 Cultural Variations in Panic Disorder

distress" (Nichter 1981) in one region than in another, leading to its more frequent "embodiment."

Gender Differences in Rates of Panic Disorder in Thailand: Community Versus Psychiatric-Clinic Samples

With a few exceptions (such as Spanish-speaking populations), women in Western countries appear to have higher rates of PD than men, with the ratio ranging anywhere from 2:1 to 3:1 (Amering and Katschnig 1990). One community survey of PD in Thailand revealed a similar ratio: the one-month prevalence rate of PD was 0.6 percent among women and 0.2 percent among men (Udomratn 2006).

In Thailand, however, men and women receiving care at psychiatric clinics demonstrate similar rates of PD, with the female-to-male ratio ranging from 0.67:1 to 1.45:1 (see Table 8.2) (Udomratn 2000). Of note, many patients at psychiatric clinics are referred from general doctors and medical specialists at other clinics, and are most commonly patients who went to those settings fearing they had a dangerous medical condition.

Why in Thailand should the female-to-male ratio of PD differ so much in community compared to psychiatric-clinic samples? One possible explanation would be gender differences in the local cultural syndromes that guide how panic attacks are experienced, reacted to, treated, and viewed. In the Thai context, the panic syndromes vary by gender. A male form of panic exists that is not highly stigmatized, thereby facilitating a Thai male's reporting panic symptoms and seeking services from a physician; the syndrome allows the enactment of panic as masculine—but it also generates considerable catastrophic cognitions.[1]

Table 8.2 The female-to-male ratio in rates of panic in Thai psychiatric clinics

Hospital	Year of Study	Number of Females	Number of Males	Female:Male Ratio
Ramathibodi	1988	14	21	0.67:1
Ramathibodi	1986–1990	67	53	1.26:1
Songklanagarind	1986–1987	17	13	1.31:1
Songklanagarind	1990–1991	40	40	1:1
Saraburi	1991–1993	77	53	1.45:1
Saraburi	1997–1998	9	12	0.75:1

Southern Thai Illness Syndromes that Overlap with Panic Disorder

Upon experiencing a panic attack, Thais often attribute their symptoms to one of three local syndromes: (1) "weak heart illness" (*rook prasard hua jai oon*),[2] (2) "wind illness" (*rook lom*), or (3) "upsurge illness" (*rook wuup*). In most instances, someone who is self- or other-labeled as suffering one of these three syndromes would be diagnosable as having PD according to the *DSM–IV*. The main focus of the present chapter is two of these illness syndromes: *lom* illness ("wind illness," *rook lom*) and *wuup* illness ("upsurge illness," *rook wuup*). *Lom* illness is more commonly found in women than in men. Two prominent complaints are gastrointestinal distress and dizziness. Laypersons consider the disorder to be treatable—although it may be fatal in some cases—with an important psychological component. *Wuup* illness is usually a male disorder, with two prominent complaints: the sudden onset of severe dizziness and a sense of imminent loss of consciousness. Laypersons usually assume the condition to be a dangerous form of *lom* illness, or to be caused by another menacing, underlying medical illness.

Case Examples

The patients described here were treated by the first author at a psychiatric clinic in the Songklanagarind Hospital. The clinic is located in the city of Hat Yai in the Southern Thai province of Songkhla and is part of the Prince of Songkla University. Patients come to the clinic in multiple ways, including walk-ins and referrals from medical clinics in the hospital and in the community.

Case 1: Somsee—A Case of 'Lom' Illness   Somsee, a married twenty-four-year-old woman, had a three-year-old daughter and a four-year-old son. Every morning, Somsee and her husband awoke at 2 A.M. in order to prepare for work. They tapped rubber trees, later delivering the sap to a merchant and earning about 150 baht (five dollars) each day. Somsee was considered a hardworking housewife and rarely took a nap during the day. In a typical daily routine, Somsee helped her husband tap trees until 6 A.M. and then returned home to prepare breakfast for the family. Somsee's two children often quarreled with one other; this incessant bickering made her angry, and quite frequently she lost her temper and struck them. A few months before her panic attacks started, Somsee's father died because of the sudden rupture of a cerebral aneurysm; other than suffering recurrent headaches for six months prior to his demise, Somsee's father had been quite healthy and had never been admitted to the hospital.

One morning a few months after her father's death, Somsee had her first *lom* attack while tapping rubber trees. The initial symptom she felt was *lom* moving upward in her abdomen. She pushed down on her abdomen in an attempt to force the *lom* out, but this only minimally reduced her distress. Somsee felt nauseous; saliva spilled out of her mouth (a common complaint during gastrointestinal-distress episodes among Thai, and Cambodian, panickers), and her heart was pounding fast and hard. Images of her father's death came into her mind, conjuring fears of having an aneurysm or some other disorder: "I have not had a medical checkup since the birth of my last child. Do I have some severe illness? Am I going to die?" She asked for protection, entreating out loud, "Oh! Lord Buddha, please. My children are still young. Please, help me!" Somsee desperately looked around for her husband, Noi, who normally tapped trees near to her, but she could not see him. "He must have gone to tap some distance away," she thought, so Somsee shouted even louder, "Help! Help! Noi! Please help me!" A short while later Noi returned to the area; he found Somsee sitting on the ground and breathing deeply. When they reached their home, Somsee asked Noi to make "*lom* medicine" (*yaa lom*) and massage her abdomen. After drinking the medicine, she burped several times; a feeling of abdominal relaxation ensued and her symptoms began to abate. Somsee and Noi attributed the episode to *lom* illness.

The attacks recurred frequently; Somsee became too afraid to go to the rubber plantation and stayed at home with her children. Owing to the chronicity of the problem, Noi consulted a "spirit doctor" (*mor phi*, in which *mor* means "doctor" and *phi* means "demons, supernatural beings, and the ghosts of the deceased") about the cause of his wife's illness. The spirit doctor ascribed the illness to a transgression against a deceased ancestor; as treatment, he recommended addressing prayers to Somsee's ancestors and offering food to Buddhist monks during the daily morning merit-making ceremony at the temple. (Merit has a protective power and can be earned in many ways: through specific Buddhist rituals, by giving donations to monks, or by doing any good deed.) If the condition still did not improve, the spirit doctor recommended performing the Nora dance ceremonial (*rum Nora long khru*), a healing ritual based on a Southern Thai classical dance, and dedicating the performance to Somsee's ancestor.

Despite offering prayers to the ancestors and "making merit" at the temple, Somsee's condition did not improve, but the couple could not afford the Nora dance ritual. Consequently, they decided to seek Western-type medical help, consulting Dr. Udomratn. After medical treatment that included a discussion about Somsee's grief over her father's death, reassurances about the health of her heart, education about the impossibility of dying from rising abdominal vapors, and the administration of anxiety medication, she had no more *lom* attacks.

Case 2: Samorn—Another Case of 'Lom' Illness   Samorn, a married twenty-six-year-old woman, had a spontaneous abortion at ten weeks of gestation. A physician attributed the miscarriage to overwork; Samorn's mother thought the cause to be a deficiency of blood. Upon becoming pregnant again, Samorn followed strictly the instructions of her physician (that is, to exert herself minimally) and those of her mother (to drink each morning and night an herbal medicine for "blood promotion," *yaa bumroong leod*, an aggregate of bark, roots, and leaves from several types of trees, boiled in water and then sipped after cooling). Her mother also advised Samorn to avoid eating mushrooms and a certain kind of shellfish—namely, cockles—because they cause "spoiled blood" (*leod seai*). The birth of a healthy daughter made both Samorn and her husband very happy.

Three months after delivery, Samorn still had not menstruated. Her obstetrician ascribed this problem to a hormonal imbalance produced by the excessive use of blood-promotion medicine (*yaa bumroong leod*); Samorn's mother agreed that the blood-promotion medicine should be stopped but gave a different diagnosis: retention of spoiled menstrual blood (*leod seai*). As further treatment, Samorn's mother bought a traditional herbal medicine, "bleeding-inducing medicine" (*yaa cup leod*), to remove bad blood until normal menstrual flow returned. After taking this medicine regularly for two weeks, Samorn's menstruation finally resumed—but she felt it was not a "good" menstruation: the color was too dark. Samorn became even more convinced that *leod seai* had been collecting in her body during the time of no menstrual flow, and that some spoiled blood remained in her uterus.

Two weeks later, Samorn prepared a lemongrass soup (*tom yum*) for her family; she added mushrooms, one of her husband's favorite foods. While eating the soup with her husband, Samorn remembered her mother's words: "Both mushrooms and cockles are not good for women who have spoiled blood." But Samorn thought to herself, "It should be all right, because some of the spoiled blood came out two weeks ago." After eating a little more soup, she had sensations in her stomach of heat, churning, and bloating, and attributed those symptoms to *lom* moving around in her belly—a *lom* produced by the interaction of mushrooms and *leod seai*. She berated herself: "Why didn't I follow my mother's advice?" Next she felt *lom* moving upward into her chest, causing even greater shortness of breath. Finally she had a full-blown panic attack. Samorn could not finish her dinner and asked her husband to take her to bed and prepare *lom* medicine for her to drink.

Case 3: Somchai—A Case of 'Wuup' Illness   Thirty-two-year-old Somchai, a married Thai-Muslim male, experienced his first episode of *wuup* illness at his temple's Friday-morning prayer session. While standing and praying at the central mosque, he suddenly felt as if his body were leaning abnormally far forward; he feared fainting and thought, "I must have *wuup* illness. Maybe I will have a stroke." He looked around the mosque at the people who were still standing and praying. Somchai considered sitting on the floor, but only an ill or weak Muslim was allowed to sit on the floor when praying at the central mosque. He was a teacher at the Islamic school. Somchai told himself, "I am a strong man. I should not show any sign of weakness." Time seemed to pass very slowly as the praying continued; Somchai felt dizzy, sweated profusely, worried about fainting.

After this event, Somchai lost self-confidence. When he resumed teaching on the following Monday, he felt too afraid to stand in his usual spot in front of the desk; instead, he stood next to it and clutched it firmly to prevent a sudden fall to the floor. He also had a further plan: if he felt faint or dizzy, which would indicate the commencement of an episode of *wuup* illness, he would teach his students while sitting in a chair. A few days later, while performing Friday prayer during the weekly ceremony at the mosque, a prayer requiring bending over and touching the ground and then standing upright, he felt dizzy and feared fainting. Praying alone in his house usually did not cause such symptoms. Although he wanted to avoid attending the weekly prayer ceremony at the central mosque, he could not do so without being accused of being a poor role model.

Somchai worried that his episodes of *wuup* illness resulted from a dangerous medical condition—a surge of *lom* and blood toward the brain. He sought out many general practitioners and internists, but did not improve. Somchai was told he did not have any illness and was given vitamins and tranquilizers. After treatment with the first author, who explained the nature of PD and reassured Somchai that he did not suffer from *wuup* illness or any other serious medical disorder, Somchai quickly improved.

The Southern Thai Conception of 'Lom' Flow in the Body: The Ethnophysiology of Panic Symptoms

The belief that a windlike substance may move upward from the abdomen to cause damage by compressing the heart and other organs is found in many Asian countries—Cambodia (Hinton et al. 2001a, 2001b), Laos (Hinton 1999), India and Sri Lanka (Leslie 1992; Tabor 1981), Thailand (as discussed in this chapter), and Tibet (See Chapter 10). (In the Korean illness *hwa byung*, a rising mass and heat is feared [Lin 1983].) In these countries, this ethnophysiology often creates hypervigilance to abdominal sensations as well as to symptoms such as dizziness associated with an upward rising of wind, and high rates of stomach-focused panic. In the Southeast Asian countries that were strongly influenced by the cultural practices of India, such as Cambodia, Laos, and Thailand, this wind ethnophysiology probably derives from the Ayurvedic tradition (Leslie 1992; Tabor 1981).[3]

According to traditional Southern Thai belief, the human body is composed of four elements: earth, water, wind (*lom*), and fire. Many Thais, especially those with minimal education, explain symptoms in terms of the *lom* physiology. In the healthy state, *lom* flows downward through the gastrointestinal tract to be expelled from the body,[4] and it flows continuously downward along the arms and legs to exit the body through the hands and feet. *Lom* can also escape through the skin pores.

In pathological states, the *lom* may move progressively upward in the body, as occurs in *lom* illness, or it may suddenly ascend directly to the head, as in *wuup* illness. If the downward flow of *lom* is blocked at the stomach or the limbs, it then moves upward in the body, resulting in various serious problems (see Figure 8.1). As it rises, the *lom*

- Hits the diaphragm, impairing inhalation and causing chest tightness
- Compresses the heart to a much smaller and thinner shape, causing it to function poorly and possibly to rip as it makes abnormal motions
- Forms a lump or mass in the throat, impairing breathing
- Enters the head, causing dizziness, blurry vision, faintness, and tinnitus (*lom ook huu*, literally translated "*lom* exiting from the ear"), potentially bringing about syncope, paralysis, or even death

To describe palpitations, Southern Thais may use the phrase "floating heart" (*jai wiew wiew*), which denotes a feeling of the heart being light and seemingly being "knocked about" by "upward-hitting *lom*" (*lom tee ud khuen bon*). Palpitations evoke fears of having a dangerous type of *lom* ascent in which *lom* compresses the heart, making it much smaller (*jai heed heed*), impairing its ability to beat normally, and causing it to beat faster in attempted compensation. Worse yet, the person may fear having "weak heart illness" (*rook prasad hua jai oon*), which when combined with a *lom* attack is especially dangerous. Because of these ethnophysiology conceptualizations, palpitations may cause a *lom*-attack sufferer to seek treatment from a physician, in particular from a cardiologist. If the *lom*-attack sufferer has head symptoms such as tinnitus, blurry vision, or dizziness, she will worry that the *lom* has traveled from the abdomen all the way up to the head, and she may well complain, "*Lom* hits upward and moves to the head" (*lom tee ud khuen hua*). Thais refer to a feeling of faintness with the phrase "afflicted by wind" (*pen lom*), further heightening fears of dizziness and related symptoms. Tinnitus is referred to as "*lom* exits from the ear" (*lom ook huu*), and having that symptom indicates that *lom* has arrived at the head; the sufferer must lie down as soon as possible to prevent any serious consequences such as a stroke.

As alluded to earlier, Southern Thais traditionally refer to menstrual blood as spoiled blood (*leod seai*) and consider its accumulation in the body to predispose the woman to *lom* illness. If a woman has anxiety symptoms or experiences panic, she may consider the cause to be *leod seai*. Some women will drink, as Samorn did, "bleeding-inducing medicine" (*yaa cup leod*), an herbal medicine, to prevent and treat spoiled blood. If menstrual flow does not occur, women often will visit a

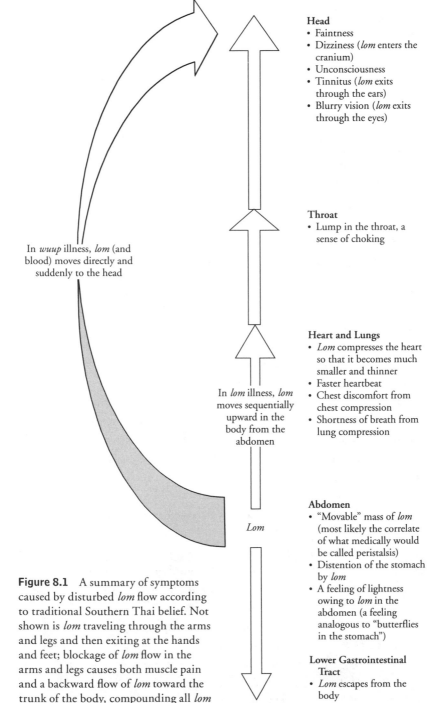

Head
- Faintness
- Dizziness (*lom* enters the cranium)
- Unconsciousness
- Tinnitus (*lom* exits through the ears)
- Blurry vision (*lom* exits through the eyes)

Throat
- Lump in the throat, a sense of choking

In *wuup* illness, *lom* (and blood) moves directly and suddenly to the head

Heart and Lungs
- *Lom* compresses the heart so that it becomes much smaller and thinner
- Faster heartbeat
- Chest discomfort from chest compression
- Shortness of breath from lung compression

In *lom* illness, *lom* moves sequentially upward in the body from the abdomen

Lom

Abdomen
- "Movable" mass of *lom* (most likely the correlate of what medically would be called peristalsis)
- Distention of the stomach by *lom*
- A feeling of lightness owing to *lom* in the abdomen (a feeling analogous to "butterflies in the stomach")

Figure 8.1 A summary of symptoms caused by disturbed *lom* flow according to traditional Southern Thai belief. Not shown is *lom* traveling through the arms and legs and then exiting at the hands and feet; blockage of *lom* flow in the arms and legs causes both muscle pain and a backward flow of *lom* toward the trunk of the body, compounding all *lom* symptoms.

Lower Gastrointestinal Tract
- *Lom* escapes from the body

clinic or a hospital physician to request medication in an oral or injected form to bring about menstruation. (Likewise, in premenstrual dysphoric disorder, which is often characterized by panic attacks [Facchinetti et al. 1992; Gorman et al. 2001; Schnall et al. 2002], the sufferer has the self-perception of being in a vulnerable state during certain points of the menstrual cycle. Such menstrual and perimenstrual panic syndromes would seem to result from the interaction of multiple processes: cognitive frames, attention, catastrophic cognitions, and hormonal shifts that produce symptoms.)

The Southern Thai ethnophysiology of emotion creates fear of *lom* disturbance. As described earlier, Southern Thais explain fear and anxiety symptoms in terms of a *lom* ethnophysiology. In addition, various *lom* idioms can be employed to describe other emotional states, and even character. One can refer to someone as being "good *lom*" (*lom dee*), meaning "good tempered," or "bad *lom*" (*lom raay*), meaning "ill tempered." When a person is ill tempered, angry, or very upset, he or she may be warned, "Be careful of upward-moving *lom*." Because of emotional expressions of this kind, some consider the word *ar-rom* ("emotion") to be formed from the word *lom*. These *lom* idioms further produce catastrophic cognitions about various emotional states, causing worry that certain emotional states correspond to dangerous physiological disturbances.

Two Southern Thai 'Lom' Syndromes: Gendered Panic

When dizziness and other panic symptoms occur, a Southern Thai frequently interprets these symptoms as being due to *lom*, but the severity of the putative *lom* illness will vary by gender. A woman with dizziness or other panic symptoms is usually thought to have *lom* illness, a condition that normally does not necessitate a trip to the hospital but can instead be treated by *lom* medicine (*yaa lom*), as Somsee did, and other home-based interventions. A man, however, with dizziness and other panic symptoms is not uncommonly thought to have *wuup* illness, a condition resulting from a dangerous pathological process, most usually a surge of *lom* and blood to the head.

The Literal Meanings of 'Lom' Illness and 'Wuup' Illness

The word *rook* means "disease" or "illness," and *lom* means "wind." As described earlier, *lom* illness (*rook lom*) denotes a disorder resulting from "wind" rising upward from the interior spaces of the body. The image is that of a passive sufferer. In *wuup* illness (*rook wuup*), the word *wuup* indicates something that suddenly increases and then rapidly decreases, a force that surges and then abruptly ends—a gust of wind or a flash followed by darkness, or most prototypically, a flame that is fanned by a wind, causing it to blaze briefly before suddenly going out. Although above we translated the word *wuup* as "upsurge" and *rook wuup* as "upsurge illness," better translations might be "surge-and-then-stop" (*wuup*) and "surge-and-then-stop illness" (*rook wuup*). The initial symptoms of an episode of *wuup* illness—palpitations and dizziness—are analogous to the surge of a wind gust or flame. The most feared symptom of an episode of *wuup* illness is syncope, a loss of all force and a fall to the ground, followed by the sudden stoppage of that force, like the subsiding of a gust or the blowing out of a flame.

The Sound-Symbolic and Articulatory Iconicism of the Words 'Lom' and 'Wuup'

The terms *lom illness* and *wuup illness* have *sound-symbolic iconicism*, that is, the sound of the term evokes its meaning, and they have *articulatory iconicism*, that is, the mouth motions made upon saying the terms mirror their meaning. As a result, the described illnesses seem more real, and take on more affective power.

In the phrase *lom illness*, the word *lom* is soft, flowing, and strongly vibrational. It begins with the liquid *l*, creating a buzzlike sound; next the mouth opens slightly, with the lips still rounded, to make the vowel sound *o*, resulting in the continuation of the buzzing sound produced by the vocal cords; and the last sound is the consonant *m*, so the vocal cords continue to oscillate, creating a humming effect. The humming vibration, or oscillation, suggests inconstancy and conjures images of passivity—being moved by an outer power, like a leaf in the wind or a reed in a tube, as in a flute. The word *lom* also has a level middle tone, further suggesting steady flow, analogous to the flow of wind.

As mentioned earlier, the word *wuup* means to surge and stop like a windblown flame. The word *wuup* not only acts as an abstract signifier, but also iconically evokes the sense of surge and stop by sound symbolism (making it a sound-symbolism icon) and oral kinesthetics (making it a kinesthetic icon).[5] When one articulates the initial sound, *wuu*, a burst of air emerges from the mouth. In fact, the phrase *wuu wuu* is used to describe the movement of wind. After articulating the initial *wuu*, the lips close in a diminishing circle to form a final *p*, which is a stop, causing all flow to cease suddenly. The tone of the word *wuup* is that of a slow rise of pitch followed by a sudden tonal fall. (Thai is a tonal language, with five tones—low, mid, rising, high, and rising-and-then-falling.) According to both sound iconicism (including tonal motions) and articulatory iconocism (mouth motions), the word *wuup* evokes a strong wind (*wuu wuu*) that suddenly stops in its flow (the final *p*), evoking what purportedly occurs in *wuup* illness: *lom* and blood moving upward from the belly and then stopping as they hit the confines of the cranium—a surge of symptoms followed by a collapse.

As can be seen in this linguistic analysis, the words *lom* and *wuup* perpetuate ideas about gendered panic, creating a word game that matches the supposed reality. Iconically, the word *lom* suggests softness (through the soft vowel), a steady flow of wind (through its constant middle tone), inconstancy (through its vibrational oscillation), and passivity (through its strongly experienced vibration). Iconically, the word *wuup* creates a sense of dramatic onset (through a burst of air) and crescendo (through its rising tone), analogous to the onset of a gust of wind or a rising flame fed by wind, and then a sense of sudden ending, a fall (through its falling tone and final consonant stop). Through sound-symbolic and mouth-movement iconicism, the word *wuup* gives a feeling of active force, of a surge followed by a fall.

The Symptoms and Treatment of 'Lom' Illness

Upon experiencing the sudden onset of multiple anxiety symptoms, a Southern Thai woman will usually consider it to be a bout of *lom* illness and will treat the illness by taking one of various *lom* medicines, such as *yaa lom*, rather than consulting a physician. If a woman has symptoms such as dizziness that are considered serious, then often another woman in the house (such as her mother, one of her children, or a live-in maid) but sometimes her husband will help her into bed and prepare *lom* medicine. To prepare *lom* medicine, one spoons the powder, which comes in a small glass vial, into a drinking glass and then pours in hot water and stirs with a spoon. After the liquid cools, it is slowly sipped. If a husband devotes much time to taking care of his wife—preparing *lom* medicine and massaging her—his mother may suspect the daughter-in-law of feigning illness to get his attention. A woman who has frequent *lom* attacks may request Thai traditional massage,[6] and if massaging causes burping, as often occurs, it will confirm the sufferer's concern that the symptoms were caused by excessive *lom* in the stomach.

   If severe bouts of *lom* illness recur frequently despite taking *lom* medicine, the sufferer will seek the advice of a native healer. Practitioners of Thai traditional medicine often diagnose disorders according to a complex humoral system that is strongly shaped by Ayurvedic concepts, utilizing herbal medicines to correct imbalances. Fortune tellers may ascribe the disorder to being under the influence of a certain planetary conjunction (such as *rahoo*, an inauspicious astrological sign, depicted as a demon) and suggest a ritual with Buddhist monks. In one typical rite, the ill person gives eight black objects to the monks, thereby ridding the body of bad luck. Some *lom*-attack victims may consult a spirit doctor (*mor phi*), as did Somsee's husband Noi.[7] The spirit doctor often asserts that the person offended an ancestor and that rituals—such as the special Nora dance ritual (*Nora long khru*)—must be conducted to appease the offended spirits.[8] A visit to a physician is resorted to only after all other treatment modalities have failed.

As discussed earlier in the section on ethnophysiology, the symptoms of an episode of *lom* illness are thought to vary depending on the amount of *lom* accumulation and the degree to which it has ascended in the body. An individual having gastro-intestinal symptoms along with minor panic symptoms—such as slight dizziness and minimal palpitations—may self-diagnose the condition as uncomplicated *lom* illness and treat it by taking one of the various *lom* herbal remedies. If the symptoms worsen, a traditional healer may be consulted. However, certain *lom* symptoms will cause the person to seek medical treatment. Symptoms such as startle and easily induced palpitations suggest the diagnosis of weak heart. If the person fears having weak heart, then treatment with a physician will be quickly sought; the enervated heart is particularly at risk during *lom* attacks. Also, if symptoms indicating that *lom* has ascended into the head—such as tinnitus, blurry vision, and dizziness—are noted, a physician may be consulted rather than a traditional healer.

The Symptoms and Treatment of 'Wuup' Illness

If a Southern Thai male suffers a panic attack, he tends to seek medical attention immediately, worrying that the disorder may be caused by *wuup* illness. The dis-order can occur in both men and women, but it is much more frequent among men. As already described, it is thought to result from a sudden and dramatic rise of *lom* (and blood) upward in the body. Sufferers worry that the *lom* (and blood) surge may bring about a stroke or other neurological disorder. *Wuup illness* is a relatively new term, becoming popular only in 1989 after a prominent Thai news-paper used it to describe what occurred to a famous Thai boxer during a fight to defend his championship title. On October 18, 1989, only two minutes into the first round, Thai-boxer Khaokor Galaxy received an uppercut from his Filipino challenger, Luisito Espinosa; although initially minimally affected by the blow, he collapsed about twenty seconds later. Lying on the tarp, Khaokor Galaxy remained in a semi-unconscious state for several minutes. Much debate ensued concerning the cause of the collapse.[9] Subsequently, Thais came to believe that a bout of ill-ness resembling Khaokor's fall, referred to by the neologism *wuup illness* or *upsurge illness*, necessitated a full physical examination.

Faintness during a *wuup* episode is considered to be a serious symptom, often leading to falling down and not uncommonly to stroke. In a bout of *wuup* illness, the sufferer sometimes collapses and remains in a semi-unconscious state for a few minutes. While on the ground, the eyes may be closed in an attempt to lessen diz-ziness, but the individual does not lose consciousness; the afflicted can hear those around him or her speaking but may be unable to make gestures or speak.[10] After recovering the power of speech and movement, the person is supposed to lie down in bed for a time in a position facilitating breathing and recuperation.

A Comparison of 'Lom' and 'Wuup' Illness: Gendered Panic

Panic varies by gender in the Southern Thai context. Men tend to have *wuup* illness, women tend to have *lom* illness. For women, dizziness and other panic symptoms evoke images of *lom* rising upward from the abdomen, of spoiled blood, and of blocked menses; for men, dizziness and other panic symptoms may evoke the image of the famous boxer who suddenly fell over in a faint. The main differences between *lom* illness and *wuup* illness are summarized in Table 8.3. One may hypothesize that as a result of gender differences in the perceived dangerousness of panic symptoms, Thai men present more often than women for medical treatment of panic. Due to ideas about *lom* and its origins in the abdomen, it seems that Southern Thai women would experience more gastrointestinal symptoms during panic attacks than Southern Thai men. In contrast, the American (U.S.) National Comorbidity Survey found a different symptom—namely, shortness of breath—to be more prominent among women during panic attacks than among men (Sheikh et al. 2002).

Conclusion

Panic disorder takes on various forms, differing by culture, subculture, historical period, and gender. We have seen how culture profoundly shapes the experience of acute anxiety in Southern Thailand, where illness syndromes and ethnophysiology (particularly that of *lom*) greatly influence panic phenomenology, experience, and meaning. How a group believes anxiety-type somatic sensations are produced must be understood in order to perform an analysis of that group's anxiety ontology and mode of panicking.

In *lom* illness there is prominent abdominal distress, which is attributed to stomach *lom* (as in Case 1, Somsee, and Case 2, Samorn). Gastrointestinal symptoms were not included in the original *DSM–III* list of panic symptoms (APA 1980). Seven years later, in *DSM–III–R*, gastrointestinal symptoms (including nausea and abdominal distress) were officially recognized as panic attack criteria (APA 1987). From the Thai perspective, this is a strange omission, because gastrointestinal complaints are a prominent aspect of panic in Thailand. One study in Thailand found that 26.7 percent of PD patients who visited a psychiatric clinic had prominent gastrointestinal symptoms (Udomratn et al. 1988). Many Asian groups appear to have more dizziness and nausea during panic attacks (see Hinton and Hinton 2002), and studies show Asian populations to be more sensitive to motion sickness (for a review, see Hinton and Hinton 2002). The reasons for this predisposition to dizziness and nausea may be cultural frames or physiological differences across groups, or a combination. In particular cultures, as a result of manner of upbringing, inherited nervous system, or cultural-generated expectation—or most likely a

Table 8.3 A comparison of *lom* illness and *wuup* illness

Variables	Illness type	
	Lom *Illness* (Wind Illness)	Wuup *Illness* (Upsurge Illness)
Sex	More women than men	More men than women
Onset of symptoms	Rapid escalation	Sudden, more rapid onset
Most prominent symptoms	GI symptoms: • Abdominal distress • Movable mass in the abdomen • Feeling of air moving upward from the stomach	Neurological symptoms: • Dizziness • Faintness • Feeling unsteady • Being unable to stand without support
Other common symptoms	Faintness	Sweating
Protective behavior and self-treatment	• Sitting upright in bed to decrease the upward movement of *lom* and to ease breathing • Walking around to promote *lom* movement • Expelling *lom* from the stomach by massage and other means • Using *lom* medicine ("sniffers," ointments, and oral medicine)	• Sitting on a chair or lying on a bed • Using special medicinal "sniffers" to decrease *lom* in the head • Rubbing a medicinal ointment on both temples to decrease *lom* in the head
Traditional belief about severity	Usually a transient condition with a psychological basis	Likely to have an underlying medical cause and so requires an examination
Help-seeking behavior	If it occurs frequently or is not relieved by *lom* medicine, requires treatment by a traditional healer (medical care is sought only as a last resort)	Will usually immediately seek medical attention, often going to the emergency room
Medical specialists consulted	An internist, a gastroenterologist, or a cardiologist	An internist or a neurologist
Diagnosis frequently given by the physician	Non-ulcer dyspepsia	Cerebrovascular insufficiency

combination of all of these factors—nausea and dizziness may be more prominent in panic attacks.

This chapter shows that the experience of panic varies greatly by gender in Southern Thailand. In other parts of Thailand, there are other gendered forms of panic. To give one example, there is a panic form that seems to be unique to men in Northeastern Thailand. In nocturnal panic, an individual awakens from sleep in a state of panic, usually with extreme shortness of breath. (For a discussion of the difference between *nocturnal panic*, *nightmare*, and *sleep paralysis*, see Hinton et al. 2005.) In Northeastern Thailand, almost exclusively among young men, there is a high rate of sudden, unexplained nocturnal death (Munger et al. 1986). North-eastern Thais attribute these deaths to the attack of a fiendish female spirit, a kind of vicious succubus; after having intercourse with a young man, she kills him. If several young men die in a village within a short time, the surviving males resort to various means to protect themselves, such as wearing woman's clothing to bed and setting up large wooden phalluses around the house. Because of unexplained nocturnal death and related beliefs, Northeastern Thai men greatly fear sensations of shortness of breath upon awakening; if this fear reaches unreasonable levels, laypersons refer to it as "fear-of-sudden-unexplained-nocturnal-death illness" (*rook klua lai tai*). In the first author's clinical experience, fear of nocturnal death gener-ates high rates of nocturnal panic among Northeastern Thai males. In this case, the biology of panic, gender construction, biological gender differences, and culturally generated fears are in dynamic interaction.[11]

In Southern Thailand, as revealed in the present study, a woman's having *lom* illness leads to important effects within the family and on her life trajectory. If a woman's *lom* illness is treated by the traditional musical healing (which almost oc-curred in one of the cases described in this chapter; for a description of this type of healing, see endnote 8), the explanation presented by the spirit medium and what is said by the afflicted during the ritual may have direct effects on the com-munity (Hinton 1999).

One must ask the following questions: Does *lom* illness serve as a collective representation that perpetuates the marginalization of women, or does it serve as a way to resist various forms of abuse?[12] Does *lom* illness provide a narrow way out, a small amount of wiggle room, or a small field of action, which for lack of better alternatives is embodied and performed? These questions need to be fur-ther investigated. (Lewis 2002 asks these same questions about possession rituals, using the terms *central* versus *peripheral possession cults* to contrast these two very different effects, and to contrast what might be called *center-consolidating* versus *center-challenging practices*.)

Gulf War syndrome, multiple chemical sensitivity, hypoglycemia, premenstrual dysphoric disorder, *spasmophilie*: gender and history and cultural context and scientific discovery, in dynamic interaction, continually constitute new illness syndromes, with these emergent syndromes creating new sayabilities, doabilities, and code complexes that individuals in specific interpersonal and financial localities embody and enact (Foucault 1971). That is, illness forms such as *lom* or *wuup* illness create specific sayabilities, doabilities, and code complexes that individuals in specific interpersonal and financial localities embody and enact. These illnesses are collective representations of what it means to be distressed, and their origins and preferred treatments will be hotly debated in a high-stakes game of definition. How an illness is *physiologized* is often a key part of this high-stakes game (Foucault 1986:107), as would seem to be the case in Southern Thailand, a context in which panic's physiology varies by gender.

More generally, the current chapter raises the question of how panic, and fear in the broad sense, differs by gender. This topic might be investigated by researching some of the following areas: cultural ideas about how biological vulnerability and susceptibility to fear vary across genders; differences in the biology of fear and the induction of symptoms (such as by hormonal shifts during the menstrual cycle producing symptoms) across genders; how fears vary in type and intensity across the genders; how the triggers of anxiety and panic vary across genders; and how the semantic networks of anxiety symptoms (dizziness, palpitations, and cold extremities) vary across genders in terms of trauma associations, catastrophic cognitions, and metaphoric associations. In addition, studies should examine whether women in a particular society have more actual sources of fear than men, as in fewer economic and work options, greater threats of violence, and a history of more trauma.

One fertile area for the study of gendered panic has been agoraphobia (Capps and Ochs 1995; Davidson 2003; Milun 2007), a type of panic that is much more common among women than men in the contemporary United States. Previous forms of gendered panic in the West also warrant further research, for example, the form of female panic common in the eighteenth and nineteenth centuries, *hysteria*, in which the rising womb or vapors rising from the womb oppressed the heart and caused suffocation could be compared to that period's frequent form of male panic, *hypochondriachal melancholy*, in which vapors rising from the spleen and other abdominal areas assaulted the heart, lungs, and head (Blackmore 1729; Micale 1995; Veith 1965; Wenegrat 2001). Studies also need to examine shifts, new "representations," in these gendered categories through time—such as the shifts produced by Charcot's investigations of hysteria at the end of the nineteenth century (Didi-Huberman 2003)—which created new social imaginaries and constellations of power, truth, and knowledge. Gender construction, the production of disorder

by gender stereotypes, challenges against gender ideals, the use of gendered stereotypes in specific social situations to gain specific means, and the consequences of
embodying gender stereotypes in certain social situations—panic and its associated
illnesses often play a key role in these areas.

Notes

1. In the present-day United States, English-speaking male panickers frequently present
with fear of heart attack, resulting in extensive medical workups; also, certain syndromes,
such as Gulf War syndrome and multiple chemical sensitivity, allow a man to seek medical
services (and disability benefits) without fear of being labeled mentally ill. Formerly, in both
the United States and Europe, male panickers might cast themselves as suffering neurasthenia, as exhausted through overindustriousness, as tragic heroes.

2. *Weak heart* is a panic syndrome that seems to be most elaborated in Northeastern
Thailand (Hinton 1999), with a sufferer focusing on fears of cardiac death during palpitations. As we will see, fears of weak heart are also prominent in *lom* illness.

3. The wind ethnophysiology of traditional Chinese medicine also had an important
influence in Southeast Asia, most particularly in Vietnam (see Hinton et al. 2003).

4. Cirrhosis-caused ascites, a serious medical condition in which the abdomen becomes
distended due to an accumulation of fluid, is mistakenly thought by many Southern Thais
to result from an accumulation of *lom*. Catastrophic cognitions about abdominal sensations
are further produced by the well-known Buddhist story of *Choo Chok*, who died of a ruptured abdomen after eating excessively.

5. For further discussion of these terms, see Hinton et al. 2004.

6. Thai traditional massage is believed to expel *lom* from the body. The treatment is
based on the idea that blockage of *lom* in any part of the body can cause illness. *Lom* may ac-
cumulate in the abdomen, and pressing on certain parts of the back, shoulders, or abdomen
can expel the *lom* by bringing about burping or by forcing the *lom* out along other routes.

7. In the past, when there were no Western-style doctors in Thailand, people usually
sought out a spirit doctor for treatment. Some spirit doctors would pray to the ancestors of
the dead person and then channel one of them while in a trance in order to determine what
must be done to appease them.

8. For a description of how a music-based dance ritual in Northeastern Thailand may
cure psychiatric disorders, including panic disorder, see Hinton (1999). The Nora dance,
a traditional Southern Thai classical dance also known as the Thai Manohra dance, is the
oldest surviving Thai dance-drama and is frequently performed in Southern Thailand. It
concerns Prince Suthon and his adventures as he tries to rescue the kidnapped Manohra, a
princess who is half bird and half human.

9. Galaxy underwent tests at Phya Thai Hospital the next day. The medical director of
the hospital, Dr. Surapong Ampanwong, asserted that dehydration caused by drastic weight
reduction could have caused Khaokor's black out; Khaokor had been overweight before the
fight and had to lose a lot of weight to qualify for it. A different medical opinion was given
by Dr. Roongtham Ladplee, a prominent Thai neurosurgeon, who said it could have been
either a mild form of epilepsy or poor cerebral circulation.

10. Mutism is also observed in the Cambodian illness syndrome called "wind overload"

(Hinton et al. 2001a, 2001b). To what extent the phenomenon is generated by cultural frames or biological processes is unclear. In this last regard, it should be noted that one of the questions on the Acute Panic Inventory (Liebowitz et al. 1984) asks the extent to which the person finds it difficult to speak.

11. For a discussion of nocturnal panic, see Craske (1999) and McNally (1994). For a review of the cognitive model of the generation of nocturnal panic, see Craske (1999:189–193) and McNally (1994:111–114).

12. Clearly, such questions might also be asked of various distress syndromes prominent among women in certain historical periods in the West, such as hysteria in the nineteenth century (Micale 1995; Veith 1965; Wenegrat 2001).

References

American Psychiatric Association (APA). 1980. *Diagnostic and Statistical Manual of Mental Disorders*. 3rd ed. [*DSM–III*.] Washington, DC: American Psychiatric Association.

———. 1987. *Diagnostic and Statistical Manual of Mental Disorders*. 3rd ed., rev. [*DSM–III–R*.] Washington, DC: American Psychiatric Association.

Amering, M., and H. Katschnig. 1990. Panic Attacks and Panic Disorder in Cross-Cultural Perspective. *Psychiatric Annals* 20:511–516.

Blackmore, R. 1729. *A Treatise of the Spleen and Vapours; or Hypochondriachal and Hysterical Affections*. London: Pemberton.

Bunditchate, A., P. Saosarn, P. Kitiruksanon, and W. Chutha. 2001. Epidemiology of Mental Disorders Among Thai People. *Journal of the Psychiatric Association of Thailand* 46:335–343.

Capps, L., and E. Ochs. 1995. *Constructing Panic: The Discourse of Agoraphobia*. Cambridge, MA: Harvard University Press.

Craske, M. C. 1999. *Anxiety Disorders*. Boulder, CO: Westview Press.

Davidson, J. 2003. *Phobic Geographies: The Phenomenology and Spatiality of Identity*. Lancaster, UK: Ashgate.

Didi-Huberman, G. 2003. *Invention of Hysteria: Charcot and the Photographic Iconography of the Salpêtrière*. Cambridge, MA: MIT Press.

Facchinetti, F., G. Romano, M. Fava, and A. Genazzani. 1992. Lactate Infusion Induces Panic Attacks in Patients with Premenstrual Syndrome. *Psychosomatic Medicine* 54:284–296.

Foucault, M. 1971. *L'ordre du discours*. Paris: Gallimard.

———. 1986. *The Care of the Self: The History of Sexuality*, Vol. 3. New York: Random House.

Gorman, J., J. Kent, J. Martinez, S. Browne, J. Coplan, and L. Papp. 2001. Physiological Changes During Carbon Dioxide Inhalation in Patients with Panic Disorder, Major Depression, and Premenstrual Dysphoric Disorder: Evidence for Mechanisms. *Archives of General Psychiatry* 58:125–131.

Hinton, D. E. 1999. Musical Healing and Cultural Syndromes in Isan: Landscape, Conceptual Metaphor, and Embodiment. Ph.D. dissertation, Department of Anthropology, Harvard University.

Hinton, D. E., P. Ba, and K. Um. 2001a. *Kyol Goeu* ("Wind Overload") Part I: A Cultural Syndrome of Orthostatic Panic Among Khmer Refugees. *Transcultural Psychiatry* 38:403–432.

———. 2001b. *Kyol Goeu* ("Wind Overload") Part II: Prevalence, Characteristics, and Mechanisms of *Kyol Goeu* and Near-*Kyol Goeu* Episodes of Khmer Patients Attending a Psychiatric Clinic. *Transcultural Psychiatry* 38:433–460.

Hinton, D. E., and S. D. Hinton. 2002. Panic Disorder, Somatization, and the New Cross-Cultural Psychiatry; or the Seven Bodies of a Medical Anthropology of Panic. *Culture, Medicine, and Psychiatry* 26:155–178.

Hinton, D. E., T. Pham, H. Chau, M. Tran, and S. D. Hinton. 2003. "Hit by the Wind" and Temperature-Shift Panic Among Vietnamese Refugees. *Transcultural Psychiatry* 40:342–376.

Hinton, D. E., A. Chea, P. Ba, and M. H. Pollack. 2004. Olfactory Panic Among Cambodian Refugees: A Contextual Approach. *Transcultural Psychiatry* 41:155–195.

Hinton, D. E., D. Hufford, and L. J. Kirmayer. 2005. Introduction to Culture and Sleep Paralysis. *Transcultural Psychiatry* 42:5–10.

Leslie, C. 1992. Interpretations of Illness: Syncretism in Modern Ayurveda. In *Paths to Asian Medical Knowledge*. C. Leslie and A. Young, eds. Pp. 209–224. Berkeley: University of California Press.

Liebowitz, M., A. Fyer, J. Gorman, D. Dillon, I. Appleby, G. Levy, S. Anderson, M. Levitt, M. Palij, and S. Davies. 1984. Lactate Provocation of Panic Attacks. I. Clinical and Behavioral Findings. *Archives of General Psychiatry* 41:764–770.

Lewis, I. M. 2002. *Ecstatic Religion*. London: Routledge.

Lin, K. M. 1983. Hwa-Byung: A Korean Culture-Bound Syndrome. *American Journal of Psychiatry* 140:105–107.

McNally, R. J. 1994. *Panic Disorder: A Critical Analysis*. New York: Guilford Press.

Micale, M. 1995. *Approaching Hysteria: Disease and Its Interpretations*. Princeton, NJ: Princeton University Press.

Milun, K. 2007. *Pathologies of Modern Space: Empty Space, Urban Anxiety, and the Recovery of Public Self*. New York: Routledge.

Munger, R., G., B. Weniger, S. Warintrawat, P. Kunasol, H. van der Werff, G. van Bruggen, C. Paquet, and N. R. Holtan. 1986. Sudden Death in Sleep of South-East Asian Refugees. *Lancet* 2:1093–1094.

Nichter, M. 1981. Idioms of Distress: Alternatives in the Expression of Psychosocial Distress: A Case Study from India. *Culture, Medicine, and Psychiatry* 5:379–408.

Nilchaikovit, T. 1988. Round Table Discussion on Panic Disorder. In *Symposium Proceedings and Panel Discussion on "Panic Disorder: An Update."* Pp. 15–28. Hong Kong: Excerpta Medica Asia.

Schnall, S., A. Abrahamson, and J. Laird. 2002. Premenstrual Syndrome and Misattribution: A Self-Perception, Individual Differences Perspective. *Basic and Applied Psychology* 24:215–228.

Sheikh, J. I., G. Leskin, and D. F. Klein. 2002. Gender Differences in Panic Disorder: Findings from the National Comorbidity Survey. *American Journal of Psychiatry* 159:55–58.

Silpakit, C., and P. Sukanich. 1992. Panic Disorder: Diagnosis and Treatment by Non-Psychiatrist Physicians. *Journal of the Psychiatric Association of Thailand* 37:182–190.

Tabor, D. C. 1981. Ripe and Unripe: Concepts of Health and Sickness in Ayurvedic Medicine. *Social Science and Medicine* 15B:442–457.

Udomratn, P. 2000. Panic Disorder in Thailand: A Report on the Secondary Data Analysis. *Journal of the Medical Association of Thailand* 83:1158–1166.

————. 2004. Panic Disorder. In *Epidemiology of Mental Health Problems and Psychiatric Disorders in Thailand*. P. Udomratn, ed. Pp. 165–184. Songkhla, TH: Lim Brother Press.

————. 2006. Epidemiology of Mental Disorders in Thailand. *ASEAN Journal of Psychiatry* 7:22–25.

Udomratn, P., S. Kuasirikul, and W. Tanchaiswad. 1988. Panic Disorder at Songklanagarind Hospital. *Journal of the Psychiatric Association of Thailand* 33:107–118.

Veith, I. 1965. *Hysteria: The History of a Disease*. London: Aaronson.

Wenegrat, B. 2001. *Theatres of Disorder*. Oxford, UK: Oxford University Press.

World Health Organization (WHO). 1978. *Manual of the International Statistical Classification of Diseases, Injuries, and Causes on Death*. Vol. 1. Pp. 177–213. Geneva: World Health Organization.

9

'Ihahamuka,' a Rwandan Syndrome of Response to the Genocide

Blocked Flow, Spirit Assault, and Shortness of Breath

Athanase Hagengimana and Devon E. Hinton

But the fact is that most of the massacres were carried out using more basic weapons: machetes, knives, axes, hoes, hammers, spears, bludgeons, or clubs studded with nails (known as *ntampongano* or "without pity"). I don't need to dwell on the horror of these deaths, the frightful noise of skulls being smashed in, the sound of bodies falling on top of each other. Every Rwandan still has these sounds etched in their memory, and will for a long time: the screams of people being killed, the groans of the dying and, perhaps worst of all, the unbearable silence of death which still hangs over the mass graves.

Sibomana *1999:59*

ON APRIL 6, 1994, a plane carrying the Hutu president of Rwanda and several other high-level Hutu leaders was shot down over the Rwandan capital of Kigali (Straus 2006). The next day the genocide began. Hutu hunted down and killed Tutsi, often using crude instruments such as machetes and nail-studded clubs, at other times killing by drowning and other methods, such as throwing grenades into churches, schools, and other public buildings where people gathered, frequently in the thousands, for refuge, then rushing in to finish the work with handheld weapons, often in successive waves over the course of hours or days (Des Forges 1999; Gourevitch 1998; Hatzfeld 2000; Keane 1995; Sibomana 1999; Taylor 1999). Rape was also common (Straus 2006). The killing and persecution continued for almost one hundred days, stopping only after the complete takeover of the country by the Rwandan Popular Front (RPF), a primarily Tutsi military force.[1] At that point, the leaders of the genocidal regime, along with several million other Hutu, fled to neighboring countries.

Tension between the Hutu majority and the Tutsi minority had long simmered in Rwanda, with periodic interruptions of violence, even though the two groups speak the same language (Kinyarwanda) and have the same myths and the same traditions (Straus 2006). Historically, the Tutsi had been pastoral, raising cattle, and had been the ruling class, whereas the Hutu were traditionally farmers and of lower class. There were certain racial stereotypes: Tutsi were considered to be taller and lighter skinned, and to have narrow rather than broad noses (for a discussion of the Hutu and Tutsi differences, and of the representation of difference and its uses, see Pottier 2002, 2005; Straus 2006; Taylor 1992, 1999, 2002).

Before the genocide, Hutu comprised 84 to 90 percent of Rwanda's population, Tutsi comprised 9 to 15 percent, and Twa comprised 1 percent. (Straus 2006). During the genocide, about 500,000 Tutsi were killed, approximately 75 percent of the Tutsi population. It is estimated that 250,000 rapes occurred. During the three-month campaign to take control of the country, the RPF killed 25,000 to 60,000 Hutu. (For a review of theories of why the genocide occurred, see Straus 2006.)

Not surprisingly, given this horrific trauma, many Rwandan genocide survivors have severe posttraumatic stress disorder (PTSD) symptoms and panic attacks (Hagengimana et al. 2003). This chapter focuses on a disorder that multiple authors have identified as the main presentation of trauma-related disorder in Rwanda following the genocide. *Ihahamuka*, which literally means "without lungs" is characterized by fear and the frequent occurrence of episodes of shortness of breath (Fisher 2004; Hagengimana et al. 2003; Musabe-Ngamije 2002; Wulsin and Hagengimana 1998).

In this chapter we do a cultural analysis of *ihahamuka* and its key symptom, shortness of breath, including trauma associations to, catastrophic cognitions about, and iconic resonances of shortness of breath. In the Rwandan context, through its *configuration as a back-and-forth flow*, breathing has multiple "ontological resonances" (A. Hinton 2004); acts as a key "ideogram" (Caillois 1990), that is, as an abstract image that represents multiple related meanings; and forms a "rhizome" (Guattari and Deleuze 1987), joining multiple cultural domains: social process, the representation of what constitutes beauty and health, how the most horrid abuse is perpetrated, how trauma is experienced, and the experiencing of particular types of bodily symptoms. To use Probyn's (2004) term, the chapter uses an analytic approach that might be called a *rhizo-ethnology* of the traumatized body.

Taylor (1992) demonstrates that *flow as health* dominates reasoning on multiple levels—aesthetics, ritual, cure, bodily symptoms—of Rwandan society, acting as a "root metaphor" or "generative schema," giving rise to a specific mythic or symbolic logic.[2] According to Taylor (1992, 1999, 2002), flow and blockage symbolism—the valuation of *flow* and the *open conduit*—guided Rwandans prior to the genocide on the cultural, exchange, and social levels; during the genocide, in perpetrating and experiencing the genocide; and after the genocide, in somatization, with constipation being a prominent complaint, an image of blockage of flow (Taylor 2002:165). (For a discussion of Taylor's analysis, see Baines 2003; Hoffman 2005; Scott 2005.)

As we demonstrate in this chapter, this flow and blockage symbolism resulted in another type of somatization of trauma-related distress following the Rwandan genocide. Traumatized Rwandans often had episodes of *ihahamuka*, the central symptom being severe shortness of breath. This blockage of flow on the level of the body was an icon, an analogue, a homologue, of the blockage that existed on multiple ontological levels of Rwandan society, and served as a symbolically powerful expression of distress.[3] To produce terror in the Rwandan genocide, the Hutu perpetrators targeted flow, and in the embodied response to trauma of Tutsi, blocked flow held a central place—in the form of a cultural syndrome, *ihahamuka*, which has shortness of breath as a core symptom.

The present chapter is based on data from Dr. Hagengimana's clinical experience as a psychiatrist treating patients in both urban and rural localities in Rwanda. He took extensive notes on certain cases. Dr. Hagengimana came to Harvard on a fellowship to study trauma. He and Dr. Hinton decided to write a chapter on a distress syndrome that Dr. Hagengimana had found to be common among Rwandan genocide survivors, namely, *ihahamuka*. Dr. Hagengimana described the cases to Dr. Hinton, who typed them up. The two then met several times to discuss the cases. Dr. Hinton then wrote a draft of the chapter, which Dr. Hagengimana read and commented on before Dr. Hinton prepared a final version.

Cases

The following cases were seen by Dr. Hagengimana in 1997 and 1998 while he worked as a psychiatrist at the outpatient clinic at the Neuropsychiatric Hospital in Kigali and at the University Hospital Clinic in Butare. More than 80 percent of the patients met PTSD criteria. Many of the referrals came from doctors at medical clinics for somatic symptoms that seemed not to have any medical basis.

Case 1: Mary

In the 1994 genocide, a Hutu soldier killed Mary's parents by bashing in their skulls with a club. He then struck the eighteen-year-old Mary on the neck with a machete.[4] Presuming her to be dead, the soldier threw Mary's limp body into a latrine.[5] Corpses were tossed into the hole beside her; within a few days, maggots grew in the corpses. Mary survived by eating avocados that had fallen beside her from a tree growing at the side of the latrine. Following several days living like this, someone finally rescued her.

After the genocide, Mary was adopted by a family member. While at boarding school, about three times a month she had episodes of *ihahamuka*, during which she fell to the ground due to extreme shortness of breath and nausea. The episodes were triggered by hearing a loud noise or by entering the school's dining room when rice or avocados were being served. Upon collapsing to the ground, she would cry out for help. The nurse and other students would rush to her aid; one of the students would place a hand on her chest to secure her heart. On the ground, her shortness of breath and palpitations continued, and Mary smelled feces and urine, worsening her nausea, sometimes to the point of vomiting. The symptoms lasted about twenty minutes, during which she feared dying of asphyxia or from her heart jumping out of her chest. In about a quarter of the episodes, images of past traumas came into her mind. The nurse at the school suspected the cause to be asthma or a heart disorder, but neither a pulmonologist nor a cardiologist could find any abnormalities.

When no physical cause could be found for her episodes, Mary was referred to psychiatry. To get to her first psychiatric clinic visit, Mary rode a bus; as the bus passed through a grove of avocado trees, she suddenly felt short of breath and extremely nauseous. Upon arriving at the clinic, she recounted this episode to Dr. Hagengimana and told him of her other near-syncopal episodes. Diagnosing her as suffering from panic disorder along with PTSD, Dr. Hagengimana treated her with alprazolam and propranolol (both common panic medications)[6] and psychotherapy. During psychotherapy, Dr. Hagengimana identified the triggers of Mary's panic attacks and their connection to her trauma experiences. The rice reminded her of the small, white maggots in the corpses lying beside her in the refuse pit; the avocados reminded her of the avocadoes on which she survived while in the latrine; and loud noises reminded her of the sickening thud of her parents' skulls being bashed in and the yelling of the perpetrators.

As treatment, Dr. Hagengimana educated Mary about how trauma-related cues—for example, the sight of avocadoes—might recall these memories and cause shortness of breath, nausea, and palpitations by triggering a fear response, even though sometimes the trauma event might not be consciously recalled at the time. He also assured her that she was healthy, that her shortness of breath, palpitations, and nausea were not dangerous but simply resulted from fear; that her symptoms were common in trauma victims; and that she was not going crazy. He discussed with her the difficulties of emotionally adjusting to the death of her parents, of coming to terms with the horrific manner in which they were murdered. As a re-sult of these interventions, Mary dramatically improved. During the following two years she was able to perform well in school and had only one more severe episode of *ihahamuka*, triggered by a fight between her adoptive parents; their hostile ex-change evoked memories of the Hutu who attacked her and killed her parents.

Case 2: André

André, a thirty-five-year-old Hutu male, was forced to watch as his Tutsi wife and two children were murdered in front of him. Then André was instructed to say his last prayers. Next he was told by a man holding a machete to bend his head over; he awaited the blade's descent into his neck. After obeying these orders, André heard a sudden burst of laughter from the machete wielder; the assailant's companion fired a gunshot into the air and ordered André to leave. André's brother, although a Hutu, was murdered because he had the physical features of a Tutsi.

After the genocide, several times a week André relived his trauma in nightmares and awoke terrified. At other times he awoke in a panic but without the awaken-ing being caused by a nightmare; that is, he had *nocturnal panic attacks* (which are common among patients with panic disorder; see Chapter 8 for further discus-sion). Upon awakening from a nightmare or having nocturnal panic, André feared dying of shortness of breath. He experienced daytime *ihahamuka* episodes, which were triggered by several types of events: working hard in the fields, encountering one of the many Hutu whom he remembered as having perpetrated violence, or hearing a loud noise. During a daytime episode of *ihahamuka*, André had severe shortness of breath along with dizziness and palpitations, causing him to sit on the ground and to pant in an attempt to catch his breath. André feared dying from asphyxia or from his heart jumping out of his chest. During the episodes he also felt extreme heat in his head—like a boiling cauldron—which caused a headache. The heat in the head, combined with his other symptoms, made him worry about going insane. André attributed the episodes to a malevolent spirit strangling him and sending into his mind frightening images; he thought the spirit was either that of a deceased relative seeking vengeance or one sent by a sorcerer hired by an enemy. He increasingly restricted his activities, avoiding even farming for fear of triggering a symptom attack.[7]

A traditional healer attributed André's symptoms to the attacks of a disgruntled relative who had not received proper burial and instructed him to locate the corpse of the deceased and perform a burial ritual. After following the healer's suggestions, André improved but remained symptomatic; consequently, he sought treatment with Dr. Hagengimana, who prescribed both alprazolam and propranolol to treat André's panic, discussed the role of survival guilt in causing the symptoms, and educated André regarding the nature of panic attacks that occur in panic disorder and PTSD. As a result of the treatment by the traditional healer and Dr. Hagengimana, André improved and was able to perform his farm labors.

Case 3: Outbreaks of 'Ihahamuka' Among Young Female Orphans

In different parts of Rwanda during 1997 and 1998, mass burials were performed for unidentified corpses; large numbers of orphaned girls and young women attended. During the burial ceremonies, many participants suddenly became short of breath, falling to the ground and gasping for air. In an event observed by Dr. Hagengimana, a young woman felt extremely short of breath and fell to the ground upon seeing a red belt similar to one worn by her father; soon other girls and young women collapsed. In the years following the genocide, many schools had outbreaks of *ihahamuka*. In a typical scenario, an orphaned girl or young woman would fall to the ground at the sudden onset of shortness of breath, dizziness, palpitations, and fear of dying; soon others, usually also orphans, would have such episodes. At one school, out of six hundred girls and young women, sixty developed *ihahamuka*, forcing early closure of the facility, with classes recommencing the following year.

The Emergence of 'Ihahamuka' in the Postgenocide Period

Prior to the 1994 genocide, to describe a tendency to be fearful and panicked, Rwandans often used the phrase *kuba igikange* (easily threatened). In a typical scenario, a young boy might develop *kuba igikange* if his father habitually became drunk and beat him. It was thought that one should not upset an easily threatened person, because a strong emotion or noise might cause fright to the point of heart dysfunction and death. Among persons with *kuba igikange* and other anxiety disorders, according to Dr. Hagengimana's clinical experience working in psychiatry clinics before the genocide, complaints of airway-passage blockage—such as *globus hystericus* (that is, a sensation of a lump in the throat), shortness of breath, and a feeling of choking—were common, and this complaint often involved spiritually related fears such as fear of being strangled by an angered ancestor spirit or by a spirit sent by a sorcerer hired by an enemy.

After the 1994 genocide, *ihahamuka* emerged as the new term to describe fear states. Within a year, almost everyone knew this term. As already described, *ihahamuka* is a panic-like syndrome characterized by episodes of marked shortness of breath, along with palpitations and other symptoms; the person usually falls to the ground, gasping for breath, fearing asphyxia, syncope, and death.[8] During an attack, not uncommonly the person has pain and heat in the head. An *ihahamuka* attack may occur upon awakening at night, sometimes after a nightmare, sometimes when no nightmare has occurred;[9] a relative may be asked to be a sleep companion to provide assistance during these nocturnal events.

As treatment, several things may be done during the attack. The left side of the chest may be pressed with one or two hands supposedly to keep the heart from bounding out of the body. The space around the individual may be cleared of people and things to increase air availability. Water may be poured on the body to cool it and relieve sweating. Milk, considered a panacea in the Rwandan culture, may be offered; if regurgitated, death is considered imminent. (As described later, in the Rwandan context, milk is a key symbol of flow; as a treatment, it seemingly serves to restore normal flow in the individual—here the back-and-forth flow of breathing.)

Some typical triggers of *ihahamuka* episodes include witnessing or being involved in an argument, visiting the location of a loved one's murder, having a nightmare, hearing a loud noise, smelling a foul odor, experiencing any strong emotion, engaging in exertion that triggers sensations, encountering a trauma reminder, experiencing the April anniversary date of the beginning of the genocide, and thinking about a financial concern, as in the painful realization that one lacks sufficient money to pay for a child's educational fees. The list just presented indicates the importance in *ihahamuka* episodes of trauma reminders and anything that induces a strong emotion or somatic symptoms.

A Cultural Analysis of 'Ihahamuka'

In the following subsections, we perform a cultural analysis of *ihahamuka*, focusing mainly on its central symptom, shortness of breath, by performing a *rhizo-ethnology*, a semantic-network analysis (Good 1994), of shortness of breath. After analyzing the etymology of the term *ihahamuka*, we delineate the trauma associations that may be evoked during the episodes, such as those that lead to shortness of breath; the fears of bodily dysregulations during the episodes; and concerns that the episode's main symptom, shortness of breath, indicates spirit assault. In the final subsection, we examine shortness of breath from the perspective of the Rwandan root metaphor of flow and blockage as described in Taylor's work to further explore the ontological resonance of shortness of breath, that is, its affective power.

The Etymology, Sound Symbolism, and Iconicism of the Term 'Ihahamuka'

The word for *lungs* in Rwandan is *ihaha*. The syllable *ha* is iconic, sonically depicting the flow of breath. To say *ha*, one must make a strong exhalation; a vigorous sense of expiratory flow is experienced. The repetition of the syllable (*ha* + *ha* = *haha*) intensifies this effect. The Rwandan word *haha* configures the lungs as the location of inhalation and exhalation, of respiratory flow. *Muka* means "without." So, literally translated *ihahamuka* (*ihaha* + *muka*) is "without lungs," a term suggesting poor respiratory flow.

Trauma Recall Occurring During 'Ihahamuka' Episodes

For Rwandans, shortness of breath may recall events that occurred during the genocide, with such trauma recall triggering or worsening an *ihahamuka* episode; or trauma recall can cause shortness of breath, bringing about an *ihahamuka* episode. Many events that occurred during the Rwandan genocide are associated with shortness of breath as a body memory. Even if these various asphyxia-type traumas were not directly experienced, given that they are represented in the collective memory, they may be evoked upon experiencing shortness of breath; or vice versa, thinking about these trauma events, these collective memories, may cause shortness of breath.

Execution by drowning was common during the genocide (Keane 1995:75; Sibomana 1999:59), and so was hiding in confined spaces such as cellars and small roof spaces to avoid capture (Prunier 1995:253; Sibomana 1999:63). If a person experienced a trauma during which terror produced shortness of breath—such as seeing others killed or fearing that one was about to be killed upon passing through a road checkpoint—that event may be recalled when dyspnea later occurs. And as indicated in this chapter's introduction, and as is further described later, shortness of breath is culturally understood in terms of the culturally salient generative schema of flow and blockage, as an exemplar of blockage. Owing to this culture-based representation, shortness of breath may be brought about by the memory of any event marked by blockage, such as passing through one of the innumerable roadblocks where so much killing occurred (Taylor 1999:130), or being encircled and entrapped—with thousands of others in close, asphyxiating proximity—at churches and other governmental buildings, then attacked. Conversely, thinking about these traumas in blockage imagery may bring about shortness of breath.

When somatic symptoms other than shortness of breath are experienced for any reason—such as upon becoming anxious or angry, when climbing stairs, or upon smelling a bad odor—they may trigger trauma memories and cause great distress, thus starting an *ihahamuka* episode; or if those symptoms occur in the context of an *ihahamuka* episode, they may trigger trauma recall and worsen the episode. As one example, nausea would be expected to encode genocide memories, due to so many bodies being left unburied where they were slain, thrown into latrines, and dumped in rivers (Keane 1995:75, 78; Prunier 1995:255). Any of various somatic symptoms other than shortness of breath—such as tinnitus, cold extremities, or dizziness—may also be linked to the memory of nearly being killed or of witnessing the death of a relative, thus causing horror, terror, and rage along with nausea and loud ringing in the ears; subsequently, these somatic symptoms become somatic markers of the event.

Concerns About Disordered Physiology During 'Ihahamuka' Episodes

Rwandans greatly fear the symptoms that occur during *ihahamuka* episodes, especially shortness of breath, which causes worry about asphyxia. The heart is considered a respiratory organ according to the traditional Rwandan ethnophysiology (Lestrade 1955:66); consequently, irregular heart motions, such as palpitations, conjure fears of impaired respiration and increase asphyxia fears. Also according to the traditional Rwandan ethnophysiology, the heart moves progressively upward from the abdomen during states of trepidation; if it rises too high, death will result from the impairment of breathing or from the heart becoming dislodged, even leaving the body.[10]

In keeping with this ethnophysiology, many of the Rwandan expressions used to describe fear refer to the rising heart, with the location of the heart—low in the belly or rising upward and threatening to leave the body—indicating the degree of fright. Let us examine some of these fear expressions (for more on the following examples, see Jacob 1983; Kagame 1956:213): "To have the heart in the lower abdomen" is to have a "calm character." A person with "a heart in one place" (*gushyita umutima hamwe*) has "a calm character." "To have the heart in the head" (*kugira umutima mu mutwe*) is to be "in a state of fright." "The heart is getting out of me" (*umutima uramiriyeme*) or "the heart is outside of me" (*gukuka umutima*) indicates "a state of terror," whereas "to have the heart return to the belly" (*gusubuiz umutima munda*) means "to return to a state of calm after a period of terror."

These expressions describing fear are often meant literally, not metaphorically. In the Rwandan context, fear is physiologized (Foucault 1986:107), and pathophysiologized, that is, considered capable of producing a dangerous physiological disturbance. These emotional expressions increase the belief in the ethnophysiology, naturalizing it; increase catastrophic cognitions about anxiety states; may lead to anxious states being somatized as palpitations, because the patient expects to have palpitations during anxiety states; and may lead to anxious states being somatized as shortness of breath, because the rising (and palpitating) heart is associated with shortness of breath.

Although shortness of breath and palpitations may initially predominate in an episode of *ihahamuka*, other symptoms, such as tinnitus and cold extremities, may emerge; and if there are catastrophic cognitions regarding those symptoms, escalation to panic will be accelerated. Typical examples include ear buzzing, interpreted as an inauspicious sign—warning of, for example, an imminent attack by an enemy or the death of a family member (Lestrade 1955:52)—and heat in the head, construed as indicating the onset of malaria or insanity (as per Dr. Hagengimana's clinical experience).[11] (Upon seeking help at a medical facility, *ihahamuka* sufferers are often misdiagnosed as having illnesses, such as asthma, because of prominent shortness of breath, or a heart condition, because of prominent palpitations. Upon reporting to a healthcare provider the symptom cluster of dizziness, severe headache, and a feeling of heat in the head, the *ihahamuka* sufferer may well be prescribed a malaria medication; upon reporting nausea, the sufferer may be given pills for treating an infestation of the gastrointestinal tract by worms.)

'Ihahamuka' Episodes Attributed to Spirit Assault

On their own, or after consultation with a traditional healer, patients and their families often decide that the *ihahamuka* episode is caused by a *strangulation assault*—most commonly by the spirit of a vengeful dead relative infuriated that he or she did not receive proper burial, or less commonly by a spirit sent by an enemy. The majority of genocide victims were never located, making it impossible to perform burial rituals. In the Rwandan context, elaborate burial rituals establish a new, special relationship with the deceased, a reciprocal relationship marked by back-and-forth exchange. Later in this chapter we describe traditional Rwandan burial rites and then review writings by clinicians that reveal the importance of addressing the issue of burial rites in promoting recovery among Rwandan refugees. We do so in order to explore the affective meaning connected with not burying a relative in the prescribed manner, to explicate the affective power connected with the idea that a relative is enraged to the point of attempting to kill by strangulation, and to explore how burial rites are understood in terms of the cultural logic of flow and blockage—namely, as key actions in the maintaining of a healthy back-and-forth level within society and between the living and the dead. (Likewise, Faust [2008] demonstrates that in the antebellum period in the United States, there existed a well-developed "concept of the Good Death," a veritable *ars moriendi*, which was part of popular culture [see also Schantz 2008]. Faust [2008] argues that in the American Civil War, a war resulting in the death of about 2 percent of the population, the emotional hardship resulting from those deaths was greatly increased by the contrast of the manner of death to the cultural ideal: so many were shot in the head or lungs or guts on the battlefield, dying in no man's land between the lines; so many—probably more than 300,000—were buried in anonymous graves, not uncommonly mass graves. Faust [2008] discusses the importance of post–Civil War representations of death, of interments and reinterments, of spiritualism used to contact the dead through the Ouija board, of religious literature, in coming to terms with that emotional trauma.)

The anthropological literature asserts that burial ceremonies are not for the dead but for the living, "serving as a way to adjust to a death" (Hertz 1960; see also Spijker 1990:104–107); that the rites transform the corpse into a new entity, transform my memory of *my-uncle-as-a-living-being,* just dead, remembered in the throes of death, into *my-uncle-as-a-benevolent-being,* dwelling in another realm— that there is a ritually enacted transformation of memory, from a "salientized" frightening image, as in the corpse or the person during dire illness or death throes, into a reassuring and nurturing image, such as a beneficial being with whom exchange has been established. If a death is sudden and tragic, societies frequently make the burial rites more elaborate in order to facilitate the adjustment for the living—a key "work of culture" (Obeyesekere 1990).[12] Ritual, acting as a form of *poesis*—meant here in the sense of creating imagery and meaning associations to an object, event, or person—transforms the memory of the person: the deceased acquires a new set of attributes, becoming a transcendent, content, and beneficent being (Hertz 1960; Spijker 1990:104–107). Burial injunctions have important psychological consequences. On the positive side, if they are performed correctly, they aid psychological adjustment; on the negative side, if the rituals cannot be performed, the person experiences a feeling of failure and terror.

According to Rwandan tradition, the deceased should be buried on the day of death, preferably within four hours (Spijker 1990:53). Ideally, the still-warm body should be folded into a ball-like shape by crossing the arms on the chest, placing the hands on the clavicles, and positioning the chin and knees against the chest (Spijker 1990:54). If burial is postponed beyond the onset of swelling, it is an abomination; if the body's swelling results in bursting, it is considered a great dishonoring. Enraged, the deceased will return to harm the negligent, living relatives (Pauwels 1958:89). If a relative is murdered without burial, it is considered to be a great humiliation; inevitable calamities must follow, such as discord, war, and the assault of the deceased on the living (Dufays and de Moor 1938:186).

Rwandan burial rituals are elaborate (see Spijker 1990). After the body is placed in the ball-like shape just described, into the deceased's right hand are placed several objects that represent gentleness, such as wool from a sheep, while also proclaiming the power of the objects to pacify the deceased's spirit; to render the deceased's spirit incapable of returning to harm its children, spouse, or cows; and to make the deceased's spirit benevolent to the living so that when invoked the deceased's spirit will provide aid and succor. If the deceased is a man, the body should be laid on the right side, with the lance or fighting hand under the body so that the lance cannot be used against living relatives. Next the feet and thighs are to be anointed, all the while enjoining the deceased not to torment the living but rather to promote prosperity, to assure a prosperous rapport among Hutu, Tutsi, and Twa (Spijker 1990:58).

The deceased should be buried near the house, ideally at the perimeter of the compound; frequently the deceased individual will have indicated the preferred location for burial. Following completion of the burial rites, the spirit of the deceased can be invoked at a time of need and asked for blessings by pouring libations of beer and presenting other offerings (Adekunle 2007; Spijker 1990:84). In this way, a contract of positive exchange is established with the deceased.

In contrast to these cultural ideals, during the Rwandan genocide bodies were abandoned to the elements, became infested with maggots, were surrounded by the buzzing of flies, and emitted a stench. Many corpses were thrown into the river; the bodies swelled and decomposed as they floated along. In most cases, a relative's body could not be found; and if it was located, the rites had been delayed significantly beyond the indicated time. Rwandan genocide survivors receiving psychiatric treatment speak with great distress about the inability to perform the traditional burial ceremonies for the deceased (Uwanyiligira 1997). Their distress is magnified by the thought that the relatives died a "bad death," a horrible and frightening death (Uwanyiligira 1997:88). These genocide survivors fear that not having received the burial rites needed to ensure passage to the state of benevolent ancestor, the deceased may be enraged and attack surviving relatives, causing illness and other calamities (Bagilishya 2000; James 1997:110; Uwanyiligira 1997:88).

As suggested by Bagilishya, a Rwandan psychologist who treats Rwandan refugees in Canada, failure to complete burial rituals increases survival guilt and leads to unresolved bereavement. He presents a traditional tale that articulates the "devastating effects of the inability to mourn on the physical and psychological integrity of the survivors of traumatic loss" (2000:347):

> A couple had five children. One day, the parents were chased from their homes by assailants who then killed them some distance away. Upon entering the home, the children could not find them anywhere. The first lost his appetite and turned into a wasp with a pinched abdomen. The second ran wildly from place to place seeking information about them, and like a rabbit with long ears, he is still running. The third searched for his parents underground and was transformed into a mole. The fourth tried to follow the tracks of death like a scent of a polecat. The first orphan was the most desperate; he rolled himself in the dust and feathers appeared all over his body; and because of all his pouting, he grew a beak, long and curved, and we can still hear the plaintive cry of the bronzed ibis in the marshes. [Bagilishya 2000:347]

Experts working with these populations suggest that, as a therapeutic intervention, the traditional burial rites should be discussed (Bagilishya 2000; Uwanyiligira 1997:101–102), and that enacting some aspect of them—or a new version—may be therapeutic. Bagilishya, who himself lost a son in the genocide, states that burial rituals help a patient to adjust to a loved one's death; that through the rites the deceased are transformed into heroic and beneficent ancestors, "are remade as heroes" (Bagilishya 2000:343); and that placing the body of the deceased in the fetal position described earlier symbolizes, enacts, and brings about the desired rebirth after death (Bagilishya 2000:345). The burial rituals assuage survivor guilt and create a sense of resolution and well-being by transforming the deceased into benevolent beings (Bagilishya 2000).

As this section shows, in the Rwandan context the effect of the genocide on the survivor, and on the victim, may be cast in a spiritual idiom—as when *ihahamuka* is attributed to spirit assault. Through proper burial, a Rwandan promotes smooth interchange among the Hutu, Tutsi, and Twa, and establishes a new "contract" with the deceased. In the new contract, a back-and-forth exchange occurs in which offerings are given to the deceased and blessings are received by the living. On a meta-level, this relationship mirrors ideal reciprocal relationships among the living. Among genocide survivors, therapy should take into account local ideas about the meaning of death and the culturally sanctioned means to transform memory in order to ensure the spiritual fealty of the living and of the dead.

Shortness of Breath in Episodes of 'Ihahamuka': A Resonating Icon of Blockage in the Realm of the Body

As documented by Taylor (1992, 1999, 2002), the master trope of health and prosperity in Rwandan society is *flow*, from the level of the body to that of social relationships, with the concept of flow uniting into one network of meaning seemingly disparate phenomena: (1) menstrual regularity; (2) the lactation of women; (3) cow's milk;[13] (4) rain from the sky; (5) agents to induce sweating and bowel movement in cure (Taylor 1992:191); (6) birth rituals; (7) a codified system of reciprocal exchange between Hutu and Tutsi, configured as a back-and-forth flow; (8) the king, icon of the kingdom, maintaining proper egress in his corporal conduits to symbolize—and bring into being—proper flow at all levels of the kingdom, as in taking a laxative every morning to ensure free flow in both his body and the kingdom (Taylor 1992:34);[14] and (9) in the traditional economy, the back-and-forth exchange of goods and services between the Hutu and Tutsi, which maintained the very life of the society (Taylor 1992:34).

The prominence of obstructed flow as the image of the dysfunctional and pathological in Rwandan society is exemplified by the semantic network of the word *blockage* (Taylor 1992:10, 159, 172; 1999:110–128): (1) to plug, fill up, obstruct, to fill a hollow or empty space; (2) to erase; (3) to decimate, to eliminate, to make something disappear; (4) to hoe the earth without taking care to remove weeds; (5) to reduce an adversary to silence by irrefutable argument; (6) to be obstructed, as in a pathological state of the mammary glands; (7) to become covered with plants, when speaking of a path; (8) to lose a daughter to death before marriage, because the marriage of a daughter to another family makes possible various elaborate exchanges resulting in a "path" with another family; (9) to harm someone, described as "blocking" them; (10) to be ill, in the general sense, configured as blockage;[15] and (11) to be an evil doer and thereby be a "blocking being," most quintessentially, a witch. The metaphorization of evildoer as a "blocked being" guided pregenocide methods of punishment. If someone stole cattle—a sacred animal that provided milk flow and acted as the essential gift item to maintain reciprocal relationships (such as matrimonial ties)—he or she would be impaled from the anus to the mouth and publicly displayed; the blocking being, the destroyer of flow, was shown to be this very sort of being by the manner of execution—by undergoing blockage in both the gastrointestinal tract and respiratory tubes (Taylor 1999:139).

The generative schemas of flow and blockage guided the means of harassment, torture, and murder during the genocide (Taylor 1999:105, 137–139; 2002): (1) cutting the Achilles tendon of both cattle and people, leaving the victims to die (the Achilles tendon allows mobility, with ambulating serving as the animal and human equivalent of flow); (2) penile resection (that is, truncating the male procreative tube); (3) breast resection (that is, truncating the female lacteal tube); (4) evisceration (rendering digestive flow impossible); and (5) impaling men and women from the lower body orifices to the mouth (that is, blocking the gastrointestinal and respiratory tubes). Through the method of mutilation (such as by cutting the breasts, emasculating, or impaling), Tutsi were transmogrified into publicly visible blocked beings, made into analogues of such pathological beings as the witch and the cattle thief. Likewise, emphasizing the collective representation of Tutsi as blocking beings, as a menace to society, they were often metaphorized as weeds blocking a path that needed to be "cleared away" (Taylor 1999:142; 2002:169).

During the genocide, roadblocks put up by Hutu genocide perpetrators were omnipresent—placed across even small paths—sometimes located just a hundred yards apart; a Tutsi might have to pass through a hundred or more such barriers before escaping (Taylor 1999:130). At the Hutu-guarded barriers, the person wishing to pass through had to undergo an interrogation. If identified as Tutsi, torture and death were the meted fate; if not considered to be a Tutsi, the person might nevertheless have to give money or other belongings, and in some cases, to kill a Tutsi, in order to pass through the barrier (Taylor 1999:158, 160; compare Karemano 2003; Pottier 2005). One of the main forms of murder also involved blockage imagery, and asphyxia. All across the country Tutsi gathered at schools, churches, and governmental offices, not uncommonly at the top of hills, to seek safety (Des Forges

1999). Often thousands were gathered, sometimes ten thousand or more. They would then be surrounded, blocked off, and killed over hours or days by grenades and by waves of assaults with machetes and clubs.

Additionally, as we have already argued, another form of torture was rendering impossible the performance of traditional burial rites, thereby preventing the establishment of the reciprocal interchange of offerings and blessings with the deceased, who as a palpable image of this lack of flow come to strangulate the living (also, the burial rituals are said to promote smooth interchange among the Hutu, Tutsi, and Twa). Finally, the genocide was a traumatic blockage on a social level: it signaled the end of the traditional reciprocal relationship of exchange between Hutu and Tutsi (Taylor 1999:105, 137–139; 2002).

Following the genocide, Taylor (2002:165) noted that large numbers of Rwandans complained of constipation, and he hypothesized that this somatizing of psychological distress resulted from the Rwandan idealization of the "open conduit" at multiple ontological levels, including the body; that blockage in the body reflected—and was caused by—blockage at other levels of the Rwandan ontology, as experienced by particular actors and subjectivities; that through this complaint the individual embodied and articulated a general ontological distress, that is, the blockage at the level of the body reflected blockages at the level of the psychological state (a state of all paths being blocked, of desperate hopelessness), of personal memory (such as memories of genocide atrocities enacted in blocking imagery), of the social state (a breakdown of smooth, reciprocal flow between groups), and of the political state (its state of crisis represented in blocking tropes). Similarly, we would argue that the act of breathing is another domain in which the drama of blockage and flow, of the idea of the open conduit, plays out; that breathing, in the healthy state, represents the ideal of continual exchange, a smooth and constant inflow and outflow. Breathing is the most lived and constantly experienced domain of flow, a process of constant inflow and outflow, the very foundation of life. It embodies and naturalizes the symbolic logic of *flow and exchange as health* and *blockage as dysfunction*.

In certain cultural groups, particular physiological processes would seem to serve as, to be elaborated as an icon, a homologue of cultural, economic, and social processes. For Rwandans, smooth breathing evokes health-and-prosperity-bestowing flows, as in menstruation, human lactation, the flow of milk from the udder of a cow, rainfall, a healthy king, and auspicious social relationships; blockage of breathing as in shortness of breath evokes disease-and-disaster-causing blockages, as in irregular or stopped menstruation, lack of milk from mother and cow, drought, an ill king, and a breakdown of social relationships. Shortness of breath's centrality in the syndrome of *ihahamuka* that constitutes a key aspect of the Rwandan response to the genocide—a genocide resulting from the breakdown of the traditional reciprocal relationship between Hutu and Tutsi, a genocide that involved such acts as the erecting of road barriers, a genocide in which the techniques of torture and the methods of killing made the victim into a blocked being—can be understood only in the context of the meaning of *flow* (of exchange and the open conduit) in the Rwandan experience.

The Generation of Episodes of 'Ihahamuka'

To summarize, several processes seemingly interact to generate an episode of *ihahamuka* among Rwandan victims of trauma. Aspects of daily living such as poverty, crime, and the ever-present threat of intra-ethnic violence heighten anxiety and so predispose Rwandans to experiencing somatic symptoms and panic. An episode of *ihahamuka* may begin when a somatic sensation is triggered by any of many causes: a worry episode, anger, exertion, hyperventilation,[16] anxiety, or thinking about a trauma, which may occur either out of the blue or for some specific reason, such as encountering reminders of the trauma—perhaps seeing a perpetrator, smelling an odor that conjures the images of corpses, or hearing a loud noise that cues the memory of heads being bashed in, grenades exploding at a school where Tutsi were gathered, or mortar shells exploding (Taylor 1999:17, 33). The experiencing of an emotion, such as fear or anger or disgust, may also directly recall trauma memories, due to that emotion having occurred during the actual trauma, or due to that emotion having become associated with personal and collective memories of the genocide in the period following the genocide; recall of the trauma memory, of the genocide, and the associated emotion will soon produce somatic sensations.

Once somatic sensations are triggered, those sensations may give rise to a bout of *ihahamuka*. Also, the somatic sensations will activate trauma associations, catastrophic cognitions, concerns about spiritual assault, and iconic resonances, all of which will lead to more anxiety; and that increased anxiety will further increase the likelihood of the person worrying about the onset of an episode of *ihahamuka*. If shortness of breath occurs, escalation to panic may soon follow, because that symptom has extensive trauma associations, gives rise to catastrophic cognitions, evokes fears of spiritual assault, and has extensive iconic resonances related to the generative schemas of flow and blockage.

Shortness of breath may bring to mind a trauma memory—such as witnessing a relative being killed and being helpless to do anything; or running at full speed, out of breath, while being chased by a Hutu holding a machete—and thereby cause extreme terror and a feeling of asphyxia. It may conjure the image of a heart that rises dangerously upward and fails to draw in the breath (as noted earlier, the heart is considered a respiratory organ). It may be attributed to a vengeful relative who, angry at not receiving proper burial, throttles one's throat. And it may evoke all the images coded as blockage within Rwandan experience: the breakdown of the back-and-forth flow of exchange between Hutu and Tutsi, the breakdown of the normal reciprocal relationship between the living and dead due to not performing burial rituals, the lack of a sense of well-being and prosperity, and all the traumatic events perpetrated by the Hutu during the genocide that are configured in terms of the root metaphor of flow and blockage—cutting of the Achilles heel, impaling through the gastrointestinal tract, breast and penile resection, entrapment and slaughter at churches, and the innumerable barriers where so much killing occurred.

Conclusion

"Human responses to war are not analogous to physical trauma: people do not passively register the impact of external forces (unlike, say, a leg hit by a bullet) but engage with them in an active and problem-solving way," as Summerfield (1999:1454) notes. Summerfield goes on to explain the dangers of ignoring the meaning and social context in which trauma occurs:

> Suffering arises from, and is resolved in, a social context, shaped by the meanings and understanding applied to events. The distinctiveness of the experience of war or torture lies in these meanings and not in a biopsychomedical paradigm. This is not just a conceptual issue, but also an ethical one, given the danger of misunderstanding and indeed dehumanizing survivors via reductionist labeling. Helping agencies have a duty to recognize distress, but also to attend to *what people carrying the distress want to signal by it.* [Summerfield 1999:1454; italics added]

In this chapter we investigated the panic-like syndrome *ihahamuka*, examining in detail its central symptom, shortness of breath. Through such an approach we performed an exegesis of *ihahamuka*, "lungs without breath," and explicated "what people carrying the distress want to signal by it."[17] The methods of harassment (such as roadblocks) and mutilation (such as cutting the Achilles tendon), and the embodiment of trauma in the form of constipation and the syndrome of *ihahamuka* with its emphasis on shortness of breath are symbolically resonant homologues in Rwandan experience, a subjectivity profoundly shaped by the symbolic system of flow and blockage.

To explicate the emotional salience of shortness of breath in *ihahamuka*, we delineated iconic relationships, the complex field of homologues—in memory, body, economic experience, linguistic space, ritual, social memory, and traumatic memory—on the basis of a key *ideogram* (Caillois 1990), that is, an abstract image that represents multiple related meanings, the ideogram of flow. An ideogram of this kind, in its multitude of iterations, gives rise not only to the *hyperreal* (Baudrillard

1994), but also to the *hyperfelt*. It is not simply a game of fetishization, creating a certain *habitus* (Bourdieu 1979), a feeling of naturalness and epiphany; the same principles produce a particular type of disordered body, an image of the game gone terribly awry. In Rwanda, flow is *hypersemiotized*, and so is shortness of breath, an icon of blocked flow.[18]

This chapter indicates that to explore symptom complaints in a traumatized population, to investigate how trauma is perpetrated and experienced, one must delineate the cultural context—including its root metaphors, its key generative schemas. Only in this way can one understand and investigate the reticulum that unites the traumatic events, the aesthetic system, the images of greatest horror, the society, and the body—what might be called the *trauma-somatic reticulum*, the symbolic bridges, metaphors, and other meanings and processes that join trauma to personal experience, to bodily experience, to somatic symptom; a reticulum that encompasses social processes, ritual action, metaphor, ethnophysiology, and symbol (compare Kleinman's notion of the *sociosomatic reticulum* in Kleinman and Kleinman 1985).

This exploration might be called *trauma-somatics*, the study of the way in which trauma results in particular symptoms, of the cultural and social links between trauma and bodily state (compare Kleinman's notion of *sociosomatics* in Kleinman and Kleinman 1985). Only through a delineation of the trauma-somatic reticulum can the manner to heal be understood and sensitively undertaken, such as in attending to burial concerns among Rwandan refugees. Just as a symbolic logic guides the perpetrating of violence and the embodying of symptom, that same symbolic logic can be used to bring about cure, empowerment, and well-being, to bring about a *poesis* that heals. In Rwanda, flow and blockage symbolism shapes ritual, aesthetics, ideas about well-being, stigmatization, the manner in which violence is perpetrated, the somatization of distress, and what are appropriate techniques of cure—for example, attempts to bring about cure and recovery through images of flow in psychological discourse, rituals (such as those honoring the dead), and the memorialization of genocide events.

In the same way that Schepher-Hughes and Lock (1987) show that the "upright" posture has complex and resonant meaning from the level of the body to morality to cure (chiropractics) to aesthetics to architecture,[19] this chapter's analysis—building on Taylor's writings—reveals that two symptoms (constipation and shortness of breath) each have linkages to multiple ontological levels. This chapter's analysis suggests that to investigate a symptom complaint, one must determine whether that symptom is cognized and configured, represented, as an exemplar of a generative schema, for example, flow and blockage; and if it is, one must investigate the ontological resonances of the symptom created by that generative schema, the ontological domains—from ethnophysiology to traumatic memory—that the somatic symptom evokes through its connections to root metaphors. Such a *multilevel ontological analysis* needs to be researched to investigate a complaint's meaning.[20] Understanding and empathy begin with an exploration of these levels. Cure may involve an intervention at any one of these levels.

Notes

We would like to thank Christopher C. Taylor for his comments on the current chapter.

1. It has been estimated that the RPF was 70 to 80 percent Tutsi, the rest mostly Hutu (C. C. Taylor, personal communication). Many Hutu, especially from the south, opposed Habyarimana and his northern dominated regime; in 1973 he had overthrown a central-southern regime.

2. In the Rwandan context, abnormal flows of all types are also devalued, but there is a special emphasis on maintaining proper flow (*isibo*), on preventing blockage.

3. Put another way, the chapter explores the dynamic interpretants of flow and blockage, one of which, we argue, is shortness of breath. These other dynamic interpretants are evoked during shortness of breath. That is, we explore the dynamic interpretants of flow and blockage that are icons. For a discussion of Peirce's notion of dynamic interpretants, see Chapter 3.

4. This method and the bludgeoning of the head with a club were two of the most common ways of killing in the genocide.

5. Hutu frequently threw their victims into latrines, a disposal method aimed at enacting the rhetoric that configured Tutsi as "trash."

6. At present, a person with *ihahamuka*—or with more general panic attacks—is frequently treated with generic Valium, alprazolam, and propranolol. These medications are readily available and inexpensive in Rwanda. Valium is a benzodiazapine that would be effective for panic disorder and associated panic attacks (see D. Hinton et al. 2000). Propranolol has been found to be effective for panic and has been utilized for trauma victims (Kinzie and Leung 1989).

7. It is common for panic disorder patients to have panic attacks caused by exertion. The exertion causes such symptoms as shortness of breath and palpitations; these symptoms then activate fear networks and thereby initiate a spiral of panic.

8. The term *ihahamuka* is considered to be specific to the genocide. If a Rwandan visiting another country suffers a trauma (such as a car accident or a severe beating) and then develops various panic symptoms, this would not be called *ihahamuka*. *Ihahamuka* results from having lived through the genocide. At present, the diagnosis of *ihahamuka* has started to become stigmatized as a sign of weakness; almost all Rwandans suffered through the genocide, so Rwandans ponder why only some individuals develop symptoms.

9. Nocturnal panic attacks are common in panic disorder patients. They cause a patient to awaken with shortness of breath and other symptoms. In the Rwandan context, events of nocturnal panic seemingly give rise to *ihahamuka* episodes, and no doubt such episodes result in more nocturnal panic. See Chapter 8 for further discussion of nocturnal panic.

10. In fact, modern studies of respiration reveal that the heart does indeed move upward during states of anxiety; consequently, when anxious, a Rwandan's heart may actually move

upward, increasing fear. The heart rests on the diaphragm, a sheet of tissue that divides the thoracic cavity from the stomach, which stretches across the thoracic cavity at the level of the lowest rib. One can breathe by movements of the chest wall or of the diaphragm. In relaxed inhalation, the diaphragm drops downward, causing an actual rise of the abdomen, and because the heart rests on the diaphragm, the heart actually descends with the diaphragm. In a state of distress, breathing occurs mainly with the ribs of the thoracic cavity, so the diaphragm—and heart—minimally descend, and consequently the heart remains higher in the chest (Barlow and Craske 1994:57–63; Otto et al. 1996:41–42).

11. Malaria causes a high fever. Rwandans may associate heat in the head with insanity because during the hot portion of a malarial attack delirium is common.

12. As an example, among Laotians, if a person dies in a tragic accident, such as a car crash, the person's body must be placed in a temporary grave for several years. Then, after about two years, the rites of death and cremation may take place. If the transitional period before cremation is not observed in cases of tragic demise (such as a car accident), the cremation will result in a maleficent "heat" engulfing the whole village when the corpse is burned; here "heat" is meant symbolically, with "bad luck" configured as a "heat," a commonly drawn analogy in Laotian ritual.

13. Traditional Rwandan society has been classified as a *bovine culture* because of its ritual, aesthetic, and economic emphasis on cattle and their products (Evans-Pritchard 1956; Smith 1985).

14. The word for *king, mwami,* is derived from the term that means both "to lactate" and "to prosper" (*kwamira*) (Taylor 1999:122).

15. Taylor summarizes key aspects of the Rwandan cultural logics of flow and blockage:

> In the unfolding of human and natural events, flow/blockage symbolism mediates between physiological, sociological, and cosmological levels of causality. Popular healing aims at restoring bodily flows that have been perturbed by human negligence and malevolence. Bodily fluids such as blood, semen, breast milk, and menstrual blood are a recurrent concern as is the passage of aliments through the digestive tract. Pathological states are characterized by obstructed or excessive flow and perturbations of this sort may signify illness, diminished fertility and death. [Taylor 1999:111–112]

16. For example, when anxious for any reason, a Rwandan may hyperventilate, bringing about many of the anxiety symptoms observed in *ihahamuka*: shortness of breath, chest tightness, dizziness, cold extremities, and lightheadedness (Barlow and Craske 1994:57–63; Otto et al. 1996:41–42).

17. Soon after the genocide, an international agency arrived in Rwanda with the intent of addressing the psychological repercussions of war. As a first intervention, these foreigners planned to make educational announcements over Rwandan radio to inform the general public of the following: that the atrocities of the genocide would result in PTSD symptoms—for example, flashbacks and startle—and that such reactions and symptoms were "a normal reaction to an abnormal event." Rwandan health care personnel, including Dr. Hagengimana, strongly opposed this approach, because they felt it would be ineffective. Dr. Hagengimana and his colleagues counseled the officials about what they considered to be the most crucial information to be disseminated: the nature of panic attacks, including the typical symptoms (sudden onset of shortness of breath, palpitations, fear, chest tightness, a feeling of choking, cold or hot extremities, dizziness, faintness, and nausea); how

panic attacks result from trauma and can be elicited by a noise, trauma reminders, or strong emotion; that panic attack symptoms such as palpitations and shortness of breath will not result in asphyxia or heart arrest; that the panic attacks might be accompanied by images of past trauma events; that bouts of *ihahamuka* are panic attacks triggered by strong emotions or trauma reminders that are accompanied by fear of death from the symptoms; that unresolved grief may be embodied by shortness of breath; and that an avenging relative is not the cause of the sudden shortness of breath and other symptoms, but rather the cause is a panic attack, which will not cause physiological dysfunction. As Dr. Hagengimana explained to the officials, the prime concern of Rwandans is that they will die during a panic attack; he explained that even if the Rwandan public is told that the symptoms are a normal reaction to an abnormal event, they will still fear death because of the palpitations and other symptoms. Discussions with this major international agency became quite heated. Rwandans organized several conferences to discuss these issues. Finally, after protests, the leader from the international agency was replaced and the radio announcements were made according to some of the recommendations of Dr. Hagengimana and his fellow Rwandan health care professionals.

18. One could also refer to exemplars displaying these resonances, analogous relations, as "simulacrum" (Baudrillard 1994). That is, there is a basic repeating form that informs all levels of a particular society, a form that exists in multiple copies, or simulacra, creating a field of iconic resonances. Baudrillard uses the term *simulacrum* to describe the almost fetishistic importance of circulation in Western society—an image of capitalism, the game of the maximal circulation of goods, as in the form of Disney rides (mainly built on a circle, such as the roller coaster), or the Pompidou Center, again with the celebration of circuits, of circulation, in its design (Baudrillard 1994).

Other thinkers have also written on the importance of the repeating form as a key organizer of cultural domains. Deleuze (1993) demonstrates that in the baroque, "the fold" served as a key form, from the level of body decoration (ruffles and tresses and ribbons) to that of musical form (the continuo base) and philosophical meditation (the psychophysics of sensation). D. Hinton (1999) describes a leitmotif-like form (a flexible longitudinal member, such as the rice stalk bent over with grain, moving in the wind) within Isan society that formed the basis of the aesthetic system. Bourdieu reveals the central importance of the repeating imagery of the rigid upright in Kabyle culture (1977, 1998). Foucault (1983) contrasted the meaning of *similitude*, based on an abstract form uniting a series of things, to that of *resemblance*, the attempt to represent a specific object; the surrealist explored similitudes, or put another way, explored ideologics in the pictorial realm.

19. On such an analysis in respect to the notion of the "upright" structuring the experience of dizziness and orthostatic panic in the trauma-related experiencing of Vietnamese refugees, see D. Hinton et al. (2007).

20. Such an analysis could be done to analyze the meaning of certain panic symptoms—such as cold extremities—in a society having prominent cold and hot symbolism, a cold and hot humoralism. As an example of such an analysis, Jenkins and Valiente (1994) link the complaint of "heat in the body" among Salvadorean refugees to ethnophysiology, emotion, interpersonal contexts, trauma history, and political context; or in Nigeria, "heat in the head" is a common complaint in anxiety, and that complaint can be adequately analyzed only in relationship to the culture's configuration of the head as highly sacred, to its focus on the head in ritual action, and to the culture's elaboration of an "aesthetic of the cool," an

aesthetic that shapes ethnopsychology, dance aesthetics, and the conceptualization of the ideal person (Ebigo 1982; Thompson 1973, 1975; for a review, see D. Hinton 1999).

In a culture, if a central somatic complaint during panic is considered to implicate a specific organ of the body (such as palpitations implicating the heart and shortness of breath implicating the lungs), or if a central emotion during panic is considered to implicate a certain organ (such as "fear" implicating a dysfunction of the "kidney," as seen in Chapter 7 of this volume), one should investigate whether semantic networks extend from that organ to the level of ethnophysiology (that is, the role of the organ in that culture's ethnophysiology), metaphor (for example, organ metaphors used to describe feeling and social relationships), ritual, social relationships (which occur due to the configuring of relationships and emotions in organ metaphors), cosmology, political order (for example, the ruler or the political structure metaphorized in organ imagery), and cure (for example, the focus on the organ in curing ritual). That is, one should perform what might be called an organ-focused multilevel ontological analysis.

To illustrate such an organ-focused multilevel ontological analysis, let us take the example of the German "heart," the *Herz*. The *Herz* is a zone of great hypervigilance, giving rise to the term *Herzphobie*, "heart phobia," a frequent panic presentation (Eifert 1992; see also Condrau and Gassmann 1989; Payer 1988). The *Herz* has a special place in iconography. It is linked to the cult of the machine (a source of cultural pride, with Carl Benz of Mercedes-Benz fame, for example, being the inventor of the car engine—along with Daimler, another German—and of the first gas-propelled car [Adler 2006]). It is the central image in metaphors having to do with feeling and love, it evokes the idea of warmth (in a country that has a very cold climate and that gives heat a wide range of meaning resonances), and it has a key place in the language and imagery of Christian religion and ritual, as in the Sacred Heart of Jesus (on these issues in the German imagination and identity, see Condrau and Gassmann 1989; Eifert 1992; Geerlings and Mügge 2006; Nager 1993; Payer 1988).

Pioneering works of multilevel ontological analysis include Bachelard's (1964) exploration of fire and Barthes's (1972) investigation of mythologies associated with objects, including food. Among more recent work using such an approach, Devisch (1984) reveals the importance of the symbolic logic of flow and blockage among the Yaka of Zaire; Heritier (1984) examines hot and cold symbolism among the Samo of the Ivory coast; Classen (2005) explores hot and cold symbolism in Mayan society; and D. Hinton (1999) investigates the cultural representation of flexibility and rigidity among Northeastern Thais.

References

Adekunle, J. 2007. *Culture and Customs of Rwanda.* Westport, CT: Greenwood Press.

Adler, D. 2006. *Daimler and Benz: The Complete History. The Birth and Evolution of the Mercedes-Benz.* New York: HarperCollins.

Bachelard, G. 1964. *The Psychoanalysis of Fire.* Boston: Beacon Press.

Bagilishya, D. 2000. Mourning and Recovery from Trauma: In Rwanda, Tears Flow Within. *Transcultural Psychiatry* 37:337–353.

Baines, E. 2003. Body Politics and the Rwandan Crisis. *Third World Quarterly* 24:479–493.

Barlow, D. H., and M. C. Craske. 1994. *Mastery of Your Anxiety and Panic.* San Antonio, TX: Therapy Works.

Barthes, R. 1972. *Mythologies.* New York: Hill and Wang.

Baudrillard, J. 1994. *Simulacra and Simulation.* Ann Arbor: University of Michigan Press.

Bourdieu, P. 1977. *Outline of a Theory of Practice.* Cambridge, UK: Cambridge University Press.

———. 1979. *La distinction.* Paris: Éditions de Minuit.

———. 1998. *La domination masculine.* Paris: Éditions du Seuil.

Caillois, R. 1990. *The Necessity of Mind.* Venice, CA: Lapis Press.

Classen, C. 2005. McLuhan in the Rainforest: The Sensory Worlds of Oral Cultures. In *Empire of the Senses: The Sensual Culture Reader.* D. Howes, ed. Pp. 147–163. Oxford, UK: Berg.

Condrau, G., and M. Gassmann. 1989. Das *Verletze Herz.* Zürich: Kreuz Verlag.

Deleuze, G. 1993. *The Fold: Leibnez and the Baroque.* Minneapolis: University of Minnesota Press.

Des Forges, A. 1999. *"Leave None to Tell Their Story": Genocide in Rwanda.* Paris: International Federation of Human Rights.

Devisch, R. 1984. *Se recréer femme: Manipulation sémantique d'une situation d'infécondité chez les Yaka du Zaïre.* London: Routledge.

Dufays, F., and V. de Moor. 1938. *Les enchaînées.* Paris: Librairie Missionnaire.

Ebigo, P. O. 1982. Development of a Culture Specific (Nigeria) Screening Scale of Somatic Complaints Indicating Psychiatric Disturbance. *Culture, Medicine, and Psychiatry* 6:29–43.

Eifert, G. H. 1992. Cardiophobia: A Paradigmatic Behavioural Model of Heart-Focused Anxiety and Non-Anginal Chest Pain. *Behaviour, Research, and Therapy* 30:329–345.

Evans-Pritchard, E. E. 1956. *Nuer Religion.* Oxford, UK: Clarendon Press.

Faust, D. G. 2008. *This Republic of Suffering: Death and the American Civil War.* New York: Knopf.

Fisher, S. 2004. Tuning into Different Wavelengths: Listener Clubs for Effective Rwandan Reconciliation Radio Programs. Paper presented to the Fourth International Conference on Entertainment-Education and Social Change, Cape Town, South Africa, September 26 to 30, 2004.

Foucault, M. 1983. *This Is Not a Pipe.* Berkeley: University of California Press.

———. 1986. *The Care of the Self: The History of Sexuality,* Volume 3. New York: Vintage Press.

Geerlings, W., and A. Mügge. 2006. *Das Herz: Organ und Metapher.* Zürich: Kreuz Verlag.

Good, B. J. 1994. *Medicine, Rationality, and Experience: An Anthropological Perspective.* Cambridge, UK: Cambridge University Press.

Gourevitch, P. 1998. *We Wish to Inform You That Tomorrow We Will be Killed with Our Families: Stories from Rwanda.* New York: Picador.

Guattari, F., and G. Deleuze. 1987. *Thousand Plateaus: Capitalism and Schizophrenia.* Minneapolis: University of Minnesota Press.

Hagengimana A., D. E. Hinton, B. Bird, M. H. Pollack, and R. K. Pitman. 2003. Somatic Panic-Attack Equivalents in a Community Sample of Rwandan Widows Who Survived the Genocide. *Psychiatry Research* 117:1–9.

Hatzfeld, J. 2000. *Life Laid Bare: The Survivors in Rwanda Speak.* New York: Other Press.

Heritier, F. 1984. "Stérilité, aridité, sècheresse: quelques invariants de la pensée symbolique." In *Le sens du mal.* M. Augé and C. Herzlich, eds. Pp. 123–154. Paris: Editions des Archives Contemporaines.

Hertz, R. 1960. *Death and the Right Hand*. Glencoe, IL: Free Press.

Hinton, A. L. 2004. *Why Did They Kill? Cambodia in the Shadow of the Genocide*. Berkeley: University of California Press.

Hinton, D. E. 1999. Musical Healing and Cultural Syndromes in Isan: Landscape, Conceptual Metaphor, and Embodiment. Ph.D. dissertation, Department of Anthropology, Harvard University.

Hinton, D. E., P. Ba, S. Peou, and K. Um. 2000. Panic Disorder Among Cambodian Refugees Attending a Psychiatric Clinic: Prevalence and Subtypes. *General Hospital Psychiatry* 22:437–444.

Hinton, D. E., Pollack M. H., and L. Nguyen. 2007. Orthostatic Panic as a Key Vietnamese Reaction to Traumatic Events: The Case of September 11th. *Medical Anthropology Quarterly* 21:81–107.

Hoffman, D. 2005. Violent Events as Narrative Blocs: The Disarmament at Bo, Sierra Leone. *Anthropology Quarterly* 2:328–353.

Jacob, I. 1983. *Dictionnaire Rwandais-Francais*. Paris: INRS.

James, F. 1997. Groupe de patients Rwandais traumatisés après le génocide. *Nouvelle revue d'ethnopsychiatrie* 34:105–116.

Jenkins, J., and M. Valiente. 1994. Bodily Transactions of the Passions: *El Calor* Among Salvadoran Women Refugees. In *Embodiment and Experience: The Existential Ground of Culture and Self*. T. J. Csordas, ed. Pp. 163–182. Cambridge, UK: Cambridge University Press.

Kagame, A. 1956. *La philosophie Bantu-Rwandaise de l'être*. Brussels: Académie Royale des Sciences Coloniales.

Karemano, C. 2003. *Au-delà des barrières: dans les méandres du drame rwandais*. Paris: L'Harmattan.

Keane, F. 1995. *Season of Blood: A Rwandan Journey*. London: Penguin Classics.

Kinzie, J. D., and P. Leung. 1989. Clonidine in Cambodian Patients with Posttraumatic Stress Disorder. *Journal of Nervous and Mental Disorder* 177:546–550.

Kleinman, A., and J. Kleinman. 1985. Somatization: The Interconnections in Chinese Society Among Culture, Depressive Experiences, and the Meanings of Pain. In *Culture and Depression: Studies in the Anthropology and Cross-Cultural Psychiatry of Affect and Disorder*. A. Kleinman and B. J. Good, eds. Pp. 429–490. Berkeley: University of California Press.

Lestrade, A. 1955. *La médecine indigène au Rwanda*. Brussels: Académie Royale des Sciences Coloniales.

Musabe-Ngamije, J. 2002. Which Program to Be Elaborated in Order to Teach Character to Rwandan Children After Genocide? *Info* 5:15–34.

Nager, F. 1993. *Das Herz als Symbol*. Basel: Editiones Roche.

Obeyesekere, G. 1990. *The Work of Culture: Symbolic Transformations in Psychoanalysis and Anthropology*. Chicago: University of Chicago Press.

Otto, M. W., J. Jones, M. C. Craske, and D. H. Barlow. 1996. *Panic Control Therapy for Benzodiazepine Discontinuation*. San Antonio, TX: Graywind.

Pauwels, R. 1958. *Imana et le culte des mânes au Rwanda*. Brussels: Academie Royale des Sciences Coloniales.

Payer, L. 1988. *Medicine and Culture*. New York: Henry Holt.

Pottier, J. 2002. *Re-Imagining Rwanda: Conflict, Survival and Disinformation in the Late Twentieth Century*. Cambridge, UK: Cambridge University Press.

———. 2005. Escape from Genocide: The Politics of Identity in Rwanda's Genocide. In *Violence and Belonging: The Quest for Identity in Post-Colonial Africa*. V. Broch-Due, ed. Pp. 195–213. London: Routledge.

Probyn, E. 2004. Eating for Living: A Rhizo-Ethnology of Bodies. In *Cultural Bodies: Ethnography and Theory*. H. Thomas and J. Ahmed, eds. Pp. 215–240. Malden, MA: Blackwell.

Prunier, G. 1995. *The Rwanda Crisis: History of a Genocide*. New York: Columbia University Press.

Schantz, M. S. 2008. *Awaiting the Heavenly Country: The Civil War and America's Culture of Death*. Ithaca, NY: Cornell University Press.

Schepher-Hughes, N., and M. Lock. 1987. The Mindful Body: A Prolegomenon to Future Work in Medical Anthropology. *Medical Anthropology Quarterly* 1:6–41.

Scott, M. W. 2005. Hybridity, Vacuity, and Blockage: Visions of Chaos from Anthropological Theory, Island Melanesia, and Central Africa. *Comparative Study of Society and History* 11:190–216.

Sibomana, A. 1999. *Hope for Rwanda*. London: Pluto Press.

Smith, P. 1985. Aspect de l'esthétique au Rwanda. *L'Homme* 96:7–22.

Spijker, G. 1990. *Les usages funéraires et la mission de l'église*. Kampen, NL: Academisch Proefschrift.

Straus, S. 2006. *The Order of Genocide: Race, Power, and War in Rwanda*. Ithaca, NY: Cornell University Press.

Summerfield, D. 1999. A Critique of Seven Assumptions Behind Psychological Trauma Programs in War-Affected Areas. *Social Science and Medicine* 48:1449–1462.

Taylor, C. C. 1992. *Milk, Honey, and Money: Changing Concept in Rwandan Healing*. Washington, DC: Smithsonian Institution Press.

———. 1999. *Sacrifice as Terror: The Rwandan Genocide of 1994*. Oxford: Berg.

———. 2002. The Cultural Face of Terror in the Rwandan Genocide of 1994. In *Annihilating Difference*. A. Hinton, ed. Pp. 137–178. Berkeley: University of California Press.

Thompson, R. F. 1973. An Aesthetic of the Cool. *African Arts* 1:40–43, 64–67, 89.

———. 1975. Icons of the Mind. *African Arts* 8:52–89.

Wulsin, L., and A. Hagengimana. 1998. PTSD in Survivors of Rwanda's 1994 War. *Psychiatric Times* 15:4:3–6.

Uwanyiligira, E. 1997. La souffrance psychologique des survivants des massacres au Rwanda: Approches therapeutique. *Nouvelle revue d'ethnopsychiatrie* 34:87–104.

Panic Illness in Tibetan Refugees

Eric Jacobson

AS PART OF A LARGER STUDY of psychiatric aspects of the contemporary practice of classical Tibetan medicine, I conducted interviews with six Tibetan refugees living in an urban area in northern India[1] who had been diagnosed with "life-wind illness" (*srog rlung gi nad*), a chronic affliction widely recognized by both lay Tibetan refugees and the classical physicians, or *emchi* (*'em chi*), who treat them.[2] In addition to attesting to chronic symptoms of depression and anxiety, four of the six also described episodes of acute panic that had occurred repeatedly over periods of some months. Neither the classical literature of Tibetan medicine nor colloquial Tibetan parlance has a specific term for such attacks. Patients and *emchi* alike regard them simply as transient intensifications of chronic "life-wind illnesses." A description of the Tibetan understanding of "life-wind illness" is therefore necessary to appreciate the "semantic network" (Good 1977) in which these episodes of panic occur.

In this chapter, the classical and lay Tibetan theories that apply to "wind illness" and spirit attacks are reviewed first, followed by narrative accounts of two of the four cases in which "life-wind illness" was accompanied by acute panic. The symptomatology and life events cited as having contributed to the onset and aggravation of illness in the four cases are then discussed. Next these data are compared to research on symptomatology and life events in panic disorder (PD) in the United States and Great Britain, and several points of similarity and difference are noted. The chapter closes with a comment on current prospects for the development of a biocultural interactionist view of panic illnesses.

Psychiatric Illnesses in Classical Tibetan Medicine

The symptomatology, etiology, pathophysiology, and therapeutics of "life-wind illness" are laid out in detail in the central classic of Tibetan medicine, *The Treatise of Secret Oral Precepts on the Eight-Branched Essential Elixir* (*Bdud rtsi snying po yan lag brgyad pa gsang ba man nag gi rgyud*; hereafter abbreviated *BSYB*). This work dates to at least the eleventh century C.E.[3] and is known to both Tibetan and cosmopolitan scholars as the *Four Treatises*. It does not separate out psychiatry as a special branch but recognizes both psychiatric and somatic symptoms as essential aspects of many types of illness. This approach is typical of classical Tibetan thought, which in general does not dichotomize mental and physical phenomena in the systematic way that Euro-American science does.

The *Four Treatises* for the most part assigns disorders that biomedicine would classify as psychiatric or neurological—that is, those in which disturbances of cognition, perception, or behavior predominate—to one of two broad nosological divisions: (1) illnesses caused by disturbances of a psychophysiological "wind" (*rlung*), or (2) illnesses caused by "demons" (*gdon*). (As the terms of this division suggest, classical Tibetan nosology is organized mostly according to the pathophysiology that is understood to underlie each type of illness, rather than its symptomatology.) These two etiologies are not exclusive of one another, and *emchi* often attribute chronic cases of severe mental illness to a combination of disturbed "wind" and virulent spirit attack. Patients who receive that dual diagnosis often consult *emchi* for help with their "wind" imbalance, as well as lama-exorcists for exorcism of demons, in accord with a generally recognized division of therapeutic labor. Even if ritual exorcism is successful, one's "wind" must expeditiously be rebalanced for one to be fortified against a subsequent spirit attack. The difficulty of doing this quickly enough explains the persistence of the disorder despite repeated resort to both *emchi* and exorcist. When the disorder is chronic and involves socially disruptive behavior, visits to a psychiatrist to obtain a prescription for "allopathic" (that is, biomedical) medication are often also included in the cycle along with the ministrations of *emchi* and lama.

The Tibetan word *lung* (*rlung*) the literal meaning of which is "wind," refers to a dynamic principle that functions both physiologically and pathophysiologically. It is one of the three *nyepa* (*nyes pa*, "harmful ones"), the other two being "bile" (*mkris pa*) and "phlegm" (*pan kan*), which are fundamental to Tibetan medical thought.[4] Each of the *nyepa* can either support physiological normality or give rise to pathology, depending on its quantitative balance vis-à-vis the other two *nyepa* across a complex anatomy, and depending on its proper circulation through a system of "channels" (*rtsa*).[5]

In its physiological sense, "wind" is the elemental principle of motility. The word *lung* refers also (and perhaps originally) to wind in the external environment.

The two meanings are closely related in that cold breezes are known to disturb the psychophysiological "wind"; however, the meteorological and physiological meanings of this term are otherwise distinct.[6] Because psychic functions are understood to be motile phenomena, normal perception, affect, and cognition are dependant on balanced proportions, flows, and distributions of "wind." Syndromes in which these functions are disturbed are therefore attributed, at least in part, to a disorder of "wind."

Each of the *nyepa* are disturbed by different types of "circumstantial cause" (*rkyen*) such as different types of climate, diet, and behavior. The following verse from the *Four Treatises* lists the general circumstantial causes of "wind" illnesses. Note that several types of physical, mental, and social suffering are implied, and that biomedicine subsumes many of them under the notion of "stressor."

> Wind's circumstantial causes are excessive reliance on bitter, light, and rough
>   [food],[7]
> Fatigue due to passion [that is, sexual indulgence], eating and sleeping being
>   reduced,
> Strenuous verbal and physical activity on an empty stomach,
> By having bled much, by having violently ejected vomit and diarrhea,
> Due to being blown on by a cold breeze, uncontrollable crying,
> Worrying, excessive mental physical or verbal activity,
> Taking one's fill of unnourishing [that is, spoiled] food,
> Repressing [bodily] impulses, [or] forcing [the bowels] by pressure.
> Due to these circumstantial causes [wind] at first increases and accumulates in its
>   own [that is, physiological] locations.[8] [*BSYB*, vol. 3, chap. 2, lines 14–22]

In this and other passages, the classic portrays "wind" as a pervasive pathogenic dynamic that mediates the vitiating effects of a wide range of physical and psychological stressors to specific forms of psychic and somatic illness.

From the point of view of Tibetan Buddhism, human beings are not entirely at the mercy of the environmental and social vicissitudes that may disturb "wind" and lead to illness. Both religious and medical remedies are available. The teachings of Buddhism include a variety of methods to cultivate mental composure, clarity, and compassion, thus ameliorating the impact of adverse circumstances and minimizing the consequent disruptions of "wind." But spiritual practices increase this kind of stability only gradually, over a period of years. The immediacy of illness calls for more expeditious measures, which both Tibetan Buddhism and medicine provide in various forms. Religious remedies include a wide variety of rites for gaining karmic merit[9] and for eliciting the blessings of the Buddhas and other enlightened beings. Performed either by the sick person's family or—more typically—by career monks and priests for a fee, such rituals ameliorate illnesses as well as other types of misfortune. In addition to these generic measures, Tibetan medicine provides hundreds of medications and other therapies (such as moxibustion and acupuncture) that are geared to the treatment of specific illnesses, including those caused by "wind." These remedies are available through the services of the *emchi*.

The second broad division of illnesses with predominantly psychiatric symptoms comprises those attributed to attack or possession by spirits. The *Treatises* describe these illnesses as more extreme disturbances of behavior, perception, and cognition than are typical of uncomplicated "wind" illnesses, the kinds of disorders that biomedical psychiatrists would classify as psychoses. Whereas "wind" is a pathophysiological dynamic that operates according to consistent, impersonal principles, spirits are volitional beings who may be motivated by revenge, anger, and other negative affects. Various types of spirits are apt to attack individuals who offend them or make them ill, even unintentionally, by straying into their territory, cutting down trees or polluting bodies of water in which they dwell, digging foundations, or carrying away precious stones; or who become unusually vulnerable due to some physical or psychological weakness.[10] Indeed, "wind" illnesses of the psychiatric kind are major predisposing factors to spirit attack, because they weaken the individual's powers of cognition and attention. An especially serious predisposition to spirit possession occurs when circumstantial causes force one of the *nyepa*, usually "wind," to be displaced from its physiological channels and enter a special psychic channel located in the heart that is the seat of consciousness. This circumstance is noted in a chapter of the *Treatises* devoted to illnesses caused by demons (*gdon*).

> As for the essential and circumstantial causes: due to being afflicted with feeble
> heart power,[11]
> Depression, too much mental work,
> Disagreeable diet, or demons, [all] these being circumstantial causes,
> The *nyepa* being agitated, they enter the place where consciousness runs.[12]
> (Consequently) the pathway of mind is reversed, memory weakens, and one becomes insane. [*BSYB* vol. 3, chap. 78, lines 5–9]

Once "wind" has been diverted from its physiological channels into "the place where consciousness runs," that is, the central channel of the heart, the individual becomes liable to an evil spirit "entering in" and "taking control of his or her speech and conduct."

Tibetan Buddhism is replete with methods for exorcising noxious spirits and otherwise protecting oneself from their attacks. These range from wearing protective amulets to the briefest rites of sacred recitation and throwing of blessed rice at a haunted corner in one's home to elaborate rituals that require days of preparation, the participation of numerous monks, and a week or more to perform.

Classical "Life-Wind Illness" and Colloquial "Life-Wind"

The *Four Treatises* defines "life-wind illness" as an excess of "wind" in the "life-wind plexus" (*srog rlung gi khor lo*), a psychophysiological coordinating center that it locates in the middle of the forehead. The "life-wind plexus" is ordinarily responsible for "clarifying the intellectual and sensory faculties, and supporting thought," and for regulating swallowing, breathing, salivation, sneezing, and belching. Here again, psychological and physiological functions that biomedicine would segregate are easily commingled. The *Treatises* lists the circumstantial causes and symptoms of "life-wind illness" as follows:

> [As for illnesses of the] life-sustaining [wind]: It being disturbed by a diet of
>   rough (foods), fasting and excessive work, [or] blocking [or] pushing impulses
>   [to defecate or urinate, one becomes] dizzy,
> The heart [that is, emotion][13] is unstable, it is difficult to draw in breath, and one
>   is unable to swallow. [*BSYB*, vol. 3, chap. 2, lines 161–163]

Although this verse mentions neither the affective element of "uncontrollable crying" nor the correlates of anxiety such as "worrying, excessive mental, physical, or verbal activity" that the *Treatises* list among the circumstantial causes of "wind" illnesses in general, both *emchi* and lay Tibetans understand that those more general causes also contribute to the occurrence of "life-wind illness."

Knowledge of classical medical doctrine is not confined to physicians and clerics who are schooled in Tibetan literature. Simplified versions of medical terminology and theory also appear in the discourse of lay Tibetan refugees, even though they are almost uniformly illiterate in the classical form of their mother tongue. My observations at Tibetan medical clinics suggest that this diffusion takes place when *emchi* provide truncated bits of the classical model on the infrequent occasions when patients request an explanation for their illness. This is a particularly clear instance of the impact of classical medical models on local life-worlds (Good and Good 1992).

The commonplace term for "life-wind illness" among lay Tibetans is simply "life-wind" (*srog rlung*). (In this chapter, "life-wind" indicates the lay construction of this disorder, and "life-wind illness" indicates the classical *emchi* construction.) In the course of my fieldwork, "life-wind" was one of only two common lay terms for psychiatric illnesses, each clearly derived from classical theory (the other being "demon" [*gdon*], after the classical "demonic illness" [*gdon gi nad*]). The currency of "life-wind" in lay conversation may be a consequence of "life-wind illness" being by far the most common diagnosis given by *emchi* to patients who present with affective, cognitive, or behavioral disturbances that are severe enough to impair their work or family lives but do not involve delusions, hallucinations, or incoherence, which would be attributed to spirit attack.

Lay parlance also reflects classical theory by invoking "wind" as the dynamic that mediates between the types of circumstances that are known to disrupt it and the resulting syndromes of psychosomatic suffering. Common explanations for affectively or cognitively aberrant behavior include "My wind is high today" (indicating a temporary condition of irritability or emotional lability due to difficult circumstances), and "He has wind" (for someone who is being unusually irritable).[14] "High wind" (*rlung mtho po*) indicates a hyperirritability that may be regarded as purely circumstantial or as a constitutional trait, for example, "He is always high wind." Also reflecting classical theory is the lay understanding that "wind" is increased by prolonged or intense emotional excitement; exhausting physical or intellectual work; exposure to bad weather, bad food, or severe economic hardship; or separation from or loss of family members: "Her wind is high from working too hard outside and getting cold." Explanations for recovery from such states also invoke "wind": "This medicine reduces my 'wind'"; "I heard some good news today, so my 'wind' is less"; or "I had a good time with my relatives, so my 'wind' is less."

As is obvious from these examples, there is a distinct similarity (not to deny that there are also differences) between the lay Tibetan explanatory use of "wind" and North American invocations of "stress" and "trauma" to explain emotional or cognitive disturbances, and even to attribute illnesses to certain kinds of physical and emotional experiences. This similarity in popular idioms reflects the previously noted parallel between the *Four Treatises'* explanatory use of "wind" and the biomedical concept of "stressor."

The attribution of illness to "life-wind" is somewhat stigmatizing, and many who are identified by third parties as having suffered from it will deny that it is so. Some, however, will admit to trusted individuals that they have suffered from this malady and will even discuss their symptoms and thoughts about it. In interviews I conducted with Tibetans who were willing to discuss their experience of "life-wind", they attributed a broader variety of symptoms to it than the *Treatises* lists for "life-wind illness." (The classical list may have been intended to be pathognomonic rather than phenomenologically exhaustive.) They also included symptoms that are typical of "wind" illnesses in general, especially those in which disturbances of cognition, perception, or affect predominate.[15] These symptoms included affective lability, cognitive disorientation, disturbances of heartbeat and breathing, and a variety of other somatosensory dysphorias (such as muscular tension, paresthesia, and numbness).

As part of my fieldwork, I administered Tibetan language versions of sections of a standard psychiatric diagnostic instrument, the Structured Clinical Interview for *DSM–III–R* (SCID; Spitzer et al. 1990), individually to each of six subjects who had been diagnosed with "life-wind illness" by their *emchi* in clinical encounters that I had observed. Evaluated in terms of the more recent *DSM–IV* criteria, five of these six either qualified for both major depressive disorder (MDD) and generalized anxiety disorder (GAD), or missed qualifying for both by only a single criterial symptom. In addition, they voiced a high proportion of somatosensory complaints, many of which are not included in *DSM–IV* criteria for either MD or GAD.[16]

On the basis of the symptoms reported by this very limited sample, the most fitting characterization of "life-wind" in *DSM* categories would be highly somaticized, comorbid MDD and GAD.[17] The tentative identification of this comorbid diagnosis as providing the closest fit to "life-wind illness" is not meant to force our understanding of this distinctively Tibetan illness into the mold of *DSM* categories, but rather to locate it roughly on that nosological map. Studies of Puerto Rican *ataques de nervios* have related culture-specific symptomatological data to *DSM* categories, to much the same end (Lewis-Fernández et al. 2002). This is an exercise that is not without practical value given that Tibetan refugees with a diagnosis of "life-wind illness" often consult psychiatrists for "allopathic," that is, biomedical medication. Having an approximate idea of "life-wind's" *DSM* equivalent may reduce the potential for misdiagnosis and therapeutic error in such cases.

Acute Panic in the Course of "Life-Wind Illness"

Four of the six subjects who had been diagnosed with "life-wind illness" also reported repeated episodes of acute panic. They differentiated these episodes from the more chronic aspects of their illness by their rapidity of onset, a marked intensification of both fear and somatosensory dysphoria, and brevity of duration. Just as it does for psychiatric illnesses in general, Tibetan medicine provides two alternate explanations for acute panic: (1) a transient aggravation of "life-wind illness," and (2) a form of spirit attack. The first explanation is the most commonly applied, and the latter less so. Attack by spirits is most typically invoked in cases marked by nonresponsiveness to the appropriate classical medications, by dramatic irregularity in the patient's radial pulses upon palpation by the *emchi*, or by particular portents in the patient's dreams.[18] In some cases, both types of explanation are applied, just as for psychotic illnesses in general. The afflicting spirits are understood to have targeted an individual when their cognitive and attentional powers, which may already be attenuated by a "wind" illness, are further weakened by circumstances known to disturb "wind," such as an immediate emotional upset, severe physical stress, or certain times of night.

Case Studies

The four subjects who had been diagnosed with "life-wind illness" and who also reported episodes of acute panic described experiences that varied in the extent to which they satisfied *DSM–IV* panic attack (PA) criteria. (In what follows, the *DSM*-defined disorder will be designated PA and the acute panics described by my Tibetan informants will be referred to as *episodes of panic*.) Of the two cases summarized here, the first came closest to meeting the *DSM* criteria, and the second departed most from them. (A third case from this set of four is described in Jacobson 2002.) These two accounts thus roughly bracket the range of variation present in the four cases. Even the first case, however, includes some symptoms that do not appear among the *DSM* criteria, suggesting that the features of panic illness in the Tibetan context might vary significantly from those of PA as delineated by contemporary psychiatry (APA 1987, 1994).

The narratives that follow situate the suffering of these individuals in the context of their traumatic flight from the violent Chinese occupation of their homeland, and in the subsequent stress of refugee life in northern India. The names used here are pseudonyms.

Jigmed

Jigmed was in his late fifties. Although he preferred the faded pants, old flannel shirt, and frayed denim jacket of a workman, he was actually an unusually prosperous dairy farmer who had recently moved his family into a newly constructed apartment building and begun work on a rental property in a major Indian city. He was also the patriarch of a large extended family. Yet despite his economic success, Jigmed was unusually thin, visibly fatigued, and tense all over, and spoke in a faint, extremely hoarse voice. His presenting complaints were insomnia, a burning sensation in the front of his chest, pervasive sadness, and chronic worry.

In the clinic, the *emchi*'s immediate diagnosis had been "life-wind illness" complicated by an excess of "blood." The treatment she proposed included not only medications and dietary and behavioral measures, but also moxibustion on the breastbone, a treatment that implied that Jigmed also suffered from a disorder of the "wind" plexus known as the "encompassing-wind" (*khyab byed rlung*), which is located in the cardiac region. In verses summarizing this syndrome, the *Treatises* mention psychiatric symptoms:

[As for illness of the] encompassing [wind]: it being agitated by rushing around,
  excessively vigorous playing, fear, depression [or] a diet of rough [foods],[19]
The heart having been "thrown out,"[20] one faints, talks much,

Is restless, and fear is kindled by angry [or] unpleasant [that is, critical] words.

[*BSYB*, vol. 3, chap. 2, lines 170–187]

In classical Tibetan terms, therefore, Jigmed suffered from comorbid "life-wind illness," excess "blood," and "encompassing-wind illness."

When interviewed in his home, Jigmed responded in a terse and fragmented manner, lacking any spontaneous narrative or emotional display other than the friendly smile and gentle laughter that are normative in Tibetan hospitality. His evident muscular tension (most noticeable in a profound constriction in the front of his chest), tired eyes, and breathy, rasping voice conveyed an impression of tremendous fatigue, strain, and unhappiness, yet his words and constant smile betrayed none of these.

Jigmed was born and raised in Tibet. He had never gone to school and never had any special training in religion, although he had maintained close relations with a lama whose monastery was within easy travel of his home. By the time the Chinese troops began their invasion in 1950, he had a wife and two children. As the Chinese imposed more and more control over Tibetan affairs, Jigmed became an active combatant in the guerrilla resistance. This involvement eventually separated him from his wife and children, and as events played out he was never able to rejoin them. He fought as a guerilla for the next seven years as the Chinese escalated hostilities and consolidated their control of the country. In the course of combat he killed numerous Chinese soldiers and even some Tibetan collaborators. In 1959, at the height of the conflict, he immigrated to India but was quickly arrested by Indian military police and deported back to Tibet, he believes at the request of Chinese authorities. He was held in Tibet only briefly, however, and soon allowed to return again to India. Despite his prolonged combat experience, at the time of our interviews Jigmed neither displayed nor reported flashbacks or other hallmark symptoms of posttraumatic stress disorder (PTSD).

Since he had come to India, his only occupation—one at which he had been financially successful—was dairy farming. In the mid-1970s he had met and married a second wife, with whom he had several children. Jigmed identified the unexpected death from illness of an eight-year-old son as having precipitated his "life-wind illness" twelve years earlier. Upon hearing the news, he had immediately experienced a pain between two of his ribs, which he described as "piercing like a hook." The pain then intensified and began to move around his upper body. Other initial symptoms were an overall tightness in his chest and a consequent difficulty breathing, which frightened him. (According to the *Treatises*, pains that move around the body and a concentration of symptoms in the upper torso are typical of "wind" illnesses.)

Over the succeeding years this affliction waxed and waned. Episodes of aggravation were typically precipitated by brooding over his son's death and other losses, worrying about family finances, or receiving depressing news about relatives or friends. These episodes would lead to deepening sadness, feelings of loneliness, loss of appetite, fatigue, and a sensation of accelerated heartbeat. Other symptoms included restlessness (pacing uncontrollably and going in and out of his house repeatedly), and insomnia that kept him awake most of the night.

Since a spate of additional deaths among his relatives (all at relatively young ages) beginning six years previously, Jigmed's illness had worsened. At the time of our interviews he suffered from almost complete nocturnal insomnia, and slept "only for an hour" during the day. This syndrome continued to wax and wane in intensity. Periods of worsened symptoms often lasted two or three weeks, and sometimes longer. Good news about family or friends would temporarily alleviate these exacerbations and reduce their frequency.

When his "life-wind" symptoms would worsen, Jigmed would begin to feel pains moving around the front and back of his chest, which would gradually become tighter and tighter. The tension would eventually make his breathing difficult, which frightened him. Most of his episodes of acute panic occurred when his breathing became very difficult in the middle of insomniac nights. At those times he would experience intense fear of impending death, disorientation ("I don't know where I am"), and an inability to think coherently—symptoms that closely approximate *DSM–IV* criteria for PA. Unfortunately neither Jigmed nor the other subjects were asked to estimate the time of onset for their attacks, so I cannot gauge how closely they meet the *DSM*'s criterion of ten minute onset to peak intensity. My impression from his account, however, was of a more gradual onset over a period perhaps as long as an hour.

In addition to recounting these episodes of panic, Jigmed also described periods of heightened irritability "even at tiny things" that would occur most often when his anxious and depressive symptoms were at their worst. At those times he could become suddenly angry if he overheard argumentative or abusive conversations, or saw people arguing or fighting, even if only on television. His anger would last for one or two hours and would be accompanied by some of the same somatic symptoms that accompanied his episodes of panic: tightness in the chest, rapid heartbeat, and pains in the upper back. These attacks conformed in general to the lay Tibetan category of "high wind" (*rlung mtho po*), an episodic hyperirritability that is attributed to excessive "wind." They did not, however, involve fear of imminent death (lay Tibetans do not generally regard "high wind" as life-threatening), and Jigmed clearly distinguished them from his episodes of panic .[21]

Additional symptoms elicited by the SCID diagnostic questions included lack of interest in ordinary activities, inability to take pleasure in anything, loss of both appetite and weight, fatigue, feeling that his life was meaningless, guilt at having killed people (during his time as a guerrilla combatant) and animals (in the course of dairy farming), and difficulty concentrating. (Killing sentient beings is included on a list of ten sins that is a commonplace teaching of Tibetan Buddhism.) Despite the apparent severity of his illness, Jigmed denied suicidal ideation or ever having been disabled from his dairy farming or other business activities. On the whole, he easily qualified for MDD and just narrowly missed the criteria for GAD. In addition to all of this, Jigmed also acknowledged two types of delusions: (1) delusions of reference (that is, that street signs and television and radio shows had special messages for him) and (2) delusions of persecution (that is, that people were spying on his every activity and gossiping about him behind his back, and that local civic organizations were plotting to cause him trouble). These views were rather mildly held, however, in that he volunteered that they were probably incorrect estimates of the actual situations, and had never acted on them. They are therefore more accurately classified as ideas of reference and persecution than as frank delusions.

When asked for the initial cause of this illness, Jigmed cited his reaction to his eight-year-old son's death, and worry about his ability to provide for the financial needs of his wife, children, and extended family. In light of his evident affluence, Jigmed's worry about finances might be regarded as excessive and as a typical symptom of GAD. However, these explanations are entirely consistent with lay understandings of the circumstantial causes of "life-wind," and with the classical account from which the lay understandings derive. As already noted, these causes include both "severe crying" and "excessive mental work," the latter of which is widely understood to include chronic worrying of just the kind Jigmed described.

We cannot conclude this discussion of Jigmed's illness without commenting on the potential relevance of PTSD. Jigmed's extended combat experience must certainly have included episodes of extreme violence that would meet the PTSD's etiological criteria for that disorder. Although he did describe cognitive impairment ("inability to think anything at all") as typical of the peak of the episodes of panic, neither flashbacks nor intrusive thoughts or imagery (which are key *DSM–IV* criteria for PTSD) were evident in Jigmed's account of his functioning at the time of our interviews. I was not able to evaluate the extent to which they may have been present in the years immediately following his combat experience.[22]

Jampa

I first learned of Jampa's illness one afternoon when her teenage daughter came into the clinic where I was observing to refill for her mother a prescription that had originally been written by another *emchi* in a nearby town. In response to questioning by the present *emchi*, the daughter explained that her mother had suffered from insomnia for six months; was at present able to sleep only very little, and then only lightly; and complained of a strong burning sensation in her stomach. In response to the *emchi's* question, "Does your mother dream?" the daughter described repetitive dream motifs that her mother had recounted to the family: "Somebody throws water on her, also somebody throws rocks. She dreamed two, three times of small children—that she is going to wash a small child."

Upon hearing this, the *emchi* immediately diagnosed the cause of the mother's insomnia as "excessively strong 'wind' combined with demons—so many demons!" In addition to classical medications, the *emchi* recommended that the family have special offering rituals performed to banish the demons, including an offering that is specific for a particular class of spirits, the *theu rang* (*the 'u rang*), whose involvement was indicated by the mother's dreams about small children.[23] The daughter explained that her family had already obtained divinations from priests and had paid monks to perform each of the several different types of exorcism rituals that had been recommended on the basis of those divinations, which had included those now recommended by the *emchi*. None of those measures, however, had alleviated her mother's suffering.

The mother, Jampa, was fifty years old and lived with this daughter and her husband in a small two-room apartment in a large center for Tibetan refugees on the edge of the city where the two parents had long worked as rug weavers. When I interviewed Jampa and her husband in their apartment, Jampa's stuporous demeanor immediately suggested a serious mental disturbance. Sitting up in bed, she stared blankly into space with a stunned look, only occasionally peering at the other people in the room. Her mouth was never fully closed, even between her extremely brief, faint utterances. When she did speak, she gestured not toward me or anyone else in the room but to the floor, to the space in front of her, or to nothing at all. She often held one hand to her head in the way that Americans may when they have a bad headache, and at times rubbed it back and forth across her forehead while squeezing her eyes tightly shut. When I asked if at those times she was experiencing the headache and buzzing sound she described as prominent symptoms, she said yes. Around her neck hung four *srungma* (*srung ma*, "protectoress")[24] amulets, each of a different color and size, a traditional and common measure to ward off noxious spirits.

In an attempt to make up for the extreme brevity of his wife's responses, Jampa's husband began explaining to me what Jampa was trying to say. Soon he was simply answering all my questions himself, even though I continued to direct them pointedly to Jampa, hoping to elicit more of a response from her. The account that she and her husband provided was highly fragmented and chronologically scrambled. It was only later that I assembled a coherent narrative by reordering the transcribed fragments.

Jampa was born in Tibet, where her family members were farmers and had maintained a religious affiliation with the head of one of Tibetan Buddhism's major sects, who had a monastery in their area. No one else in the family had ever had the type of illness that troubled her now. In 1960 she came with her family to India, fleeing the violent consolidation of Chinese control over Tibet. There they first made their living by gathering firewood, and reestablished their connection with the same religious hierarch they had venerated in Tibet, who had also fled to India.

After completing grade school through the seventh class, Jampa was sent to an especially hot region of southern India for a course in textile weaving. While there she fell ill with episodes of fever that were severe enough to keep her out of class. During these times she complained that her body felt very light. Because of those fevers, Jampa returned home to live with her parents after completing only one year of her weaving course. When a local biomedically trained Tibetan physician was consulted, he said it was only a fever and gave her some tablets to take, but offered no more specific diagnosis or explanation. Every three or four years since then the fevers returned. At the worst Jampa would feel extremely hot, her teeth would clench, and her entire body would shake so much that those in attendance would have to hold her down on the bed.[25]

Soon after returning home from school, Jampa met and married her current husband. They decided to live in the refugee center, where she initially worked making clothes but was soon trained in carpet weaving, which was the center's primary industry. Subsequently both she and her husband worked in the carpet factory for about twenty years, until her current illness forced her to stop, seven months prior to our interviews.

About two years ago, at the age of forty-eight, Jampa had experienced an episode of dizziness during which "everything went dark." It was unclear from her account whether she had gone completely blind or suffered only a marked reduction in vision. Because the condition had spontaneously remitted after four days, she had neither consulted a doctor nor taken any medication. (This may have been a mild stroke, but because she had not been examined at the time, there was no way to check that possibility. The possibility of psychogenic conversion may also be considered, although this seems to have been her only episode of blindness.) Other than that, Jampa had not been sick at all in the months immediately prior to the onset of her current illness. She had generally been healthy except for an occasional sensation of burning in her stomach that would cause her to forego eating. She had suffered from this, however, for many years, and did not regard it as a symptom of serious illness.

Her current illness had begun when the older of her two daughters, whom Jampa "loved very much," was given an opportunity for training as a lab technician at a school in a distant part of India. (The Central School for Tibetans, of which the daughter had attended a local branch, often arranges such opportunities for its graduates.) Out of attachment to this daughter, Jampa had asked her not to go, but the girl was determined to take the opportunity. Within a month, even before the daughter had actually left for school, her mother became increasingly upset about her impending departure and developed symptoms. She ate less or not at all, and complained more often of the burning sensation in her stomach and of dizziness. In addition, Jampa's sleep became disturbed and her body often felt abnormally light. However, because she had generally been healthy of late, the family was not too concerned at first. They consulted an "allopath" (that is, a biomedical physician) only about the burning sensation in her stomach, for which he prescribed some medicine.

Two weeks after her daughter's departure, Jampa's affliction was aggravated by a further emotional shock, the death of an old woman who lived in the apartment next door, whom Jampa had been looking after on a daily basis. Jampa reported having few friends outside of her immediate family, and her friendship with this neighbor seems to have been one on which she was somewhat dependent. At the old woman's death Jampa's symptoms worsened markedly. Her insomnia in particular became much more severe. She would lie in bed all day, unable to sleep except for brief periods of no more than a quarter to a half hour. Often she did fall asleep in the early evening, but would wake up at midnight and be unable to sleep for the remainder of the night. Her husband began to stay up all night to comfort her. He soon took leave from his job at the carpet factory to care for her full-time, but after two months had to return to work out of economic necessity. Jampa described what little sleep she had as "strange" (perhaps hypnagogic) and recounted the same repetitive dream motifs that her daughter had reported to the *emchi*. Because repetitive dreams are often taken as indications of affliction by specific types of spirits, the family had consulted various lama-exorcists. A local one advised them that a harmful spirit, *nyanpo* (*gnyan po*, "harmful one"), was contributing to her illness. He had not specified whether or not this was the ghost of the deceased neighbor, but the family recognized that as a possibility because spirits of the recently deceased are known to be *nyanpo*.[26]

As her symptoms grew worse, Jampa's body began to feel lighter and lighter. Soon she began to fear that she might float away. Occasionally this apprehension became so intense that she would shout out in alarm, calling for her husband and children to hold her down, which they did in order to calm her. (She had also panicked at the sensation of floating away during the bouts of fever she had suffered intermittently over the past thirty years.) From an American point of view, the sensation of increasing bodily lightness is a highly unusual focus for PA. (As discussed in Chapter 3, the association of "lightness" with fear states also occurs in other Asian contexts that have a "wind"-based ethnophysiology.) Nevertheless, Jampa described it as the most alarming of her acute symptoms, an immediately threatening, potentially catastrophic loss of control. Accordingly, the episodes she described had all the essential elements of our current notion of PA: an acute, relatively brief episode of extreme fear related to a catastrophic expectation (that is, of floating away into the sky) that arises in response to a disturbing alteration of somatic or cognitive experience (that is, her sensation of extreme bodily lightness), over which the subject experiences a lack of control.

In response to the SCID diagnostic questions, Jampa and her husband together also acknowledged all the criterial items for MDD. Those that had been present daily since her daughter left for the training program included depressed affect, lack of interest in former activities, anhedonia, insomnia, retarded speech and movement, fatigue, thinking her life was useless, and suicidal ideation. At the illness's onset she had lost her appetite (as during previous episodes of the burning sensation in her stomach), and this had led to a weight loss of three to four kilograms. At the time of our interview, her appetite had improved a bit but was still not back to normal. She also reported the daily occurrence of racing thoughts, particularly when she was alone. From a psychodynamic point of view, Jampa's distress at her daughter's departure for school and at her neighbor's death, and her fear of "floating" away, that is, departing from the social world, are all consistent with a disabling intense fear of abandonment.

Jampa also reported other somatosensory dysphorias: burning and "buzzing" feelings in her feet, feeling hot, headaches accompanied by a "buzzing" tinnitus, and what Jampa called "beating of the channels." It was difficult to obtain a clear description of this last symptom. The term *channel* (*rtsa*) refers alike to blood vessels, lymphatic ducts, motor and sensory nerves, and the pathways through which the "wind" circulates. Her husband explained it as a "hot feeling" in her "channels," but her use of the word *beating* indicated a discomforting pulsation as well.

In addition to her chronic symptoms and her acute panics about "floating away," Jampa also acknowledged periods of markedly heightened irritability. These had begun with her daughter's actual departure. They typically had a sudden onset and could last for up to half a day. As in Jigmed's case, these episodes corresponded to the lay Tibetan construct of "high wind."

Jampa acknowledged only two items on the SCID Psychosis Screen. The first item was the hallucinatory buzzing in her ears. Her husband said, "She hears rainfall even when it's not raining." ("Buzzing" sounds are included in the *Treatises* list of general "wind illness" symptoms.) The second was the perception, occurring at the same time, that her body had changed in a "strange" way that she could not describe. These symptoms were both rather benign in that neither led to any particular behavior on Jampa's part. Her perception of her body becoming so light that it was about to float away might be regarded as a psychotic hallucination. However, to do so could be construed as psychopathologizing the foci of her panic simply because it is aberrant from a North American perspective. We count the conviction of our homegrown PD patients that they are experiencing heart attacks or the onset of insanity not as psychotic hallucinations but rather as "catastrophic misinterpretations," and this view is clinically sustainable precisely because those beliefs are activated only during the relatively brief duration of an attack. Jampa's frightening experience of becoming so light as to "float away" was similarly confined to relatively brief episodes of panic, and was therefore entirely analogous to North American and British apprehensions of immediately impending heart attack, suffocation, or insanity.

Circumstances that alleviated her illness included being visited by pleasant company, such as her sister or other family members. If her younger daughter misbehaved or was noisy, her symptoms worsened. These effects are both congruent with the classic's account of the general features of "wind" illnesses, which specifies "pleasant conversation" as therapeutic and "harsh speech" as aggravating.

Jampa and her husband had not settled on any single explanation for her suffering, but the combination of classical medicines and religious rituals to which they had turned for relief was consistent with the general opinion of the priests and *emchi* they had consulted that her illness was caused by a combination of excessive, disturbed "wind" and affliction by harmful spirits. As noted earlier, this is a common explanation among Tibetan refugees for severe, persistent illnesses with prominent psychiatric features. Its likely provenance is the classical explanation given out to lay clients by *emchi* and exorcists that the deleterious effects of "wind" disorders on mental focus and clarity render one unusually vulnerable to spirit attack. The cyclic, alternating resort to *emchi* for medication and then to lama-exorcists for rituals is also a common pattern in such cases.

At the time of our interviews, the daughter whose departure had triggered Jampa's illness was due to graduate in the next month, and the family was anxiously awaiting her return home in hopes that the mother's condition would improve.

Relevance to Other Research on Panic Attack and Panic Disorder

The following sections review data from the four cases of "life-wind illness" I studied in which episodes of acute panic were prominent, including the two just reviewed. Comparison with recent findings on PA and PD in the United States and Great Britain brings to light a number of significant similarities and a few significant differences.

Symptoms Conforming to 'DSM' Criteria

These Tibetan subjects' accounts of their episodes of panic bear most of the hallmarks regarded as essential in the *DSM–IV* definition of PA: "discrete period of intense fear or discomfort"; "sudden onset"; severe disturbances of somatic sensation or cognition or both; individually stereotypical focus of apprehension on particular somatic sensations of distress (most often respiratory or cardiac) or on cognitive dysfunctions; stereotypical interpretation of such sensations or dsyfunctions as boding either imminent death, insanity, or extreme social embarrassment; perceived lack of control over these symptoms; and relatively brief duration (APA 1994:394–395). The fact that my field research protocol did not include a systematic evaluation for PA (I was at that time focused on the investigation of MD and GAD) makes my subjects' unprompted description of these characteristic features all the more striking.

Table 10.1 compares the symptoms of the acute episodes as described by the Tibetan subjects and the positive *DSM–IV* criteria for PA. (Exclusionary criteria are omitted.) This tabulation includes only those symptoms that occurred exclusively or that markedly worsened during their attacks; other symptoms that were chronically present as part of the underlying "life-wind illness" and did not intensify during attacks are omitted.

Table 10.1   Number of subjects meeting criteria for *DSM–IV* panic attack (*n* = 4)

A: (i) A discrete period of intense fear or discomfort	4
(ii) Sudden onset, building to a peak in ten minutes or less	?*
B: At least four of the following:	
Dizziness or lightheadedness, faintness, unsteadiness	3
Fear of imminent death	3
Palpitations, pounding, or accelerated heartbeat	3
Shortness of breath or smothering sensation	3
Derealization or depersonalization	2
Fear of losing control or "going insane"	2
Nausea or abdominal distress	2
Paresthesia	2
Chest pain or discomfort	1
Chills or hot flashes	1
Choking sensation	1
Sweating	0
Trembling or shaking	0

*One of the A criteria (indicated by a question mark) was not assessed.

Another similarity between these four cases and *DSM* PA is a high level of co-morbidity with depression and anxiety. When symptoms of my subjects' underlying "life-wind illnesses" were evaluated against *DSM* criteria, two of the four qualified fully for both MDD and GAD, and the other two each qualified for one or the other diagnosis, failing the remaining one by only a single criterion symptom. This result is consistent with findings in the United States and Great Britain that patients with PA have a 45 to 60 percent comorbidity of MDD, GAD, or both (Andrade et al. 1994; Kessler et al. 1998; Wittchen et al. 1994). In addition to having comorbid depressive, anxious, and somatosensory symptoms, some of my Tibetan subjects also reported cognitive disorganization and dissociative phenomena.

There is also significant heterogeneity in the Tibetan cases, most of which is accommodated by the *DSM* criteria. A number of symptom surveys in the United States and Great Britain have demonstrated that cases of PA may be subtyped according to the individual's stereotypical focus of alarm, that is, cardiac, respi-ratory, gastrointestinal, parathesiac, hyperventilatory, vestibular, and oculoves-tibular sensations; cognitive dysfunctions; depersonalization; or dread (Briggs et al. 1993; Cox et al. 1994; Lelliot and Bass 1990; Meuret et al. 2006; Uhlenhuth et al. 2006). Jigmed's panic (the first case reviewed earlier) focused primarily on cardiac complaints. Jampa (the second case reviewed) panicked in response to sensations of increasing bodily lightness and the anticipation of floating away. Of the two women whose cases have not been presented here, one described a primarily respiratory panic, the other focused on disruptions in both breathing and heartbeat. In three of these four cases, therefore, the focus of panic was car-diac or respiratory, the same two foci found to be most common in American and British PAs.

These subjects described their attacks as usually not triggered by particular kinds of situations, that is, by specific settings or objects. In *DSM–IV* terms these were "unprovoked" or "spontaneous" attacks. As exceptions to this generality, two subjects reported that their attacks had at some times (although not usually) been triggered by physical effort (which is also a common trigger of PA in the United States), and two reported attacks occurring most often, although not exclusively, during insomniac nights.

Symptoms Varying from 'DSM' Criteria

Table 10.2 tabulates reported attack symptoms that are not found in the *DSM–IV* PA criteria. Note that somatosensory and cognitive symptoms predominate among these. As can be seen in the table, the Tibetan episodes of panic varied from *DSM* criteria most markedly in three ways: they included a number of somatosensory and cognitive symptoms that are not listed among the *DSM* criteria, they had an

Table 10.2 Number of subjects reporting additional
symptoms of acute anxiety episodes not included in
DSM–IV panic attack criteria (*n* = 4)

Affective:	
"Agitated mind" (connotes affective suffering)	1
Cognitive:	
Difficulty concentrating or thinking	2
Disorientation	1
Mind goes blank	1
Intrusive thought to "go out at night"	1
Racing thoughts	1
Dissociative:	
Amnesia for acute anxiety episodes	1
Impaired recall of general knowledge	1
Somatosensory:	
Back pain	2
Fatigue due to difficult breathing	2
Headache	1
Sensation of increased bodily lightness	1
Special senses:	
Impaired vision, "like dust in my eyes"	1

apparently slower rate of onset, and there were no attempts to flee the locale of the attack.

As a group, the four subjects endorsed somatosensory symptoms as typical of their attacks a total of twenty-seven times, for an average of 6.75 somatosensory symptoms per case.[27] Despite this result, none of the met the *DSM–IV* criteria for somatization disorder.[28] The variety of somatosensory symptoms was also significant. In spontaneous descriptions of their attacks (as distinct from their responses to the SCID questions) each of the four subjects reported some somatic symptoms that do not appear among the *DSM–IV* criteria. Both Jigmed and Jampa (whose cases have been described herein) described intensifications of localized pain that were also, at lower levels of intensity, chronic features of their underlying "life-wind." Jigmed had a burning pain that moved around the front and back of his rib cage; Jampa suffered from a burning sensation in her stomach.

In the descriptions of the chronic "life-wind" that constituted the background

of these attacks, somatosensory symptoms were also more numerous and prominent than the *DSM* criteria for MD or GAD suggest (although quantitative data
on the occurrence of such symptoms in cases of comorbid MD and GAD are not
evident in the psychiatric literature).

In recorded clinical meetings with their *emchi*, these subjects mentioned somatosensory symptoms far more often than they mentioned dysphoric affects, although
this tendency was not as marked in the longer interviews I conducted with them
outside of the clinic. This outcome suggests that a somaticizing style of clinical
presentation may be characteristic of Tibetan refugees who suffer from "life-wind."
If confirmed in a larger sample, this tendency would parallel the somaticizing clinical style of neurasthenia patients in Taiwan and China (Kleinman 1980, 1982, 1986;
Lee 1998), and would be congruent with other research suggesting a more broadly
Asian tendency to emphasize somatic complaints when presenting illnesses that
include affective suffering (Farooq et al. 1995; Hsu 1999; Lin et al. 1985; Tseng et al.
1990). However, unlike the cases described by Kleinman (1982, 1986), my Tibetan
subjects also spoke explicitly about their emotional distress, albeit outside the clinic.
Three described themselves as pervasively sad, and the fourth said she suffered from
"agitated mind" (*sems 'khral*), which in colloquial Tibetan connotes affective suffering. Moreover, all four subjects were able to attribute their emotional distress to
specific losses, making it difficult to argue that the prominence of somatosensory
symptoms in their clinical presentation constituted somatization in the sense of a
psychodynamic defense, that is, focusing on somatosensory dysphorias or dysfunctions as a way of deflecting awareness from dysphoric affects.

Neither does the fact that these individuals adopted a somaticizing style in their
clinical (and perhaps social) presentation of "life-wind" necessarily imply that they
did so in the service of negotiating social or financial advantages, an interpretation
that is prominent in early accounts of somaticized "idioms of distress" (Kleinman
1982; Nichter 1981). Jigmed had continued to work, travel, and head his extended
family throughout his illness. Of the two women whose cases have not been presented here, one kept up a regular routine of domestic duties—cooking, cleaning
and looking after her grandchildren while their mothers were at work—and the
other fared for herself, living alone, with only a single neighbor to "look after" her
occasionally. Jampa was the only one of the four whose illness had elicited a leave
from work and extensive compensatory support from a relative (her husband).
None of the other three subjects seemed to have won any significant decrease in
their duties or gained any increase in social support by presenting their illnesses
in a somaticized idiom.

Symptoms of cognitive disruption that are not included among the *DSM* criteria were reported a total of six times by three of the four subjects, for an average of

1.5 such symptoms across the group of four as a whole. Most of these symptoms were varieties of general cognitive disorganization or suspension (for example, "My mind goes blank"). The intrusive thought to "go out into the night" that was reported by one subject (the case presented in Jacobson 2002) is understood in refugee culture to be a particularly dangerous form of spirit attack. Individuals who yield to that impulse are sometimes found later in wilderness areas in a stuporous state, and in some cases are said to have thrown themselves off of cliffs or into rivers.

I did not obtain a quantitative assessment of the typical rate of onset for these attacks, but my impression in each case was that onset was longer than the ten minutes specified in the *DSM–IV* criteria. This duration may be a significant distinction between Tibetan panic illness and *DSM* PA. Alternatively, this disparity might be cited as a reason to classify these episodes as anxiety attacks rather than as PAs. The force of that argument, however, is mitigated by Manson's (1985) singling out of duration as one of the symptomatological parameters that is most likely to vary for similar psychiatric disorders between Euro-American and other cultural settings.

Another departure from *DSM* criteria was that none of my Tibetan subjects reported a desire to flee the locale of their attack. In two cases this may have been because their attacks most often occurred late at night, when they were at home trying to sleep, and being at home at night is definitely safer, from a Tibetan refugee point of view, than going outside in the night, which is known to invite attack by malevolent spirits.

Despite these three disparities—the number and variety of somatosensory symptoms, an apparently slower rate of onset, and the absence of an urge to flee the locale of their attack—each of these four subjects satisfied all of the other *DSM–IV* criteria for PA. In view of this, the episodes they described deserve to be regarded as examples of a Tibetan refugee variant of panic illness.[29] This coincidence of hallmark features of PA with significant departures on some points suggests, as do Hinton's similar findings for Khmer panic illness (Hinton 2002; Hinton et al. 2001a, 2001b, 2001c, 2002), that in order for *DSM* criteria to detect panic attack disorders more adequately across cultures, they must embrace a wider range of symptomatic variation, especially with respect to somatosensory symptoms and temporal parameters.[30]

Distressing Life Events as Triggering Periods of Increased Frequency of Attacks

Another significant point of cross-cultural comparison is variation in the frequency of attacks. In the Tibetan refugee cases, the frequency waxed and waned in concert with fluctuations in the severity of the individual's underlying "life-wind." This result is consistent with Amering and Katschnig's (1990) finding that alternating periods of relapse and remission were reported to be typical in 24 percent of the long-term studies of PD in different cultures.

Table 10.3 gives the frequencies with which the four subjects discussed here cited various types of distressing events as having triggered periods of worsened "life-wind" and more frequent episodes of panic.[31] Many of these varieties of suffering are accommodated by implication in the *Four Treatises'* list of the "circumstantial causes" of "life-wind illness" (see earlier discussion of these causes). Each subject also identified specific distressing events that had initiated their illnesses. Jigmed's initial episode occurred when the death of his young son brought on an intense, worsening chest pain. In Jampa's case, her daughter's decision to leave home for vocational training at a remote school triggered an agitated depression that worsened dramatically when a neighbor-friend unexpectedly passed away, initiating a prolonged period of severe "life-wind" that was complicated by spirit attack. Of

Table 10.3 Distressing experiences identified as contributing to periods of aggravated "life-wind illness" and increased frequency of panic attack ($n = 4$)

Flight from Tibet and refugee relocation	4
Financial:	
Anxiety about family finances	3
Loss of family capital	2
Death, illness, and separation:	
Death of child	2
Separation from child	2
Death of spouse	2
Prolonged illness of spouse	2
Absence of care by relatives	2
Death of parent	1
Permanent separation from spouse	1
Death of sibling or other relative	1
Death of neighbor	1
Personal illness or injury:	
Major physical illness	2
Major physical injury	1
Other:	
Capture by Chinese military	1
Extensive combat experience	1
Jailed	1

the two women whose cases have not been reviewed in detail here, the "life-wind illness" of one began when, having recently lost two young children to illnesses, she learned of yet another daughter's death. The other women's first episode was triggered when her husband was robbed of his entire stock-in-trade by Chinese troops, and her illness markedly intensified when he later fell ill and died.

In addition to undergoing these comparatively recent familial catastrophes, each of these four subjects, like all other refugees who fled Tibet in the 1950s and 1960s, had survived a brutal military invasion in which separation from family members, friends, and neighbors, or their violent death, was commonplace. Estimates suggest that as many as 900,000 Tibetans, roughly one-sixth of the entire population, perished during the nine years of that conflict (Hutheesing 1960; Kumar 1994). Some years later in India, these same refugees learned of the wholesale destruction of Tibetan monasteries by the Red Guard during Mao's Cultural Revolution. Considering the deep faith and devotion that virtually all Tibetans, especially those raised in Tibet, hold for their homeland and religion, this latter event must be counted among the most painful of their loses.[32] These familial and collective traumas surely predisposed this refugee population to the spectrum of anxious and depressive illnesses that has been noted in other groups of Asian refugees (Carlson and Rosser-Hogan 1991; Eisenbruch 1991; Kroll et al. 1988; Lin et al. 1985).[33]

The types of loss that my Tibetan subjects cited as having provoked their "life-wind" and accompanying episodes of panic are also congruent with studies in the United States and Great Britain that have identified similar events as the most common antecedents to both depressive episodes and PA. These events include separation from spouse or family, death of a family member or close friend, difficulty at work, and loss of employment, material possession, physical health, or a cherished ideal (Brown et al. 1987; Eifert and Forsyth 1996; Jacobs et al. 1990).

Toward a Biocultural Interactionist View of Panic Illnesses

The numerous parallels reviewed here between the episodes of acute panic that sometimes accompany "life-wind" in Tibetan refugees and PD as it has been documented in the United States and Great Britain add to the growing record of significant similarities across cultural variants of panic illness. As has been widely recognized, these similarities suggest a common underlying pathophysiology with a significant biological component to account for the cross-cultural similarities. At the same time, the significant variation in panic illnesses found across cultural settings (Amering and Katshning 1990; Cross-National Collaborative Panic Study 1992; Hinton et al. 2001a, 2001b) makes it clear that there must be some provision for the influence of cultural learning and experience on the expression of whatever underlying pathomechanic is proposed.

The leading candidates for a biological pathomechanic in recent years have been neurophysiological theories of dysfunction in a brain "fear network" (Coplan and Lydiard 1998; Gorman et al. 2000; Krystal et al. 1996; Sinha et al. 2000). The two most widely supported mechanisms for the observed cultural differences are "catastrophic misinterpretation" of somatic and mental symptoms (Clark 1986, 1988; Cox 1996; see also the closely related concept of "anxiety sensitivity" in Cox et al. 1996; Lee et al. 2006; McNally 2002; Reiss et al. 1986; Taylor 1995; Taylor and Cox 1998) and traumatic conditioning of a panic response to interoceptive cues (Bouwer and Stein 1997, 1999; Breslau and Davis 1987; McNally 1994). Given that "catastrophic misinterpretation" is acknowledged to be influenced by ethnotheories, and that the traumatic experiences of refugee groups are often suffered collectively, either of these models would plausibly accommodate the cultural variation in some features of panic illnesses.

The research literatures supporting each of these proposed mechanisms—dysfunctions of fear circuitry in the brain, cognitive misinterpretation, and traumatic conditioning of interoceptive cues—are now robust enough that they are likely to continue to advance our ability to account for both the core and culturally heterogeneous features of panic illness for some time to come. It is likely that there are several ways in which these three models might be integrated to accommodate the accumulating evidence of both variation and similarity in panic illnesses across cultures (see, for example, Middleton 1998). A vigorous debate between competing integrative hypotheses might propel the anthropology of anxiety illnesses more fully into the arena of biocultural interaction that was recommended more than twenty years ago (Carey 1985; Good and Kleinman 1985).

Notes

The research on which this chapter is based was supported by grant 1 F31 MH10087 from the National Institutes of Mental Health. It has benefited from the thoughtful suggestions of Byron Good, Alan Harwood, David Healey, Devon Hinton, Roberto Lewis-Fernández, Jamie McGuire, and Yangga Trarong.

1. These interviews were conducted between 1990 and 1996 with patients recruited as a sample of opportunity in the course of observing in classical Tibetan medical clinics. The study also included original translations of portions of the Tibetan medical classic (*BSYB* n.d.) and fieldwork in Tibetan refugee communities in three cities. It was supported by grant 1 F31 MH10087 from the National Institutes of Mental Health, and by a dissertation travel grant from Harvard University. Other publications based on data from this study are Jacobson (2002, 2007).

2. On their initial occurrence, Tibetan medical terms are given as English glosses enclosed by quotation marks, followed by their Roman transliteration according to the convention of Wylie (1959). English glosses are also placed in quotes on every subsequent appearance in order to remind the reader that the Tibetan medical concepts to which they

refer, although in some instances overlapping those of the corresponding American words, nevertheless differ in important ways. For instance, the classical Tibetan concept of "blood" (*khrag*) overlaps but is not conceptually identical with the biomedical term *blood*. Where a Tibetan word is used as such, it appears as a phonetic approximation and is placed in italics, such as *lung* for "wind" (*rlung*).

3. The *Four Treatises* is attributed by many Tibetan scholars to a miraculous teaching of the Medicine Buddha. According to that account, female religious spirits (*Mka' 'gro ma*) wrote down the teaching and it was subsequently translated into Tibetan in the eighth century C.E. Shortly thereafter, it was miraculously concealed in a pillar of Samye monastery in Lhasa, and then recovered *circa* 1038 C.E. A competing strain of Tibetan scholastic opinion regards it as a brilliant synthesis of earlier Ayurvedic and other materials by the physician Yuthog Yonten Gonpo the Younger (*Gyu thog gsar ma yon tan mgon po*, 1126–1202 C.E.).

4. The three *nyepa*—"wind," "bile," and "phlegm"—correspond respectively to the *tridosa* of *vata*, *pitta*, and *kapha*, which are central to the theory of the Ayurvedic medical texts that were the major, though not the sole, source for the Tibetan classic (Jacobson 2000; Meyer 1996).

5. The Tibetan *tsa* (*rtsa*, "channel" or "vein") is applied alike to blood vessels, nerves, lymphatic ducts, and the conduits of "wind" (the latter having no clear parallel in Euro-American anatomy). The *Four Treatises* describe a number of different types of "wind" channels.

6. See Kuriyama (1994, 1999) for discussions of the historical development of the analogous ancient Chinese medical concept of *ch'i* from its original signification of meteorological wind. Like the Tibetan *lung*, *ch'i* is a dynamic agent that is fundamental to both physiology and pathophysiology.

7. A "rough diet" is one disproportionate in foods that have the quality of "roughness" (*rtsub*), one of seventeen "qualities" (*yon tan*) that constitute one aspect of the *Four Treatise*'s multidimensional classification of the varying physiological effects of foods. Examples of "rough" foods include strong tea, certain uncooked vegetables, and goat meat. Spoiled food is also "rough."

8. Words placed in brackets in this and the other translated verses are my own interpolations, the accuracy of which were confirmed by my tutors in the *Four Treatises*—Lama Jinpa and Drupgyur, Rinpoche, both faculty members of the Chakpoori Institute for Tibetan Medicine.

9. The doctrine of "karma" (*las*), which is fundamental to all strains of Buddhism, posits a causative dynamic through which the moral valence of one's conduct affects the ongoing circumstances of one's life, sometimes at a temporal delay that may even stretch from one lifetime to another (via reincarnation). Undertaking acts of great positive moral merit such as the performance or sponsorship of religious rituals and offerings is consequently a common response to illness, on the reasoning that improved karma may ameliorate or cure the illness.

10. The third volume of the *Four Treatises*, the *Treatise of Oral Precepts*, includes chapters devoted to illnesses caused by each of a number of specific types of spirits: "elemental spirits" (*'byung wa*), "spirits who afflict children" (*byis pa'i gdon*), serpent spirits (*klu*, equivalent to the Sanskrit *naga*), "sky spirits" (*gza*), and "demons" (*gdon*). Each of these spirits has a different habitat, sensitivity, and capacity to cause harm. This list should not be taken as comprehensive; Tibetan demonology recognizes many other kinds of spirits and ghosts as well, some of which are also regarded as able to cause illness.

11. An *emchi* informant explained that the phrase *snying stobs zhan*, which translates literally as "weak heart power," refers here to a weakness not of the physical organ but of the "wind" that flows through the "central channel" in the heart, "the place where consciousness flows" (*rnam shes rgyu gnas*). A second *emchi* explained, "This doesn't mean that the heart organ itself is weak. It means the person is weak-minded. A weak-minded person can't tolerate even the smallest unpleasantness."

12. When "wind" or either of the other two *nyepa* are disrupted from their proper channels and enter "the place where consciousness runs," the portion of the central psychic channel that is located in the heart, illnesses that are characterized by delusion, hallucination, and disturbed conduct result. This condition also renders the individual especially liable to spirit possession.

13. According to one *emchi* informant *nying* (*snying*), the primary meaning of which is "heart," in this passage instead connotes "emotions," the heart being especially related to emotions for Tibetans as well as for Euro-Americans. "Wandering heart" (*snying 'phyo*) accordingly denotes affective instability.

14. These and the following examples of colloquial reference to "wind" as an explanation for disturbed behavior are drawn from transcripts of interviews I conducted with patients who had been diagnosed by *emchi* as suffering from "life-wind illness" and from interviews with other Tibetan refugees who did not have that diagnosis.

15. The symptoms that the *Treatises* list as typical of "wind" illnesses in general also include anger; aching in the back of the neck, chest, and jaws; dry vomiting; and pain moving around the body.

16. Several investigators have found that somatosensory complaints are also typical of depressed Asian refugees (Farooq et al. 1995; Hsu 1999; Kroll et al. 1988; Lin et al. 1985).

17. This diagnosis is congruent with findings of significant rates of comorbidity between MD and GAD in the United States, and between depressive and anxious disorders in general (Ballenger 1998; Pasnau and Bystritsky 1994; Wittchen et al. 1994). It also underlines the relevance for transcultural psychiatry of the proposed category of "mixed anxiety and depression," even though its advocates intend it for cases of comorbid anxiety and depression that are subcriterial (Guarnaccia 1997; Katon and Roy-Byrne 1991; Sartorius and Ustan 1995; Zinbarg et al. 1994). The high level of comorbidity between both fully qualified and subcriterial MD and GAD in my small sample of "life-wind illness" cases reflects the fact that Tibetan refugees who present themselves to *emchi* for treatment are generally far more depressed or anxious or both than many of those who present with milder symptoms of the same types in the United States. Tibetan refugee culture seems to require a relatively high level of severity for symptoms of these kinds before judging them to require clinical attention.

18. According to one *emchi* informant, the types of spirits most often responsible for brief, acute episodes of panic are the "king" (*rgyal po*), the "mighty" (*btsan*), and "ghosts of the dead" (*shi 'dre*).

19. On "rough" (*rtsub*) see note 11.

20. According to an *emchi* informant, the literal meaning of *spyugs*, "to throw out," is not intended here. Rather, it indicates that the "encompassing-wind" in the heart region is disturbed and not functioning properly. As a result, the heart becomes weak. It does not imply that the "encompassing wind" departs entirely from the heart; it is more likely that the "wind" is "thrown out" of its physiological channel within the heart—the departure of

any of the *nyepa* from their proper pathways being a frequently invoked pathophysiological mechanism.

21. Thanks to Devon Hinton for directing my attention to the literature documenting "anger attacks" in the United States (Fava 1998; Mammen et al. 1999; Rosenbaum 1999).

22. There is some evidence that Tibetan refugees exhibit a certain psychological hardiness vis-à-vis traumatic stressors. Crescenzi et al. (2002) found that only 20 percent of a sample of sixty-five Tibetan refugees who had been imprisoned by the Chinese before leaving Tibet met the Harvard Trauma Questionnaire criterion score for PTSD despite a large percentage of the group endorsing sixteen of twenty-seven types of traumatic events.

23. *The'u rang* are diminutive humanoids who are said to be seen only rarely. On some occasions they perform beneficial actions, but on others they can be malevolent.

24. This term is applied both to female protective deities and to amulets that are empowered with the magical diagrams and mantras that invoke the protection of these deities. Such amulets are also empowered by the blessings of the lama-exorcists who produce them.

25. In these episodes Jampa may have been suffering from relapsing malaria.

26. *Nyanpo* (*gnyan po*, "harmful" or "dangerous") refers to any spirit that is especially liable to cause injury, regardless of its demonological classification. "Ghosts of the dead" (*shi 'dre*) unintentionally harm those to whom they were attached in life when they remain in the vicinity of their former home (as some are wont to do) rather than proceeding to the "intermediate realm" (*bar do*) between death and rebirth. Even though they do so out of a positive emotional attachment, and may even attempt to actively help their former friends and relatives, their very proximity causes sickness.

27. Terheggen et al. (2001) found that on average their sample of Tibetan refugees more affirmatively endorsed symptoms of anxiety and depression that were phrased in somatic terms than they endorsed those symptoms that were phrased in psychological or affective terms.

28. On the basis of their research findings, Cox et al. (1994) suggest that despite the *DSM–IV* requirement of at least four somatosensory symptoms for a diagnosis of PA, the average patient, even in the United States, may suffer from a greater number.

29. *DSM* standards are invoked here because of their currency in biomedical psychiatry, and in the absence of any more anthropologically informed standard for the identification of cultural variants of panic illness.

30. The case for panic illness as a cross-cultural category is further supported by the Cross-National Collaborative Panic Study (1992), which found significant numbers of subjects who met modified *DSM–III* criteria for PD in fourteen countries spanning four cultural areas. Although the use of *DSM–III* criteria in that study probably biased it to exclude some cultural variants, it at least demonstrated that a version of *DSM* PD could be identified across multiple cultural settings. In their discussion of this data, Amering and Katschnig (1990) note the high correlation of symptoms across *DSM–III*-defined PA, *koro* in Southeast Asia (Bernstein and Gaw 1990), and *kayak angst* in Greenland and Polar Eskimo society (Carr 1978). They interpret these similarities as evidence of an underlying transcultural biological disease process.

31. Many of the types of stressor events that these patients described also appear in the tables of traumatic experiences reported by Tibetan refugees in Crescenzi et al. (2002:371) and Terheggen et al. (2001:397).

32. Terheggen et al. (2001) asked eleven Tibetan refugees to rank a list of twenty "traumatic experiences" according to their relative severity. The highest ranked item was "destruc-

tion of religious signs," and the third ranked item was "being forbidden to live according to one's own religion."

33. Kroll and colleagues (1988) have argued that in such populations the depressive, anxious, and posttraumatic disorders, which are described and diagnosed separately in the *DSMs*, converge into a syndrome of bereavement that so intertwines the features of all three as to deserve its own diagnostic category.

References

American Psychiatric Association (APA). 1987. *Diagnostic and Statistical Manual of Mental Disorders.* 3rd ed., rev. [*DSM–III–R.*] Washington, DC: American Psychiatric Association.

———. 1994. *Diagnostic and Statistical Manual of Mental Disorders.* 4th ed. [*DSM–IV.*] Washington, DC: American Psychiatric Association.

Amering, M., and H. Katschnig. 1990. Panic Attacks and Panic Disorder in Cross-Cultural Perspective. *Psychiatric Annals* 20(9):511–516.

Andrade, L., W. W. Eaton, and H. Chilcoat. 1994. Lifetime Comorbidity of Panic Attack and Major Depression in a Population-Based Study: Symptom Profiles. *British Journal of Psychiatry* 165:363–369.

Ballenger, J. C. 1998. Comorbidity of Panic and Depression: Implications for Clinical Management. *International Clinical Psychopharmacology* 13:S13–17.

Beckwith, C. I. 1979.The Introduction of Greek Medicine into Tibet in the Seventh and Eighth Centuries. *Journal of the American Oriental Society* 99:297–313.

Bernstein, R. L., and A. C. Gaw. 1990. Koro: Proposed Classification for *DSM-IV. American Journal of Psychiatry* 147:1670–1674.

Bouwer, C., and D. Stein. 1997. Association of Panic Disorder with a History of Traumatic Suffocation. *American Journal of Psychiatry* 154:1566–1570.

———. 1999. Panic Disorder Following Torture by Suffocation Is Associated with Predominantly Respiratory Symptoms. *Psychological Medicine* 29:233–236.

Breslau, N., and G. Davis. 1987. Posttraumatic Stress Disorder: The Etiological Specificity of Wartime Stressors. *American Journal of Psychiatry* 144:578–583.

Briggs, A. C., D. D. Stretch, and S. Brandon. 1993. Subtyping of Panic Disorder by Symptom Profile. *British Journal of Psychiatry* 163:201–209.

Brown, G. S., A. Bifulco, and T. O. Harris. 1987. Life Events, Vulnerability, and Onset of Depression: Some Refinements. *British Journal of Psychiatry* 150:30–42.

BSYB. n.d. (*circa* 11th century C.E.) *Bdud rtsi snying po yan lag brgyad pa gsang ba man ngag gi rgyud* (Treatise of Secret Precepts on the Eight-Branched Essential Elixir). Dharamsala, IN: Tibetan Medical and Astrological Institute.

Carey, G. 1985. Epidemiology and Cross-Cultural Aspects of Anxiety Disorders: A Commentary. In *Anxiety and the Anxiety Disorders.* A. H. Tuma and J. Maser, eds. Pp. 325–330. Hillsdale, NJ: Erlbaum.

Carlson, E. B., and R. Rosser-Hogan. 1991. Trauma Experiences, Post-Traumatic Stress, Dissociation, and Depression in Cambodian Refugees. *American Journal of Psychiatry* 148(11):1548–1551.

Carr, J. E. 1978. Ethno-Behaviorism and the Culture-Bound Syndromes: The Case of Amok. *Culture, Medicine, and Psychiatry* 2(3):269–93.

Clark, D. M. 1986. A Cognitive Approach to Panic. *Behaviour, Research, and Therapy* 24(4):461–470.

———. 1988. A Cognitive Model of Panic Attacks. In *Panic: Psychological Perspectives*. S. Rachman and J. D. Maser, eds. Pp. 71–89. Hillsdale, NJ: Erlbaum.

Coplan, J. D., and R. B. Lydiard. 1998. Brain Circuits in Panic Disorder. *Biological Psychiatry* 44(12):1264–1276.

Cox, B. J. 1996. The Nature and Assessment of Catastrophic Thoughts in Panic Disorder. *Behaviour, Research, and Therapy* 34(4):363–374.

Cox, B. J., R. P. Swinson, N. S. Endler, and G. R. Norton. 1994. The Symptom Structure of Panic Attacks. *Comprehensive Psychiatry* 35(5):349–253.

Cox, B. J., J. D. Parker, and R. P. Swinson. 1996. Anxiety Sensitivity: Confirmatory Evidence for a Multidimensional Construct. *Behaviour, Research, and Therapy* 34(7):591–598.

Crescenzi, A., E. Ketzer, M. Van Ommeren, K. Phuntsok, I. Komproe, and J. de Jong. 2002. Effect of Political Imprisonment and Trauma History on Recent Tibetan Refugees in India. *Journal of Traumatic Stress* 15(5):369–375.

Cross-National Collaborative Panic Study. 1992. Drug Treatment of Panic Disorder. Comparative Efficacy of Alprazolam, Imipramine and Placebo. *British Journal of Psychiatry* 160:191–202.

Eifert, G. H., and J. P. Forsyth. 1996. Heart-Focused and General Illness Fears in Relation to Parental Medical History and Separation Experiences. *Behaviour, Research, and Therapy* 34(9):135–39.

Eisenbruch, M. 1991. From Post-Traumatic Stress Disorder to Cultural Bereavement: Diagnosis of Southeast Asian Refugees. *Social Science and Medicine* 33:673–680.

Farooq, S., M. S. Gahir, E. Okyere, A. J. Sheikh, and F. Oyebode. 1995. Somatization: A Transcultural Study. *Journal of Psychosomatic Research* 39(7):35–38.

Fava, M. 1998. Depression with Anger Attacks. *Journal of Clinical Psychiatry* 59 (18):18–22.

Good, B. J. 1977. The Heart of What's the Matter: The Semantics of Illness in Iran. *Culture, Medicine, and Psychiatry* 1(1):25–58.

Good, B. J., and A. Kleinman. 1985. Culture and Anxiety: Cross-Cultural Evidence for the Patterning of Anxiety Disorders. In *Anxiety and the Anxiety Disorders*. A. H. Tuma and J. D. Maser, eds. Pp. 297–324. Hillsdale, NJ: Erlbaum.

Good, B. J., and M. J. Good. 1992. Comparative Study of Greco-Islamic Medicine: The Integration of Medical Knowledge into Local Symbolic Contexts. In *Paths to Asian Medical Knowledge*. C. Leslie and A. Young, eds. Pp. 257–271. Berkeley: University of California Press.

Gorman, J. M., J. Kent, G. M. Sullivan, and J. D. Coplan. 2000. Neuroanatomical Hypothesis of Panic Disorder, Revised. *American Journal of Psychiatry* 157(4):493–505.

Guarnaccia, P. J. 1997. A Cross-Cultural Perspective on Anxiety Disorders. In *Cultural Issues in the Treatment of Anxiety*. S. Friedman, ed. Pp. 3–20. New York: Guilford Press.

Hinton, D. E. 2002. "Wind Overload" and Orthostatic Panic Among Khmer Refugees. *Transcultural Psychiatry* 39:220–227.

Hinton, D. E., P. Ba, and K. Um. 2001a. A Unique Panic-Disorder Presentation Among Khmer Refugees: The Sore Neck Syndrome. *Culture, Medicine, and Psychiatry* 25:297–316.

Hinton, D. E., K. Um, and P. Ba. 2001b. *Kyol Goeu* ("Wind Overload") Part I: A Cultural Syndrome of Orthostatic Panic Among Khmer Refugees. *Transcultural Psychiatry* 38:403–432.

———. 2001c. *Kyol Goeu* ("Wind Overload") Part II: Prevalence, Characteristics, and Mechanisms of *Kyol Goeu* and Near-*Kyol Goeu* Episodes of Khmer Patients Attending a Psychiatric Clinic. *Transcultural Psychiatry* 38:433–460.

Hinton, D. E., S. D. Hinton, K. Um, A. Chea, and S. Sak. 2002. The Khmer "Weak Heart" Syndrome: Fear of Death from Palpitations. *Transcultural Psychiatry* 39:323–344.

Hsu, S. I. 1999. Somatisation Among Asian Refugees and Immigrants as a Culturally Shaped Illness Behavior. *Annals of Academy of Medicine Singapore* 28(6):841–45.

Hutheesing, R. 1960. *Tibet Fights for Freedom: The Story of the March 1959 Uprising as Recorded in Documents, Dispatches, Eye-Witness Accounts, and Worldwide Reactions.* Bombay: Indian Committee for Cultural Freedom.

Jacobs, S., F. Hansen, S. Kasl, A. Ostfeld, L. Berkmen, and K. Kim. 1990. Anxiety Disorders During Acute Bereavement: Risk and Risk Factors. *Journal of Clinical Psychiatry* 51:269–274.

Jacobson, E. 2000. Situated Knowledge in Classical Tibetan Medicine: Psychiatric Aspects. Ph.D. dissertation, Department of Anthropology, Harvard University.

———. 2002. Panic Attack in a Context of Co-Morbid Depression and Anxiety in a Tibetan Refugee. *Culture, Medicine, and Psychiatry* 26(2):259–279.

———. 2007. "Life-Wind Illness" in Tibetan Medicine: Depression, Generalized Anxiety, and Panic Attack. In *Soundings in Tibetan Medicine: Anthropological and Historical Perspectives.* Mona Schrempf, ed. Pp. 225–245. Proceedings of the 13th International Association for Tibetan Studies, Oxford, 2003. Leiden, NL: Brill.

Katon, W., and P. P. Roy-Byrne. 1991. Mixed Anxiety and Depression. *Journal of Abnormal Psychology* 100(3):337–345.

Kessler, R., P. E. Stang, H. U. Wittchen, T. B. Ustun, P. P. Roy-Byrne, and E. E. Walters. 1998. Lifetime Panic-Depression Comorbidity in the National Comorbidity Survey. *Archives of General Psychiatry* 55(9):801–808.

Kleinman, A. 1980. *Patients and Healers in the Context of Culture.* Berkeley: University of California Press.

———. 1982. Neurasthenia and Depression: A Study of Somatization and Culture in China. *Culture, Medicine, and Psychiatry* 6:117–190.

———. 1986. *Social Origins of Distress and Disease: Depression, Neurasthenia, and Panic in Modern China.* New Haven, CT: Yale University Press.

Kroll, J., M. Habenich, T. Mackenzie, M. Yang, S. Chang, T. Vang, T. Nguyen, M. Ly, B. Phommasouvanh, H. Nguyen, Y. Vang, L. Souvannasoth, and R. Cabugao. 1988. Depression and Post-Traumatic Stress Disorder in Southeast Asian Refugees. *American Journal of Psychiatry* 146(12):1592–1597.

Krystal, J. H., D. N. Deutsch, and D. S. Charney. 1996. The Biological Basis of Panic Disorder. *Journal of Clinical Psychiatry* 57 (Supplement 10):23–31.

Kumar, A., ed. 1994. *Tibet: A Source Book.* New Delhi: All Party Indian Parliamentary Forum for Tibet.

Kuriyama, S. 1994. The Imagination of Winds and the Development of the Chinese Conception of the Body. In *Body, Subject, and Power in China.* A. Zito and T. E. Barlow, eds. Pp. 31–41. Chicago: University of Chicago Press.

———. 1999. *The Expressiveness of the Body and the Divergence of Greek and Chinese Medicine.* New York: Zone Books.

Lee, K., Y. Noda, Y. Nakano, S. Ogawa, Y. Kinoshita, T. Funayama, and T. A. Furukawa.

2006. Interoceptive Hypersensitivity and Interoceptive Exposure in Patients with Panic Disorder: Specificity and Effectiveness. *BMC Psychiatry* 6:32.

Lee, S. 1998. Estranged Bodies, Simulated Harmony, and Misplaced Cultures: Neurasthenia in Contemporary Chinese Society. *Psychosomatic Medicine* 60:448–457.

Lelliot, P., and C. Bass. 1990. Symptom Specificity in Patients with Panic. *British Journal of Psychiatry* 157:593–597.

Lewis-Fernández, R., P. Guarnaccia, I. E. Martínez, E. Salman, A. Schmidt, and M. Liebowitz. 2002. Comparative Phenomenology of *Ataque de Nervios*, Panic Attacks, and Panic Disorder. *Culture, Medicine, and Psychiatry* 26(2):199–223.

Lin, E. H., W. B. Carter, and A. Kleinman. 1985. An Exploration of Somatization Among Asian Refugees and Immigrants in Primary Care. *American Journal of Public Health* 75(9):1080–84.

Mammen, O. K., M. K. Shear, P. A. Pilkonis, D. J. Kolko, M. E. Thase, and C. G. Greeno. 1999. Anger Attacks: Correlates and Significance of an Under-Recognized Symptom. *Journal of Clinical Psychiatry* 60(9):633–642.

Manson, S. M. 1985. Culture and *DSM-IV*: Implications for Diagnosis of Mood and Anxiety Disorders. In *Depression and Culture*. A. Kleinman and B. J. Good, eds. Pp. 99–113. Berkeley: University of California Press.

McNally, R. J. 1994. *Panic Disorder: A Critical Analysis*. New York: Guilford Press.

———. 2002. Anxiety Sensitivity and Panic Disorder. *Biological Psychiatry* 52(10):938–46.

Meuret, A. E, K. S. White, T. Ritz, W. T. Roth, S. G. Hofmann, and T. A. Brown. 2006. Panic Attack Symptom Dimensions and Their Relationship to Illness Characteristics in Panic Disorder. *Journal of Psychiatric Research* 40(6):520–27.

Meyer, F. 1996. Theory and Practice of Tibetan Medicine. In *Oriental Medicine*. J. Van Alphen and A. Aris, eds. Pp. 109–141. Boston: Shambhala.

Middleton, H. C. 1998. Panic Disorder: A Theoretical Synthesis of Medical and Psychological Approaches. *Journal of Psychosomatic Research* 44(1):121–132.

Nichter, M. 1981. Idioms of Distress: Alternatives in the Expression of Psychosocial Distress: A Case Study from South India. *Culture, Medicine, and Psychiatry* 5:379–408.

Pasnau, R. O., and A. Bystritsky. 1994. On the Comorbidity of Anxiety and Depression. In *Handbook of Depression and Anxiety*. J. A. den Boer and J. M. Ad Sitsen, eds. Pp. 45–56. New York: Marcel Dekker.

Reiss, S., R. A. Peterson, D. M. Gursky, and R. J. McNally. 1986. Anxiety Sensitivity, Anxiety Frequency, and the Prediction of Fearfulness. *Behaviour, Research, and Therapy* 24(1):1–8.

Rosenbaum, J. F. 1999. Anger Attacks in Depression. *Journal of Clinical Psychiatry* 17(2):15–17.

Sartorius, N., and T. B. Ustan. 1995. Mixed Anxiety and Depressive Disorder. *Psychopathology* 28 (Supplement):21–25.

Sinha, S., L. A. Papp, and J. M. Gorman. 2000. How Study of Respiratory Physiology Aided Our Understanding of Abnormal Brain Function in Panic Disorder. *Journal of Affective Disorders* 61:191–2000.

Spitzer, R. L., J. B. William, M. Gibbon, and M. B. First. 1990. *Structured Clinical Interview for DSM-III-R, Non-Patient Edition*. Washington, DC: American Psychiatric Press.

Taylor, S. 1995. Anxiety Sensitivity: Theoretical Perspectives and Recent Findings. *Behaviour, Research, and Therapy* 33(3):243–258.

Taylor, S., and B. J. Cox. 1998. Anxiety Sensitivity: Multiple Dimensions and Hierarchic Structure. *Behaviour, Research, and Therapy* 36:37–51.

Terheggen, M. A., M. S. Stroebe, and R. J. Kleber. 2001. Western Conceptualizations and Eastern Experience: A Cross-Cultural Study of Traumatic Stress Reactions Among Tibetan Refugees in India. *Journal of Traumatic Stress* 14(2):391–402.

Tseng, W-S., M. Asai, L. Jieqiu, P. Wibulswasdi, L. D. Suryani, J-K. Wen, J. Brennan, and E. Heiby. 1990. Multi-Cultural Study of Minor Psychiatric Disorders in Asia: Symptom Manifestations. *International Journal of Social Psychiatry* 36(4):252–264.

Uhlenhuth, E. H., A. C. Leon, and W. Matuzas. 2006. Psychopathology of Panic Attacks in Panic Disorder. *Journal of Affective Disorders* 92(1):55–62

Wittchen, H-U., S. Zhao, R. C. Kessler, and W. W. Eaton. 1994. *DSM-III-R* Generalized Anxiety Disorder in the National Comorbidity Survey. *Archives of General Psychiatry* 51:355–364.

Wylie, T. V. 1959. A Standard System of Tibetan Transcription. *Harvard Journal of Asian Studies* 22:261–276.

Zinbarg, R. E., D. H. Barlow, M. R. Liebowitz, L. L. Street, E. Broadhead, W. Katon, P. Roy-Byrne, J. Pepine, M. Teherani, J. Richards, P. Brantly, and H. Kraemer. 1994. The *DSM-IV* Field Trial for Mixed Anxiety-Depression. *American Journal of Psychiatry* 151(8):1153–1162.

Index

Figures and tables are indicated by *f* and *t*, respectively, following page numbers.

Ackerman, S., 15

Acute anxiety. *See* Panic and panic attacks

ADC. *See* Hispanic Treatment Program of the Anxiety Disorders Clinic

African Americans, 98

Agoraphobia: cues for, 10; diagnostic criteria, 12*t*; dizziness and, 124, 128*n*18; in *DSM-III*, 8; in *DSM-IV*, 10; environmental influences on, 44, 175–76; gender and, 200; learning theory and, 6–7; "no place" and, 44; panic disorder with, 10; social nature of, 44; symptoms of, 124; urban modernization and, 176

Agoraphobic Cognitions Questionnaire, 75*n*9

Allbutt, Clifford, 86, 96, 99

American Psychiatric Association, xvii

Americans, panic triggers among, 59

Amering, M., 250, 256*n*30

Ampanwong, Surapong, 201*n*9

Anger transducers, 178

Anthropology of sensations, 57–74; catastrophic cognitions perspective, 63, 65–66; descriptive perspective, 58–60; ethnophysiological perspective, 62–63; historical perspective, 72–73; landscape perspective, 69–70; memory perspective, 70–71; metaphor perspective, 66–67; physiological perspective, 61–62; sociosomatic perspective, 71–72; sound and kinetic symbolism perspective, 67–69

Antietam, Battle of, 88

Anxiety: Cambodian conceptualization of, 68; cultural history of, 21; defined, 7; etymology of, 68; function of, xiii; heart-related, 120; shortness of breath as sign of, 10, 59, 60, 68; universality of, xiii, 135

Anxiety and the Anxiety Disorders (Tuma and Maser), 4

Anxiety disorders, xix, 1; biological approach to, 4–7; cross-cultural studies of, 21; types of, 5, 7–8

Anxiety neurosis, 8, 184

Anxiety reaction, 8, 123

Anxiety Sensitivity Index, 75n9

Anxiety states, 184

Anxiety transducers, 178

Anxious fatigue, 107–8

Army of the Potomac, 87–88

Arnold, Matthew, 96

Articulatory iconicism, 67, 194–95

Articulatory kinemes, 68

Ascites, 201n4

Asians: and dizziness, 10, 61; mind-body theories of, 75n8; and motion sickness, 197; predisposition of, to panic, 75n8

Asphyxia, 60

Ataques de nervios, 135–55; cultural factors in, 48, 59; instruments for, 140–42; panic attacks compared to, 142–45, 144t; panic disorder compared to, 23, 137–55; popular vs. professional perspective on, 154; provocation of, 145–49, 153–54; psychiatric diagnoses in relation to, 137–39, 137t, 152; symptoms of, 138–39, 143–45, 146t, 148, 150–51t; treatment of, 154

Attributions, 34, 34t, 42

Automatic thoughts, 32

Autonomic arousal patterns, 24n2, 32, 61

Autonomic response specificity, 61

Autopsy, 86–87

Avoidant coping, 33

Ayurvedic tradition, 62, 72, 75n7, 190, 195, 254n3

Bachelard, G., 226n20

Bagilishya, D., 216–17

Barlow, D. H., 108

Barthes, R., 226n20

Bartholow, Roberts, 97–98; *A Manual of Instructions for Enlisting and Discharging Soldiers*, 97

Baudrillard, J., 225n18

Beck, A. T., 32–33

Beliefs, 51

Benz, Carl, 226n20

Benzodiazepines, 6, 25n6

Bereavement syndrome, 257n33

Biological approach to panic disorder, 2, 4–12, 14–15, 61–62, 120–25, 136

Biology: cultural approach combined with, 252–53; and dizziness in China, 167–73

Biolooping, 114, 126n2. *See also* Looping effect of human kinds

Blake, Caminee, xviii

Body: catastrophic cognitions and, 33; Chinese conception of, 175; cues from sensations of, 15–16, 32–33, 41; cultural influences on, 39; fear of sensations in, 63, 65; mind in relation to, 75n8, 97–98, 104–5, 171–72, 172t, 174; and sensation schemas, 33, 41; trauma and, 71, 222. *See also* Sensations

Bourdieu, P., 225n18

Breathing: meaning associated with, in Rwanda, 206, 219; mechanics of, 223n10

Brewster, Charles Harvey, 103–4

BSYB. See Four Treatises (BSYB)

Buddhist meditation, 52. *See also* Tibetan Buddhism

Burial rites, 214–17, 219, 224n12

Burnside, Ambrose E., 101, 103

Calcium, 120–22

Cambodians: catastrophic cognitions of, 25n11, 66; and dizziness, 25n11, 59–62, 70–72; ethnophysiology of, 62–63, 64f, 65; and *khyâl*, 13, 25, 59, 61–63, 65, 71, 73; and memory, 70–71; and metaphors, 67, 69; and tinnitus, 13, 66, 69; and "weak heart" concept, 72–73

Carbon dioxide, 124

Cardiac asthma, 127n10

Cardiac hyperaesthesia, 92

Cardiac neurosis, 91–92, 123

Cardiac vulnerability, 114–20

Catastrophic cognitions, xviii, 2, 14–19, 125–26; of Cambodians, 25n11, 66; cultural influences on, 63, 65–66; *lom* illness and, 201n4; and misinterpretations, 253; personal catastrophe,

33; about somatic sensations, 15–16; theoretical implications of, 16–19

Category errors, 57–58

China: case studies in, 160–66; circulation concept in, 175; dizziness in, 157–80; ethnophysiology in, 167–73; medical practice in, 157–59; and motion sickness, 61, 75n6, 176, 177; organ system in, 158, 160–70, 168t; panic in, 157–80; and Tibet, 252

Chinese Classification of Mental Disorders (*CCMD-II*), 158

Chronic fatigue syndrome, 127n9

Chvostek sign, 120–21

Civil War: death concepts, representations, and rituals after, 214; irritable heart syndrome in, 85–109, 115

Clark, D., 15

Clarke, Edward H., 86

Classen, C., 226n20

Classificatory looping, 114, 126n2. *See also* Looping effect of human kinds

Cognition: nonrational, 35; origins of panic in, 32–35

Cognitive psychology, 24n4

Cognitive theory of panic disorder, 16–19, 16f

Colonization of ontology, 72, 76n19

Comorbidity, 10

Composite International Diagnostic Interview, 185

Conceptualization of illness, 37, 40–43, 48, 49, 113–14, 126n2, 200

Constipation, Rwandan genocide and, 207, 219, 221

Control: as central factor in anxiety, 34; cultural expectations regarding, 42, 48; dizziness and, 177–78

Core symptoms, 36

Courage, 102–4, 107–8

Crampton Test, 116

Crescendo, 10, 13, 19, 145

Cross-cultural comparison strategies, 35–37

Cross-National Collaborative Panic Study, 256n30

Cues. *See* Triggers

Cultural approach to disorders: benefits of, xvii; conceptualization/construction and, 40–43, 49, 113–14, 126n2, 200; *DSM* compared to, xix, 21–23; idioms and, 42; perspectives in, 38–43; sensation and, 57–74. *See also* Cultural approach to panic disorder

Cultural approach to panic disorder: biological approach and, 252–53; case study in, 46–48; catastrophic cognitions and, 17, 19–20; conceptualization/construction and, 40–43, 48, 113–14; cross-cultural comparison strategies and, 35–37; issues in, 22–23; meanings discovered by, 3; outcomes of, 23–24; perspectives in, 2; physiology and, 61–62; and presentation of disease, 25n10; study of, xiv-xv; twentieth-century theories and, 113–26

Cultural idioms of distress, 39, 42

Culture: and beliefs, 51; bodily practices and, 39; emotion influenced by, 38–40, 38t; experience influenced by, 38; repetition and, 221–22, 225n18

Culture-bound syndromes, 39, 49

Da Costa, Jacob Mendez, 86, 88, 90–96, 99–101, 104–9, 115; *Medical Diagnosis*, 86, 90

Daimler, Gottlieb, 226n20

Darwin, Charles, xiii

Dean, E. T., 89, 90

Deleuze, G., 225n18

Depersonalization, 66, 75n3

Depression, 20–21, 49

Derealization, 66, 75n3

Devisch, R., 226n20

Diagnosis: criteria, 8–10, 8t, 9t, 11t, 12t, 147t; hierarchical model of, 8–9, 25n9; pathology-based, 90

Diagnostic and Statistical Manual of Mental Disorders (*DSM*): cross-cultural applicability of, 135; as cultural artifact, xvii

Diagnostic and Statistical Manual of Mental Disorders-I (*DSM-I*), 8, 123

Diagnostic and Statistical Manual of Mental Disorders-II (*DSM-II*), 8

Diagnostic and Statistical Manual of Mental Disorders-III (*DSM-III*): cross-cultural study involving, 256*n*30; panic disorder in, xv, 2, 4–9, 8*t*, 123–25, 197; symptom-based criteria in, 4–5; in Thailand, 184

Diagnostic and Statistical Manual of Mental Disorders-III-Revised (*DSM-III-R*): and life-wind illness, 236; panic disorder in, 9–10, 9*t*, 141, 197

Diagnostic and Statistical Manual of Mental Disorders-IV (*DSM-IV*): agoraphobia in, 12*t*; and anxiety disorders, xix; Chinese patients and, 159*t*; cultural categories compared to, xix; cultural influences on, 60; Glossary of Culture-Bound Syndromes, 153; irritable heart syndrome in, 107; and life-wind illness, 236–37, 240, 246–50, 246*t*, 248*t*; panic attacks in, 12, 136; panic disorder in, xiv, 8, 10, 11*t*, 12, 58–60, 125, 141

Diagnostic and Statistical Manual of Mental Disorders-IV-TR (*DSM-IV-TR*), 12

Diagnostic and Statistical Manual of Mental Disorders-V Work Group, 12

Disturbed thinking, 32

Dizziness: agoraphobia and, 124, 128*m*18; as Asian anxiety response, 10, 61; biology and, 167–73; as Cambodian anxiety response, 25*m*11, 59–62, 68–72; case studies in, 160–66; in China, 157–80; in contemporary syndromes, 127*n*9; environmental influences on, 174–77; ethnophysiology of, 167–73; heart syndromes and, 116; interpersonal, economic, and political effects of, 177–78; meanings of, 157; and memory, 177; metaphor and, 75*n*6, 173–74; in traditional Chinese medicine, 172–73, 179–80; transducers of, 178–79

Dominicans, 137–55

Double hermeneutic, 114

Duden, B., 86

Dunbar, H. F., 106

Dunster, Edward S., 98

Dynamic interpretants, 67, 76*n*13, 179, 223*n*3

Effort syndrome, 15, 115–16, 121, 124, 126*n*6

Emchi (Tibetan classical physicians), 230–31, 233–34, 236, 237, 240–41, 245, 249, 255*n*11, 255*n*13, 255*m*18, 255*n*20

EMIC. *See* Explanatory Model Interview Catalogue

Emotion: anthropology of, 74*n*2; cultural influences on, 38–40, 38*t*; heart as seat of, 85, 87, 99–105, 255*n*13; and irritable heart syndrome, 92–94, 106; in Thailand, 193; in traditional Chinese medicine, 171–72, 172*t*

Emotion-physiology, 24*n*2

Endocrinal states, 24*n*2

Environment: Chinese conception of, 175; dizziness and, 174–77; meaning of sensations and, 69–70. *See also* Space/place

Epidemic anxiety: communication of, 43–44; features of, 42, 43; *Ihahamuka* and, 210; space/place and, 44; workplace stress and, 45

Espinosa, Luisito, 196

Ethnophysiology, 62–63, 64*f*, 167–73, 190–93, 213–14

Exertion, heart problems and, 94–99, 116–17

Explanatory Model Interview Catalogue (EMIC), 140–42

Explanatory models, 157

Fahrenkamp, Karl, 106

Fatigue, irritable heart syndrome and, 93, 95–96, 99, 107–8

Fatigue transducers, 178

Faust, D. G., 214

Fear: *ataques de nervios* and, 143; cultural influences on, 63, 65; defined, 7; function of, xiii; universality of, xiii

Feedback loops, 18f, 34, 35, 37, 39, 42, 52

Fight-or-flight response, xiii, 61

Fisk, Wilbur, 97

Flow and blockage symbolism, 206–7

Foucault, Michel, 72, 225n18

Four Treatises (BSYB), 231–35, 237–38, 251, 254n3, 254n10

Fredericksburg, Battle of, 88, 90

Freud, Sigmund, 2, 24n1

Friedman, S., 45

Functional disease of the heart, 105

Functional disorder: defined, 126n7; irritable heart syndrome as, 86, 89, 91–93, 96, 101, 105, 108

GAD. *See* Generalized anxiety disorder

Galaxy, Khaokor, 196, 201n9

Gastric neurosis, 123

Gender: and agoraphobia, 200; male panickers in U.S. and Europe, 201n1; and panic, issues in, 200–201; and panic in Thailand, 186, 186t, 193–97, 199

Generalized anxiety disorder (GAD), 7, 184, 236, 240, 247, 249, 255n17

Genocide, 205–10, 216–20

Gestures, 68–69

Good, Byron, xvii, xviii, 21, 23, 135–36

Good, Mary-Jo, xvii

Gulf War syndrome, 127n9, 201n1

Habermas, Jürgen, 76n19

Hacking, Ian, 37, 72, 126n2

Hagengimana, Athanase, 208–10, 224n17

Handfield, Jones, Charles, 91–92, 99

Hartshorne, Henry, 86, 88, 89

Harvard Trauma Questionnaire, 256n22

Harvey, William, 175

Health, epidemic anxiety and, 45

Heart: anxiety related to, 120; conceptions of, 85, 99–105, 108; and courage, 102–4, 107–8; cultural image of, 101; life-wind illness and, 247; meanings of, in German culture, 226n20; and morality, 87, 101–2; panic disorder and, 114–18; physical conception of, 85, 94, 99–105, 114–15, 117–18; popular

concerns about, 116–18, 120; during respiration, 223n10; as seat of emotions, 85, 87, 99–105, 255n13; in traditional Chinese medicine, 164–66, 168–69; vulnerability of, 114–20. *See also* Irritable heart syndrome

Heart attack, 201n1

Heidegger, Martin, 107–8

Heritier, F., 226n20

Hess, E. J., 103

Highly sensitive persons, 127n16

Hinton, Devon E., xviii, 183, 225n18, 226n20

Hispanic Treatment Program of the Anxiety Disorders Clinic (ADC), 140

Hormones, 123

Howell, J. D., 106

Hsu, Elisabeth, 173

Hunt, Sanford B., 105

Hwa byung, 76n12, 190

Hybrid panic attacks, 12, 13, 19

Hybrid syndromes, 72

Hyperventilation, 34

Hypochondriachal melancholy, 200

Hysteria, 200

Ihahamuka, 205–23; case studies in, 207–10; cultural analysis of, 211–20; defined, 206, 223n8; emergence of, 210; epidemics of, 210; etymology of, 211–12; flow and blockage symbolism and, 207, 212, 219–20; generation of episodes of, 220–21; medication for, 223n6; physiological concerns during episodes of, 213–14; public announcements concerning, 224n17; sound symbolism of, 211–12; spirit assault as cause of, 214, 217; tinnitus and, 213–14; trauma recall during episodes of, 212–13; treatment of, during attack, 211; triggers of, 211

Illness experience, conceptual influences on, 37

Imipramine, 6, 25n7

International Statistical Classification of Diseases-9 (ICD-9), 158, 184

Irritable heart syndrome, 85–109; age and, 99; case study in, 90–91; causes of, 88, 91–96, 105–7; civilian cases of, 93–95; Da Costa and, 90–95; description and explanation of, 86–95; emotion and, 92–94, 106; exertion and, 94–99; existential perspective on, 107–8; fatigue and, 93, 95–96, 99, 107–8; first description of, 88; as functional disorder, 86, 89, 91–93, 96, 101, 105, 108, 126*n*7; industry and, 86, 95–96; interpretations of, 99–107; later interpretations of, 106–7; medical context for discovery of, 86–87, 92, 104–5; as metaphor, 108; naming of, 91; as psychiatric condition, 106–7; PTSD and, 126*n*6; symptoms of, 92; treatment of, 94; wars and, 85, 88–93, 96–97, 105–9, 115
Irritable weakness, 127*n*16

Jackson, Thomas J. "Stonewall," 90
James, William, 96, 108
Japan, menopausal experience in, 75*n*5
Jenkins, J., 225*n*20

Karma, 254*n*9
Katschnig, H., 250, 256*n*30
Khmer. *See* Cambodians
Khyâl, 13, 25, 59, 61–63, 65, 71, 73
Kidney: panic episodes and, 162–64; in traditional Chinese medicine, 169–70
Kinetic symbolism, 67–69
Kirmayer, Laurence J., xviii
Klein, D. F., 6, 123–24
Kleinman, Arthur, xvii, 21, 23, 25*n*9, 36, 135, 157, 166
Kleinman, J., 166
Klotz, H. P., 121
Koro, 43–44
Krishaber, M., 121
Kroll, J., 257*n*33
Kuba igikange, 210
!Kung, 41

Lactate, 15, 121–22, 124

Ladplee, Roongtham, 201*n*9
Laennec, René, 86
Laos, 224*n*12
Laotians, 70
Latham, Peter Mere, 87
Lee, Robert E., 87
Lee, Sing, 72
Levinas, E., 107
Lewis, I. M., 199
Lewis, T., 115
Liddell, Howard, xiii
Liebowitz, Michael, 138, 140, 141
Life-wind illness, 230; acute panic in, 236; case studies in, 237–45; causes and symptoms of, 234; in classical medicine, 231–33; defined, 234; *DSM* and, 236–37, 240, 246–50, 246*t*, 248*t*; lay knowledge of, 234–35; stigma associated with, 235; symptoms of, 235, 246–50, 246*t*, 248*t*; triggers of, 250–52, 251*t*
Linderman, G. F., 104
Linguistic objectification, 67
Liver: panic episodes and, 160–62; in traditional Chinese medicine, 167–68
Lock, M., 75*n*5, 222
Lom illness (wind illness), 187–91, 192*f*, 193–97, 198*t*, 199, 201*n*4, 201*n*6
Looping effect of human kinds, 37. *See also* Biolooping

Mackenzie, James, 106
Major depressive disorder (MDD), 236, 240, 244, 247, 249, 255*n*17
Malaria, 65
Manson, S. M., 250
Maudsley Hospital, London, 184
McClellan, George B., 87–88
McClure, J., 15, 121–22, 124
McPherson, J. M., 90
MDD. *See* Major depressive disorder
Medical anthropology of sensations, 57–74
Medical practice: in China, 157–59; objectivity in, 86–87, 100, 105
Memory: dizziness and, 177; sensations and, 70–71

Menopause, Japanese experience of, 75*n*5
Menstruation, panic episodes and, 189,
    191, 193
Metaphor: dizziness and, 173–74;
    environmental imagery and, 69–70;
    ethnopsychology and, 76*n*12; heart
    as, 87; irritable heart syndrome as,
    108; panic as, 42–43; sensations and,
    66–67
Mind-body relationship: in Asia, 75*n*8; in
    traditional Chinese medicine, 171–72,
    172*t*, 174; in United States, 97–98,
    104–5
Mini-International Neuropsychiatric
    Interview, 185
Mitchell, Silas Weir, 99
Modernity: anxiety and, 44–45; irritable
    heart syndrome and, 95–96
Morality: heart and, 87, 101–2; karma and,
    254*n*9; military fitness and, 97–98
Moral panics, 49–50
Motion sickness, 61, 75*n*6, 176, 177, 197
Multilevel ontological analysis, 223,
    226*n*20
Multiple chemical sensitivity, 127*n*16,
    201*n*1
Multiplex theory of panic, 126
Murphy, H. B. M., 44
Mutism, 210*n*10
Myers, Arthur B. R., 96

National Comorbidity Survey (U.S.), 197
National Institute of Mental Health
    (NIMH), 2, 4
Nausea, 9–10
Neo-Kraepelinian approach, 4–6, 21
Neurasthenia, 72, 99, 157, 201*n*1
Neurocirculatory asthenia, 115–16, 127*n*8
New York State Psychiatric Institute
    (NYSPI), 138, 140
New York Times, 101
Nichter, M., 39
Nietzsche, Friedrich, 72
Nigerians, panic triggers among, 59–60
Nocturnal death, 199
Nocturnal panic, 127*n*10, 199, 209, 223*n*9

Nora dance, 188, 195, 201*n*8
Nova Scotia, 45
Nyepa (harmful ones), 231–33, 254*n*4

Obeyesekere, G., 49
Obsessive-compulsive disorder, 7
Organs, 158
Orr, Jackie, *Panic Diaries*, 2, 24
Out-of-the-blue criterion, 6, 10, 13–15

Pan, xviii-xix
Panic and panic attacks: *ataques de nervios*
    compared to, 142–45, 144*t*; biocul-
    tural interactionist view of, 252–53;
    causes of, 123; characteristics of, 41;
    in China, 157–80; cognitive origins
    of panic, 32–35; and comorbidity,
    247, 255*n*17; cultural influences on,
    xiv-xv, 2; cultural-political role of,
    49–50; defined, xiii, 1; diagnostic
    criteria, 11*t*; in *DSM-IV*, 11*t*; emotion
    and, 74*n*2; etymology of, xviii-xix;
    Freud on, 24*n*1; generation of, 10, 13,
    16*f*, 18*f*; hybrid, 12, 13, 19; meanings
    of, 51; as metaphor, 42–43; models
    for understanding, 40; multiplex
    theory of, 126; panic disorder vs., 12,
    136; Rwandan genocide and, 205–23,
    224*n*17; sensations prominent during,
    58–60; spontaneity and, xiv; study
    of, xiv; as symptom, 40; as syndrome,
    40–41; temporal aspect of, 40, 145,
    250; in Thailand, 183–201; Tibetan
    refugees and, 230, 236–53; twentieth-
    century theories of, 113–26; unex-
    pected, xiv, 14, 145–47; unprovoked,
    xiv, 10, 145–48, 154
Panic disorder (PD), 247; *ataques de nerv-
    ios* compared to, 23, 137–55; biological
    approach to, 2, 4–12, 14–15, 61–62,
    120–25, 136, 252–53; causes of, 125;
    cross-cultural studies of, 22–23, 31–53,
    256*n*30; cultural history of, 20–21,
    113–26; defined, 1; definitional contro-
    versies, 13–14; diagnostic criteria, 8–10,
    8*t*, 9*t*, 11*t*, 12*t*, 147*t*; diseases related to,

2; early theories of, 2; incidence of, 1; irritable heart syndrome as, 107; medication for, 6, 25n6; onset of, 1; panic attacks vs., 12, 136; preoccupations of individuals with, 32; psychological measures of, 75n9; psychological theory of, 14–19; recent theories of, 12–19; in Thailand, 185–86, 185t; theoretical perspectives on, 20; unique features of, 6–7; universality of, 2–3, 23; unprovoked, 6; vicious circles and, 32–34, 52. *See also* Cultural approach to panic disorder; Panic and panic attacks

Paradis, C., 45

Paroxysms of fear, 123

Pathogenic mechanisms, 37

PD. *See* Panic disorder

Peirce, Charles Sanders, 76n13, 179

Peninsula Campaign, 89, 103

Phobias, 7, 25n8

Physiology of panic disorder, 61–62

Physiopsychology, 7

Pitts, F., 15, 121–22, 124

Place. *See* Space/place

Polymodal sensations, 74n1

Polythetic categories, 36–37

Posttraumatic stress disorder (PTSD): defined, 7; forerunners of, 126n6; heart syndromes and, 115–16; and life-wind illness, 240; panic disorder and, xix, 10, 12–13, 19; Rwandan genocide and, 206–8, 224n17; Tibetan refugees and, 240, 256n22; Vietnam War and, 106

Probyn, E., 206

Psychophysiologic autonomic and visceral disorders, 8

Psychophysiologic disorders, 8, 123

Psychophysiology, 24n2

PTSD. *See* Posttraumatic stress disorder

Puerto Ricans: and *ataques de nervios*, 135–55; case study involving, 46–48; panic triggers among, 59

Rabinbach, A., 95

Race: military fitness and, 97–98; in Rwanda, 206

Rape, 205–6

Rapid-crescendo criterion, 10, 13, 145

Reiser, S. J., 86

Repetition, culture and, 221–22, 225n18

Respiration, 223n10

Rhizo-ethnology, 206, 211

Richardson, Benjamin Ward, 86, 102, 105

Runaway feedback loops. *See* Feedback loops

Rwanda: burial rites in, 214–17, 219; case studies in, 207–10; ethnic conflict in, 206; ethnophysiology of, 213–14; flow and blockage symbolism in, 206–7, 217–22, 223n2, 223n3, 224n15; genocide in, 205–10, 216–20, 223n8; meanings associated with breathing in, 206, 219; panic syndrome in, 205–23

Rwandan Popular Front (RPF), 206, 223n1

Sachar, E. J., 15

Salmán, Ester, 141

Scentless public space, 45

Schemas: description of, 32; self-schemas, 34; sensation schemas, 33, 41

Schepher-Hughes, N., 222

Schizophrenia, 20

Schneider Index, 116

SCID. *See* Structured Clinical Interview for *DSM-III-R*

"Sea of Marrow," 169f

Self-schemas, 34

Sensation amplification, 74

Sensations: amplification of, 74; catastrophic cognitions and, 63, 65–66; as cues, 15–16, 32–33, 41; cultural factors in, 59; defined, 57, 74n1; environmental influences on, 69–70; ethnophysiology of, 62–63; fear of, 63, 65; historical perspective on, 72–73; inducing of, 63; linguistic objectification and, 67; local biology and, 61–62; meanings of, 74; medical anthropology of, 57–74; memory and, 70–71; metaphor and, 66–67;

polymodal, 74*n*1; prominent, during panic, 58–60; schemas of, 33, 41; sociosomatic perspective on, 71–72; sound/kinetic symbolism and, 67–69

Sensation-type category errors, 58

Separation anxiety, 38, 123

Sheehan, David, 6; *The Anxiety Disease*, 2

Shell shock, 126*n*6

Shortness of breath: as American anxiety response, 10, 59, 60, 68; *Ihahamuka* and, 206–23, 224*n*16; life-wind illness and, 247; metaphor of, 66–67; as panic disorder symptom, 124–25; as Western anxiety response, 76*n*15. *See also* Suffocation

Sibomana, A., 205

Smith, Calvin, 127*n*10; *That Heart of Yours*, 116–18, 119*f*

Social-conflict transducers, 178

Social influences: diversity of, 33; on individual identity, 43; interactional factors, 35

Socioeconomic status, 45

Sociosomatic reticulum, 71

Soldier's heart, 106, 115

Somaticization, 248–49

Sound symbolism, 67–68, 194–95, 211–12

Southern Thailand. *See* Thailand

Space/place, epidemic anxiety and, 44–45. *See also* Agoraphobia; Environment

Spasmophilie, 120–21

Spasticity, 120–22, 127*n*16

Speaking, difficulties in, 196, 210*n*10

Spencer, Herbert, 100

Sperber, D., 50

Spirit attacks/possession: in Rwanda, 214, 217; Tibetan refugees and, 233–34, 236, 241, 243, 245, 255*n*18, 256*n*26

Spirit doctors, 188, 195, 201*n*7

Spitzer, Robert, 6

Stearns, P., 100

Sterling Forest Conference, 4–5, 14, 21

Stethoscope, 85–86, 89, 92, 100, 105

Stillé, Alfred, 86, 88, 103

Strange situation, 38

Stress, Tibetan "wind" and, 232, 235

Structured Clinical Interview for *DSM-III-R* (SCID), 141–42, 236, 239, 244

Suffocation, 124. *See also* Shortness of breath

Summerfield, D., 221

Susto, 39

Symptoms: of *ataques de nervios* vs. panic episodes, 138–39, 143–45, 148, 150–51*t*; core, 36; cross-cultural comparison of, 36; *DSM-IV* on, 58–60; meanings of, 222–23, 225*n*20; panic as, 40; in twentieth-century theories, 125

Syndrome, panic as, 40–41

Taylor, C. C., 206–7, 217, 219, 224*n*15

TCM. *See* Traditional Chinese medicine

Thailand: case studies in, 187–90; cultural areas of, 183; *DSM* introduction in, 184; ethnophysiology of panic symptoms in, 190–93; gender and panic in, 186, 186*t*, 193–97, 199–201; panic in, 183–201

Thumos, 85

Tianjin Mental Health Hospital, 158–59

Tibet: conflict in, 252; lay knowledge of classical medicine in, 234; psychiatric illnesses and classical medicine in, 231–34, 236, 254*n*10, 255*n*11, 255*n*12; spirit attacks/possession in, 233–34, 236, 241, 243, 245, 255*n*18, 256*n*26; "wind" in, 231–35. *See also* Life-wind illness; Tibetan refugees

Tibetan Buddhism, 232–34, 240, 252

Tibetan refugees: case studies of, 237–45; panic illness in, 230, 236–53; psychological hardiness of, 256*n*22

Time: boundary/horizon of panic, 40; duration of panic, 145, 250

Tinnitus, 13, 66, 69, 75*n*4, 191, 213–14

Traditional Chinese medicine (TCM): case studies involving, 161–66; dizziness in, 172–73, 179–80; element interrelationships in, 170, 170*f*; element-organ relationships in, 170, 171*f*; and metaphor, 173–74; mind-body relationship in, 171–72, 172*t*, 174; organ functions and correspondences in, 167–70, 168*t*; role of, in Chinese medical system, 157–58; "Sea of Marrow" in, 169*f*; winds in, 176–77

Transducers, of dizziness, 178–79

Trauma: and body, 71; context and meanings of, 221–22. *See also* Posttraumatic stress disorder

Trauma-somatic reticulum, 222

Treadwell, Joshua B., 86, 101

Triggers: for agoraphobia, 10; bodily sensations as, 15–16, 32–33, 41; cultural context and, 17, 20, 25*n*11, 59–60; for life-wind illness, 250–52, 251*t*; panic disorder not caused by, 10, 12, 14; in twentieth-century theories, 125

Trousseau sign, 121

Udomratn, Pichet, 183, 184, 188, 190, 199

Uncanny, 75*n*10, 107–8

Upsurge illness. *See Wuup* illness

U.S. Sanitary Commission, 90, 97, 98

Valiente, M., 225*n*20

Values, moral panics and, 50

Vicious circles, 32–34, 52

Vietnamese refugees, panic triggers among, 26*n*11

Vietnam War, 106

Von Bergmann, Gustav, 106

Vulnerability, cardiac, 114–20

War: heart syndromes and, 85, 88–93, 96–97, 105–9, 115–16; trauma resulting from, 221. *See also* Genocide

Weak heart illness, 187, 191, 201*n*2

Weiss, Mitchell, 140

Wells, H. G., *The War of the Worlds*, 2

Westphal, Carl, 124

Wilks, Samuel, 86

Wind illness. *See* Life-wind illness; *Lom* illness

Winds: in Tibetan tradition, 231–35; in traditional Chinese medicine, 176–77

Wongchaowart, Boonnum, 184

Wood, Paul, 106

Workplace stress, 45

World War I, 106, 115, 126*n*6

World War II, 106, 115–16

Wuup illness (upsurge illness), 187, 189–91, 193–97, 198*t*

Zang fu, 167–74